Atlas of the Peripheral
Ocular Fundus

Atlas of the Peripheral Ocular Fundus

Second Edition

William L. Jones, O.D., F.A.A.O.

Adjunct Professor, College of Optometry, University of Houston; Adjunct Associate Professor, Southern California College of Optometry, La Jolla; Adjunct Associate Professor, College of Optometry, Pacific University, Forest Grove; Assistant Clinical Professor, School of Optometry, University of California, Berkeley; Director of Optometric Education, Veterans Administration Medical Center, Albuquerque, New Mexico

Butterworth–Heinemann

Boston Oxford Johannesburg Melbourne New Delhi Singapore

Copyright © 1998 by Butterworth–Heinemann

 A member of the Reed Elsevier group

Every effort has been made to ensure that the drug dosage schedules within this text are accurate and conform to standards accepted at time of publication. However, as treatment recommendations vary in the light of continuing research and clinical experience, the reader is advised to verify drug dosage schedules herein with information found on product information sheets. This is especially true in cases of new or infrequently used drugs.

 Recognizing the importance of preserving what has been written, Butterworth–Heinemann prints its books on acid-free paper whenever possible.

 Butterworth–Heinemann supports the efforts of American Forests and the Global ReLeaf program in its campaign for the betterment of trees, forests, and our environment.

Library of Congress Cataloging-in-Publication Data

Jones, William L., 1946-
    Atlas of the peripheral ocular fundus / William L. Jones. -2nd ed.
        p.   cm.
    Includes bibliographical references and index.
    ISBN 0-7506-9050-X
    1. Fundus oculi--Diseases—Atlases. 2. Retina—Diseases—Atlases.
I. Title
    [DNLM: 1. Retinal Diseases—pathology—atlases. 2. Retinal Vessels--pathology--atlases.   3. Choroid Diseases--pathology--atlases.   4. Vitreous Body--pathology--atlases. 5. Fundus Oculi--atlases.   WW 17 J79a 1998]
    RE545.J66   1998
    617.7'4--dc21
    DNLM/DLC
    for Library of Congress   97-26003
                                                                                    CIP

British Library Cataloguing-in-Publication Data
A catalogue record for this book is available from the British library.

The publisher offers discounts on bulk orders of this book.

For information, please write:
Manager of Special Sales
Butterworth–Heinemann
225 Wildwood Avenue
Woburn, MA 01801-2041
Tel: 781-904-2500
Fax: 781-904-2620

For information on all Butterworth–Heinemann publications available, contact our World Wide Web home page at: http://www.bh.com.

10 9 8 7 6 5 4 3 2 1

Printed in the United States of America

To my wife Siu and my daughter Yung for all their support and understanding during the writing of this book

Contents

Preface

This book was designed to be a readily available source on the peripheral ocular fundus for eye care practitioners. It covers many of the developmental anomalies of the peripheral retina, ora serrata, and pars plana, but emphasis is placed on degeneration and anomalies of the retina and vitreous, which have the potential for producing a retinal break and/or detachment. A detailed discussion of each entity includes clinical description, histopathology, clinical significance, and brief discussions of treatment.

Each condition is illustrated by photographs, most of which were taken through the condensing lens used for binocular indirect ophthalmoscopy. This technique produces a picture free of many of the distortions seen in photographs taken with a standard fundus camera. The realistic view of the peripheral ocular fundus will allow clinicians to greatly enhance their perception and understanding of peripheral fundus lesions. There are many diagrammatic representations that simplify the pathologic characteristics of each lesion and significantly enhance the reader's comprehension of their clinical and pathologic appearance. B-scan ultrasonograms are included to enhance the description of these entities. Finally, a few histologic figures aid in the understanding of the pathophysiology. Referencing is extensive and thus allows the text to be a valuable resource for additional information in the ophthalmic literature.

William L. Jones

Acknowledgments

I thank Dr. Arup Das (retinal specialist) for graciously taking time out of his busy schedule to proofread the section on the treatment of retinal detachments. I also thank my friend and colleague William Townsend for donating a slide of lattice degeneration using scleral depression. Finally, I thank Butterworth–Heinemann for their support in writing the second edition of this book.

Chapter 1

Viewing the Peripheral Fundus

Adequate viewing of the peripheral fundus requires dilation of the pupil and the use of an indirect ophthalmoscope. Good dilation is usually achieved by instilling one drop of tropicamide (Mydriacyl) 1% and phenylephrine (Neo-Synephrine) 2.5% and waiting 20–30 minutes for the drugs to take effect. An adequate view of the intraocular structures anterior to the equator requires the use of a binocular indirect ophthalmoscope. This instrument delivers a large field of view at the expense of magnification, but most lesions of the peripheral fundus can be seen easily with this method. Its other advantages are stereopsis, a bright light source, and the ability to see very peripheral lesions with the aid of scleral depression. The disadvantage of the binocular indirect ophthalmoscope is that the image produced by the condensing lens is reversed and inverted. The binocular indirect ophthalmoscope is the instrument of choice for examining the peripheral fundus.

Scleral depressors are used to indent the globe. They are constructed of stainless steel–plated metal in either a straight or curved configuration; some even have a thimble cup arrangement (Figure 1-1). Scleral depression can be done either through the lids or, after administering topical anesthesia, on the bulbar conjunctiva. It is usually not necessary to apply inward pressure; generally, all that is needed to achieve adequate depression is to insert the depressor into the orbit adjacent to the globe. The rolled end of the depressor acts as a space-occupying mass in the orbit, which results in indentation of the adjacent globe. Scleral depression through the lids usually produces little discomfort, and topical anesthesia is not required. If a metal depressor is not available, a cotton-tipped applicator is a good substitute; however, it is best not to use it directly on the bulbar conjunctiva because it causes a mild epithelial abrasion. When performing scleral depression, care should be taken not to abrade the cornea by rubbing it with the depressor. The metal depressor should be cleaned with soapy water or alcohol after each use.

Scleral depression pushes peripheral fundus structures into the viewing and illumination beams of the ophthalmoscope (Figure 1-2). With this technique, it is possible to see from the ora serrata to the tips of the ciliary processes. During the actual indenting of the globe, a roll of retina or pars plana is produced. Scleral depression does not necessarily greatly indent the globe but rather may simply flatten the eye wall, as may be seen with ultrasonography (Figure 1-3). The flattening of the eye wall may be all that is necessary to place a peripheral lesion in view. Moving the depressor back and forth causes a lesion to be moved higher or lower on the roll so that it can be viewed at different angles of illumination and on edge. This is helpful in the diagnosis of a retinal break because it allows the clinician a view of its edge (see Figures 3-68, 3-83, 5-15, and 5-19). Often, a small elevated peripheral fundus lesion, such as a limited detachment around an atrophic hole, may not be adequately seen with a binocular indirect ophthalmoscope but may be seen in greater detail with scleral depression. Scleral depression does not initiate or exacerbate a retinal tear or detachment because the usual mechanism causing retinal tears is vitreous traction, and scleral depression decreases vitreous tractional forces by indenting the globe. This is also true of retinal detachment, because vitreous traction is often the leading cause of sensory retinal separation. Also, repositioning the fluid under a detachment with scleral depression will not exacerbate the condition.

Several optical devices can be used with the biomicroscope to view the peripheral fundus, including the Goldmann three-mirror contact lens. The square mirror is used to view the far periphery and

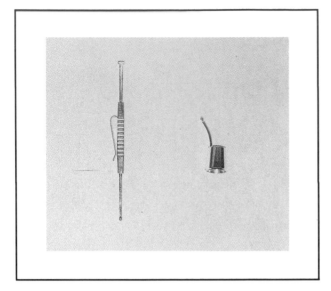

FIGURE 1-1
A straight pocket clip depressor and a curved thimble scleral depressor.

the trapezoidal mirror is used to view the mid to far periphery. Its advantages are magnification, stereopsis, and the lack of mirror-image reversing. Disadvantages are contact with the globe (requiring topical anesthesia and significant patient cooperation) and a smaller field of view.

The 60- through 90-diopter precorneal condensing lenses also can be used with the biomicroscope to view the peripheral fundus, and the view is usually just as good as that attained with the three-mirror contact lens. The advantages are magnification, stereopsis, and less discomfort to the patient. The only disadvantage is that the image is not quite as clear as with the three-mirror because of the air space between the lens and the cornea compared to liquid contact when using the three-mirror.

Ultrawide-field contact lenses also permit viewing of the peripheral fundus. The advantages are a very wide field of view (although usually not wide enough to view the area adjacent to the ora serrata), stereopsis, and easy viewing of the peripheral fundus through a 4-mm fixed pupil. The disadvantages are contact with the globe and reversed and inverted images. Ultrawide-field lenses are great for viewing large fundus lesions, such as retinal detachments, large intraocular tumors, and diffusely scattered lesions. Large retinal detachments can be easily drawn by turning the retinal drawing paper upside down and drawing the detachment just as it appears in the lens. A retinal drawing can be made in less than 10 minutes with this technique.

With all these optical devices, the peripheral view can be greatly enhanced by performing scleral depression, which requires the help of a second person to perform the depression while the observer looks through the biomicroscope.

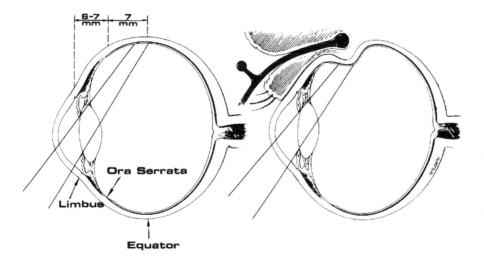

FIGURE 1-2
Scleral depression. Note that depressing the globe, through the lid in this example, indents the peripheral retina into the path of the viewing beam. (Reproduced with permission from A Cavallerano, MJ Garston. Examination of the peripheral ocular fundus. Rev Optom 1979;116:43–49.)

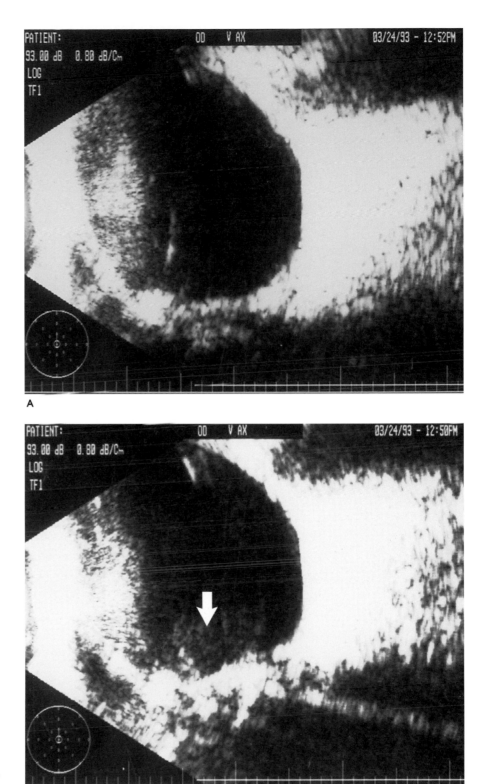

FIGURE 1-3
B-scan ultrasonograms of scleral depression. A. Scleral depressor inserted inferiorly, applying little pressure on the globe. B. Inward pressure shows as a flattening with slight convexity of the eye wall. Also note that the release of tension on the vitreous fibrils in the region being depressed causes them to become thicker and more visible on the ultrasound (*arrow*).

Chapter 2

Anatomy of the Peripheral Fundus

Retina

The retina is composed of the inner neural or sensory layers and the outer pigment epithelium (Figure 2-1). There are nine layers of the neural retina; from inner to outer they are the internal limiting membrane, nerve fiber layer, ganglion cell layer, inner plexiform layer, inner nuclear layer, outer plexiform layer, outer nuclear layer, external limiting membrane, and photoreceptors. The normal neural retina is essentially transparent except for the pigment in the blood, although it does absorb a small quantity of light passing through it. The sensory retina in the periphery is thin and relatively weak and thus is susceptible to full-thickness breaks. The degenerations of the periphery are usually trophic, related to both trophic and tractional factors, or strictly tractional.[1]

The retinal pigment epithelium (RPE) is a unilayer of polygonal cells that are fairly uniform in size and pigment content, except at the macular area and the vitreous base. Some of the main functions of the RPE are the renewal of photoreceptor outer segments and the deturgescence of the subretinal space. These cells are critical to the nourishment of the photoreceptors and for transferring waste products from the outer retinal layers. The RPE is also responsible for phagocytosis of the discarded discs of rods and cones.[2] The inner surface of an RPE cell has tiny extensions, known as microvilli, that are located between the photoreceptors. The space between the microvilli and the photoreceptors is filled with a material that has the staining properties of mucopolysaccharide,[3] and this medium serves as a weak bond between the sensory retina and the RPE. Fluid that percolates through breaks in the sensory retina may weaken this bond and may lead to a retinal detachment, but vitreous traction is more important in causing detachment. The bond is substantial, however, as demonstrated by the high occurrence of retinal breaks without subsequent retinal detachment (even a localized detachment). Therefore, this bond is significant in the formation of retinal detachment. In the presence of a retinal detachment, RPE cells can break loose from the basal lamina and float under the detachment or migrate through the retinal break to become involved in proliferative vitreoretinopathy, which can lead to a tractional retinal detachment.

The RPE is firmly attached to the basement membrane that forms the innermost layer of the basal lamina (Bruch's membrane). The basal lamina is composed of the basement membrane of the RPE, inner collagenous zone, elastic layer, outer collagenous zone, and basement membrane of the choriocapillaris.[4] The union of these layers causes the pigment epithelium, Bruch's membrane, and the choroid to bond tightly together. RPE cells are firmly attached to each other by a continuous layer of intercellular adhesions, known as the zonular occludens.[5] This layer serves as a barrier to the movement of large molecules from the choroid to the retina. The color of the RPE generally varies from light gray to jet black (as seen in Chapter 3 in the sections on Congenital Retinal Pigment Epithelium Hyperplasia and Acquired Hyperplasia of the Pigment Epithelium). Melanin is responsible for the RPE's black color, and the RPE also contains lipofuscin, a wear-and-tear pigment that has a golden orange color. In minuscule quantities, as in a blonde fundus, the pigment epithelium appears to be essentially transparent (Figure 2-2).

Choroid

The choroid is made up of many layers; the innermost is the basal lamina (Bruch's membrane), which is thin and essentially transparent. The layer below the basal lamina is the choriocapillaris, a bright red, fine meshwork of large capillaries. The layer of

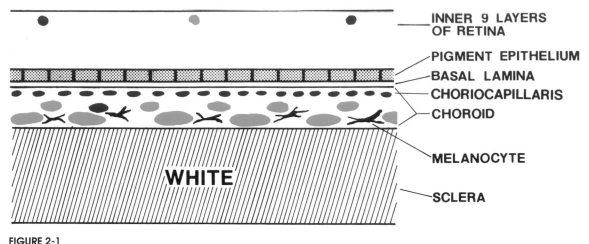

FIGURE 2-1
Diagrammatic representation of normal retina.

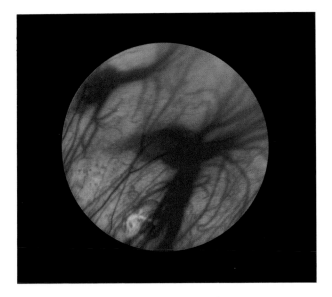

FIGURE 2-2
Vortex vein seen in a blonde fundus seen through the fundus camera. Note the tributaries, the ampulla, and the exiting vein that disappears into the sclera.

medium and large choroidal vessels lies immediately below the choriocapillaris. The vessels add to the reddish color of the choroid, but they do not form a uniform red filter, as does the choriocapillaris. Among the medium and large vessels can be found melanocytes, which give the choroid a darkish color. Again, melanin is responsible for

the black color. Finally, there is the sclera, which is white.

The bright orange to grayish color of the fundus reflex depends on hemoglobin in the blood vessels, the amount of melanin in the RPE, and the choroidal melanocytes. The appearance of many lesions of the peripheral fundus depends on which of the pigmented structures is exaggerated or missing. Close examination and understanding of Figure 2-1 will greatly enhance the clinician's understanding of diseases affecting the peripheral fundus or the posterior pole.

Equator

The equator of the fundus is approximately 14–15 mm from the limbus and can be located by finding the vortex veins (see Figure 2-2). The vortex system is composed of tributaries that vary in size and shape and generally number between four and 15.[6] They empty into the ampulla (the dilated sac of the vortex vein), which may have a pigmented crescent. The exiting vortex veins travel obliquely through scleral canals for approximately 4 mm and exit the globe posterior to the equator. There are usually four vortex veins (one per quadrant): The superior veins drain into the superior ophthalmic vein and the inferior veins into the inferior ophthalmic vein. In some instances, as many as eight to ten vortex veins are found in one eye. The equator can be visualized by drawing an

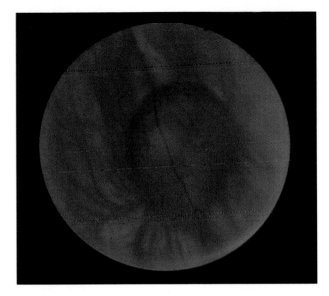

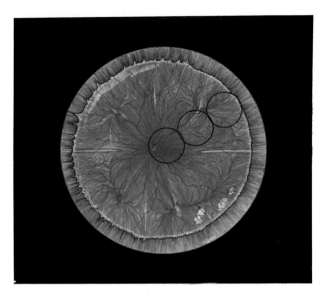

FIGURE 2-3
The dark roundish area in the center of the figure is a vortex ampulla varix as seen through the fundus camera.

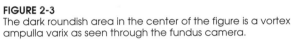

FIGURE 2-4
The peripheral fundus. The three black circles represent the views through an 18-diopter condensing lens from the optic disc to the ora serrata. The long ciliary nerves and long posterior ciliary arteries are seen at the 3 and 9 o'clock positions. Short posterior ciliary nerves are seen at 1:30, 2, 6:30, and 11:30 o'clock. A large ora tooth is at 10 o'clock, and double ora teeth are at 11 o'clock. There are five vortex veins, located at 5:30, 7:30, 10:00, and 11:30; some show pigmentation at the site of the ampulla. Peripheral cystoid degeneration is seen circumferentially next to the ora serrata. Chorioretinal atrophy is seen from 4 to 5 o'clock and white-without-pressure is seen from 9:30 to 12 o'clock. A retinal tuft with vitreous traction is seen at 8 o'clock. There is pigment cuffing of a retinal venule at 4 o'clock. The pars plana is the light brown broad ring peripheral to the ora serrata. (Reproduced with permission from A Cavallerano, MJ Garston. Examination of the peripheral ocular fundus. Rev Optom 1979;116:43–49.)

imaginary circle through the ampullae of the vortex veins. When the globe is moved into different positions during ophthalmoscopy, sometimes an exiting vortex vein may develop a stricture, which results in a venous stasis condition. The subsequent increase in venous pressure can produce a dramatic dilation of the internal ampulla, known as a varix (Figure 2-3). The varix disappears when the globe is moved into another position.[7–10] Vortex vein varices have been confused with a possible choroidal mass.[11]

Ciliary Nerves and Arteries

Long and short ciliary nerves run perpendicular to the ora serrata in the peripheral fundus (Figures 2-4, 2-5, and 2-6). They are initially seen approximately at the equator and usually disappear from view at the ora serrata. They are located in the suprachoroidal space. A long ciliary nerve is found at the medial and temporal aspects of the globe, thus dividing the fundus into superior and inferior halves. The 10–20 short ciliary nerves are found at locations in the fundus other than the 3 and 9 o'clock positions. Ciliary nerves may have pigmented margins.

The nasal long posterior ciliary artery is located just superior to the nasal long ciliary nerve, and the

temporal long posterior ciliary artery is just inferior to the temporal long ciliary nerve. The short posterior ciliary arteries are seen at other locations in the fundus. These arteries may also have pigmented margins.

Retinal blood vessels become smaller and more numerous as they travel from the posterior pole into the peripheral retina. Arterioles are smaller in caliber and lighter in color than the venules. Retinal vessels may even travel parallel to the ora serrata in the far periphery and thus are more easily involved in a peripheral flap tear formation. Most of the blood vessels seem to disappear approximately 2 mm from the ora serrata.

Anterior to the equator is the peripheral retina, which is approximately three disc diameters wide and ends at the ora serrata. Most of the peripheral

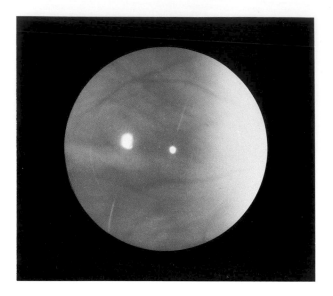

FIGURE 2-5
The temporal long ciliary nerve seen through the indirect condensing lens.

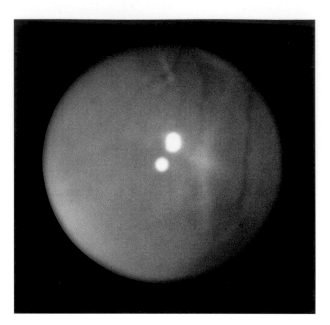

FIGURE 2-6
The short posterior ciliary nerve can be seen as a white curved line in the inferonasal quadrant through the indirect condensing lens.

retinal lesions discussed in this text are located in this zone.

Ora Serrata

The ora serrata denotes the anterior limit of the neural retina. As the neural retina approaches the ora, there are fewer ganglion and nerve fiber layers as well as photoreceptors, and the inner and outer nuclear layers merge. The inner limiting membrane interweaves with the vitreous base, and the external limiting membrane continues into the ciliary body as a junctional zone between the pigmented and the nonpigmented epithelia. The residual sensory retina continues forward as the nonpigmented epithelium. The RPE continues forward as the pigmented epithelium of the ciliary body.

The ora serrata has a scalloped appearance, serrated more nasally than temporally (Figures 2-7 and 2-8). It is 2 mm wide nasally and 1 mm wide temporally. It is slightly more anterior nasally (7 mm from the nasal limbus as compared to 8 mm from the temporal limbus). This corresponds to the insertion of the medial and lateral rectus muscles. The rounded extensions of the pars plana at the ora serrata are called ora bays, and the retinal extensions between bays are known as dentate processes or ora teeth (see

Figures 2-4 and 2-7). There are approximately 20–30 dentate processes per eye. Transillumination of the globe may allow for a view of the ora serrata and other anterior structures (Figure 2-9).

An anatomic variation of the pars plana at the ora serrata is the finding of a deep ora bay (Figure 2-10) or a large ora tooth (see Figure 2-4). Deep ora bays are found at least six times more frequently than any other variation of the ora serrata, they have a tendency to be bilateral, and they are two to four times wider than adjacent bays.[12] Generally, the temporal ora serrata has no bays and teeth, which is due to a difference in the development of the temporal pars plana as compared to the nasal half (Figure 2-11). Another developmental variation is a bridging or a tooth that does not touch the ciliary epithelium of the pars plana and thus forms a curved, bridgelike structure. It extends from the peripheral retina to as far anterior as the middle of the pars plana. It often displays a marked degree of cystoid degeneration.[12]

The transition between the more and less scalloped ora serrata is slightly temporal to the 12 o'clock meridian superiorly and slightly nasal to the 6 o'clock meridian inferiorly. A vertical line drawn between these two points, called the anatomic meridian, marks the watershed drainage of the temporal and nasal vortex vein collection systems.[12] The average ora serrata has 16 dentate processes, one

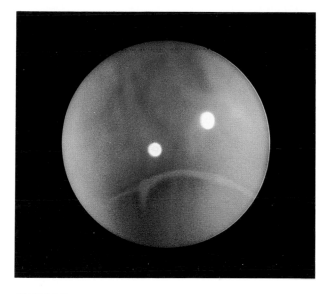

FIGURE 2-7
The superior ora serrata shows two ora bays and an ora tooth seen through the indirect condensing lens with scleral depression.

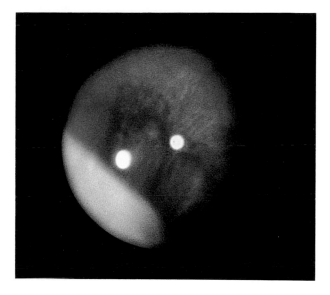

FIGURE 2-8
The superior ora serrata shows three ora bays and prominent retinal pigmentation just posterior to the ora, which denotes the location of the vitreous base (prominent vitreous base). The view is through an indirect condensing lens with scleral depression.

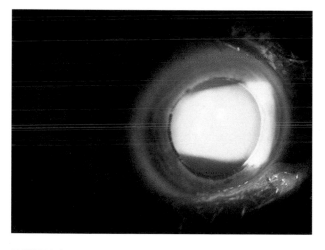

FIGURE 2-9
Transillumination of the globe shows a pigmented band just posterior to the limbus that is the base of the corona ciliaris. Next is a lighter band, the pars plana, which ends with the ora serrata. The broken lightly pigmented area posterior to the ora serrata is the prominent vitreous base.

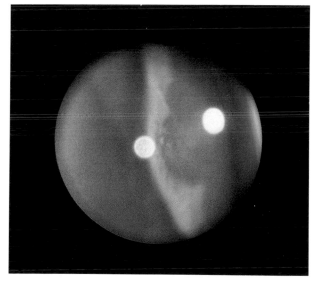

FIGURE 2-10
The nasal ora serrata shows a deep ora bay as seen through the indirect condensing lens during scleral depression.

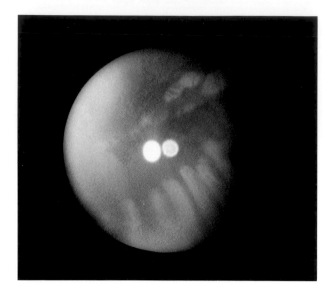

FIGURE 2-11
View of the superior peripheral fundus shows, from top to bottom, peripheral retina with paving-stone degeneration, ora serrata, pars plana, and the tips of the ciliary processes, which appear as whitish, fingerlike projections. The view is through an indirect condensing lens of an eye with a sector iridectomy.

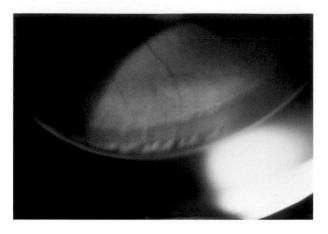

FIGURE 2-12
View of the superior peripheral fundus shows, from top to bottom, peripheral retina with cystoid degeneration, ora serrata, pars plana, and the tips of the ciliary processes (which appear as whitish, fingerlike projections). The view is through the QuadrAspheric condensing lens in an eye with posttraumatic aniridia.

large or giant dentate process, 10 ora bays, and one double ora bay.[13, 14] The ora serrata is the anterior limit of a retinal detachment.

Pars Plana

The pars plana is a broad, pigmented, chocolate-colored band that stretches from the pars ciliaris to the ora serrata (Figure 2-12; see also Figures 2-4, 2-7, 2-8, 2-10, and 2-11). It is composed of an inner nonpigmented epithelium, an outer pigmented epithelium, basal lamina, and a layer of blood vessels. The pars plana is approximately 4 mm wide nasally and 5 mm wide temporally. The nonpigmented epithelium can be detached from the pigmented epithelium, as in a pars plana cyst (see Figure 3-2).

Corona Ciliaris

The corona ciliaris is the anterior portion of the ciliary body and is approximately 2 mm wide. It contains some 60–70 ciliary processes that appear a light cream color with indirect ophthalmoscopy (see Figures 2-11 and 2-12). The color is created when the nonpigmented epithelium is seen on the internal surface of the processes with tangential illumination. Ciliary processes seen with straight-on illumination through a peripheral iridectomy or iridodialysis during biomicroscopy are brown because of the pigment epithelium under the nonpigmented epithelium. The corona ciliaris is composed of nonpigmented and pigmented epithelia, stroma, blood vessels, and smooth muscle.

Vitreous Body

Duke-Elder claimed that the first theories of vitreous structure proposed a compartment made up of "loose and delicate filaments surrounded by fluid, as described by Demours in 1741."[15] The vitreous body fills two-thirds of the globe and has a volume of 4–5 ml. The vitreous is a transparent medium that allows light to reach the retina; it probably serves as structural support for the developing retina and later may be involved in metabolic support. The vitreous body is the structure found in the cavity bordered anteriorly by the posterior lens surface, the zonules between the ciliary processes and the lens, the corona ciliaris, and the pars plana and posteriorly by the retinal surface and the surface of the optic nerve head. The axial length of the vitreous body in an emmetropic eye is approximately 16 mm. The depression just behind the lens is known as the patellar fossa, and the anterior vitreous face is attached to the posterior lens capsule at the hyaloideocapsular ligament of Weiger, which is an annular region 1–2 mm wide and 8–9 mm in diameter.[16] At the center of the hyaloideocapsular ligament is Berger's space, and arising from it is a canal that traverses the vitreous body posteriorly to the optic disc, called Cloquet's canal, which is the site of the hyaloid artery. The space where Cloquet's canal opens as it approaches the optic disc is the area of Martegiani.

The vitreous is most likely made up of collagen type II,[17–19] which is also found in cartilage, although it has some unique features that are likely related to its physiologic role in the vitreous.[20] The vitreous fibrils are continuous elements from the anterior peripheral vitreous to the posterior vitreous. The elastic nature of the vitreous seems to depend on the fact that these collagen fibrils are unbranched rather than cross-linked and are organized in a network where they are able to slide along each other.[21–23] Collagen fibrils are present in the vitreous body in the following decreasing order, according to density: vitreous base, posterior vitreous cortex adjacent to the retina, anterior vitreous cortex behind the lens and posterior chamber, and (the area of least prevalence) the center of the vitreous body and adjacent to the anterior cortical gel.[16]

The vitreous is also made up of hyaluronic acid (HA), which is a major glycosaminoglycan and appears to be synthesized primarily by hyalocytes.[24] It is believed that HA fills the spaces between the collagen fibrils and has a stabilizing effect on the collagen network.[25] Two important properties of HA contribute to the unique nature of the vitreous: (1) The HA keeps the vitreous collagen fibrils separated, which helps to minimize light scattering by the fibrils and thereby contributes to the transparency of the vitreous,[26, 27] and (2) the viscoelastic properties and mechanical functioning of the vitreous depend on the presence of both collagen fibrils and HA because fibrils would cross-link if they were adjacent to each other.[20] The HA is in the highest concentration in regions where there are the most hyalocytes and, therefore, it is theorized that they are responsible for the synthesis of HA. Other studies support this theory of HA synthesis from hyalocytes.[28–31] The level of HA is kept in equilibrium by hyalocytes, by its escape from the vitreous through the anterior segment, and by re-uptake by hyalocytes.[24, 32] It is known that changes in the vitreous environment around the HA can lead to extension or contraction of the HA molecules and thereby result in swelling or shrinkage of the entire vitreous.[33–36] The large HA molecules can bind a considerable amount of water (more than 99% of the total weight of HA molecules).[37] Ultrastructural studies have found that collagen fibrils are microscopic structures and that visible vitreous fibrils seen clinically occur due to the lack of HA, which allows for a bundling of many fibrils.[38] The vitreous body is 98% water, and even slight changes in hydration can lead to dramatic alterations in its internal morphology.[16]

There are free amino acids in the vitreous but at a level one-fifth that of plasma.[39] As the vitreous ages, the amino acid concentration increases due to plasma leakage from blood vessels of the retinal and ciliary body epithelia.[40] The levels of ascorbic acid are higher in the vitreous than in the plasma at a ratio of 9:1; these levels are believed to result from active transport via the ciliary epithelium.[41] The role of this high concentration in the vitreous body is related to its abilities to absorb ultraviolet radiation and to scavenge free radicals, which protect the lens and retina from the damaging effects of metabolic and light-induced singlet oxygen generation.[42–44]

Vitreous Cortex

The vitreous cortex is the shell of condensed vitreous that surrounds the vitreous gel. The cortex is divided into the anterior cortex (anterior hyaloid face), which starts 1.5 mm anterior to the ora serrata, and the posterior cortex, which is posterior to the ora serrata. The posterior cortex is 100–110 μm thick and is composed of dense, tightly packed collagen fibrils.[45, 46] There is no vitreous cortex over the optic disc and only thin cortex over the macula due to rarefaction of the collagen fibrils.[46] Because there is no vitreous cortex over the optic disc, a hole in the posterior cortical face occurs following a posterior vitreous detachment (PVD). If the ring of glial tissue surrounding the disc comes off and remains attached to the prepapillary hole, an annular ring floater is visible in the vitreous cavity (Vogt's or Weiss's ring). The prepapillary hole in the posterior cortex allows liquefied vitreous to enter the retrocortical space and become available to enter retinal breaks.

The posterior vitreous cortex adheres to the internal limiting membrane (ILM) of the retina, which is the basal lamina of Müller's cells. The bonding of the posterior cortex to the ILM is believed to be the result of extracellular matrix molecules.[47] Others report that vitreous cortex collagen fibrils actually insert into the basal lamina.[48] The basal lamina is usually 0.03–0.06 μm thick, but it is thinnest at the fovea and thicker in other areas of the posterior pole.[16] The ILM ends at the rim of the optic disc, but the basement membrane continues across the disc

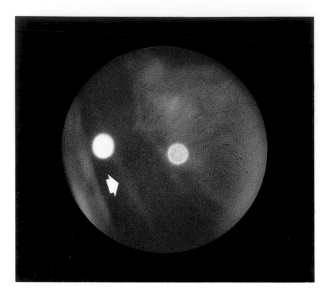

FIGURE 2-13
The anterior margin of the vitreous base can be seen as a white line halfway up the pars plana (*arrow*). The temporal ora serrata is shown through the indirect condensing lens with scleral depression.

and is known as the ILM of Elschnig. This membrane is thought to be the basal lamina of the astroglia in the optic nerve head; it is composed only of glycosaminoglycans, containing no collagen.[49] The basal lamina over the disc is 50 μm thick, but its center, known as the central meniscus of Kuhnt, is even thinner (20 μm).

The vitreous cortex has the firmest attachments at the vitreous base, the optic disc, the macula, and over retinal blood vessels. The attachments over the disc, peripapillary area, and macula are not focal but in the form of a sheet. In the macula, the ILM is thin and is purported to have attachment plaques,[47] which may explain the tendency toward traction-induced changes in this area.[50–54] Focal areas of firm vitreoretinal attachments are associated with localized vitreous traction on the retina. With age, the vitreous becomes more mobile during eye movements and is able to exert more retinal traction. When significant traction has occurred for years, the physical stimulus to the RPE may result in reactive hyperplasia, which may be seen as a pigment clump in the fundus. If this traction dramatically increases, as happens during a PVD or severe ocular trauma, a retinal tear at sites of pigment clumping may result. Pigment clumping sometimes appears on the operculum of an operculated tear or on the flap of a horseshoe tear.

Vitreous Base

The vitreous base, or vitreoretinal symphysis, is 1.5–2.0 mm anterior to the ora serrata, 1–3 mm posterior to the ora serrata,[55] and several millimeters into the vitreous body.[56] The base extends about the inner circumference of the eye and reflects the contour of the ora serrata. It straddles the ora serrata and is wider nasally than temporally. The anterior limit is sometimes seen as a whitish ridge on the pars plana (Figure 2-13). The posterior margin usually cannot be seen; however, its anterior and posterior limits are often denoted by an increase in pigmentation in the ciliary body and RPE beneath the vitreous base. This increased pigmentation is the result of vitreous traction on the base, which stimulates the underlying RPE to undergo hyperplasia, resulting in a prominent vitreous base.[56, 57] A prominent vitreous base is sometimes mistaken for lattice degeneration because it appears as a pigmented elongated area of peripheral retina parallel to the ora serrata. Lattice degeneration, however, always has some fairly normal retina between the lesion and the ora serrata, whereas a prominent vitreous base is always connected to the ora serrata. Also, lattice degeneration is often associated with white vessels, but these are not commonly seen with a prominent vitreous base (see Table 3.10). The posterior margin of the vitreous base may become visible under severe vitreous traction or on a retinal detachment and appears as a thin, elevated, whitish ridge.[7] The vitreous base is the dividing line between the anterior and posterior vitreous cortex. Condensed vitreous fibrils often appear above the vitreous base.

A dense network of vitreous fibrils originates in the base (see Figure 2-13). The fibrils penetrate to the basal lamina of the nonpigmented epithelium of the pars plana, which results in a firm union between the vitreous cortex and the pars plana. On the retinal side of the vitreous base, the ILM of the retina is absent under the symphysis and the vitreous fibrils form intricate bonds with the retinal glial cells (Müller cells).[8] The vitreous base is the most adherent location of the vitreous to the internal surface of the globe, and any attempt to pull it free results in a tearing of the nonpigmented epithelium of the pars plana or retinal tissue.[9] It requires severe blunt ocular trauma to separate the vitreous base from its underlying attachment (avulsed vitreous base). A posterior vitreous detachment stops at the posterior margin of the base and denotes its location.

Posterior to the base, the vitreoretinal adhesions are considerably weaker and are easily separated by a PVD. Even though these posterior vitreoretinal adhesions become more tenuous with advancing age, there may be focal areas of exaggerated vitreo-retinal attachments. These focal areas may demonstrate loss of the retina and inner limiting laminas with direct union between the vitreous fibrils and the retinal glia in a way that resembles attachments at the vitreous base.[58–60] These firm attachments can be associated with retinal tears following a PVD. Thus, the finding most often associated with a rhegmatogenous retinal detachment is a PVD.

With age, the posterior margin of the vitreous base may develop posterior extensions as far back as the equator, and retinal breaks can occur at these extensions. Approximately 15% of breaks are found along irregularities in the posterior margin of the vitreous base.[61] When a retinal tear occurs posterior to this margin, the physical ripping and anterior progression stops at the vitreous base and denotes its location. A PVD does not involve the vitreous base and thus, retinal tears within the base are uncommon. If they do occur, they are often related to focal traction within the base (e.g., zonular traction tufts).[1] Small retinal breaks found within the vitreous base (intrabasal) do not need to be treated due to the extreme physical adherence of the base to the underlying retina. Because there is a firm gel structure over the vitreous base, liquefaction is reduced and there is less likelihood of fluid entering an intrabasal break to cause a retinal detachment. Tears can also occur on the pars plana at the anterior margin of the base; they tend to be linear or triangular. These may lead to a detachment of the nonpigmented from the pigmented epithelium.

References

1. Straatsma BR, Foos RY, et al. Degenerative Diseases of the Peripheral Retina. In TD Duane, EA Jaeger (eds), Clinical Ophthalmology. Philadelphia: Harper & Row, 1976;26:1–30.
2. Young RW. Visual cells and the concept of renewal. Am J Med Sci 1976;272:700–725.
3. Hogan MJ, Alavarado JA, et al. Histology of the Human Eye: An Atlas and Textbook. Philadelphia: Saunders, 1971:607–637.
4. Zimmerman LE, Straatsma BR. Anatomical Relationships of the Retina to the Vitreous Body and to the Pigment Epithelium. In CL Schepens (ed), Importance of the Vitreous Body in Retina Surgery with Special Emphasis on Reoperation. St. Louis: Mosby, 1960:15–29.
5. Peyman GA, Spitznas M, et al. Peroxidase diffusion in the normal and photocoagulated retina. Invest Ophthalmol 1971;10:181–189.
6. Cavallerano A, Garston MJ. Examination of the peripheral ocular fundus. Rev Optom 1978;11:43–49.
7. Hunter JE. Vortex vein varix. Am J Optom Physiol Optics 1983;60:995–996.
8. Lopez P. Varix of the vortex vein ampulla. J Am Optom Assoc 1986;57:104–108.
9. Osher RH, Abrams GW, et al. Varix of the vortex vein ampulla. Am J Ophthalmol 1981;92:653–660.
10. Singh AD, De Potter P, et al. Indocyanine green angiography and ultrasonography of a varix of vortex vein. Arch Ophthalmol 1993;111:1283–1284.
11. da Cruz L, James B, et al. Multiple vortex vein varices masquerading as choroidal secondaries. Br J Ophthalmol 1994;78:800–801.
12. Rutnin U. Fundus appearance in normal eyes. Parts I and II. Am J Ophthalmol 1967;64:821–852.
13. Straatsma BR, Foos FY, et al. The Retina—Topography and Clinical Correlations. In New Orleans Academy of Ophthalmology: Symposium on Retina and Retinal Surgery. St. Louis: Mosby, 1969.
14. Straatsma BR, Landers MB, et al. The ora serrata in the adult human eye. Arch Ophthalmol 1968;80:3–20.
15. Demours P. Observations anatomiques sur la structure cellulaire du corps vitre. Memories de Paris 1741.
16. Sebag J. Vitreous Biochemistry, Morphology, and Clinical Examination. In WF Tasman, EA Jaeger (eds), Clinical Ophthalmology. Vol. 3. Philadelphia: Harper & Row 1992;26:1–21.
17. Stuart JM, Cremer MA, et al. Collagen following induced arthritis in rats. Comparison of vitreous and cartilage-derived collagens. Arthritis Rheum 1979;22:347–352.
18. Linsenmayer TF, Gibney E, et al. Type II collagen in the early embryonic chick cornea and vitreous: Immuno-radiochemical evidence. Exp Eye Res 1982;34:371–379.
19. Hong BS, Davidson DF. Identification of type II procollagen in rabbit vitreous. Ophthalmic Res 1985;17:162–167.
20. Sebag J. The Vitreous: Structure, Function and Pathobiology. New York: Springer-Verlag, 1989:63–64.
21. Balazs EA. Fine structure of the developing vitreous. Int Ophthalmol Clin 1973;15:53–63.
22. Balazs EA. Die mikrostruktur ind chimie des glaskorpers. In W Jaeger (ed), Bericht uber die Zusammen Kunst der Deutschen Ophthalmologischen Besemschaft. Heidelberg 1967. Munich: Bergmann Verlag, 1968:536-572.
23. Weber H, Landuehr G, et al. Mechanical properties of the vitreous in pig and human donor eyes. Ophthalmic Res 1982;14:335–343.
24. Balazs EA, Denlinger JL. The Vitreous. In H Davson (ed), The Eye. Vol 1A. London: Academic, 1984:533–589.
25. Balazs EA. Functional Anatomy of the Vitreous. In WF Tasman, EA Jaeger (eds), Biomedical Foundations of Ophthalmology. Vol.1. Philadelphia: Harper & Row, 1982:17:6–12.
26. Scott JE. Proteoglycan-collagen interactions and corneal ultrastructure. Biochem Soc Trans 1992;19:877–881.
27. Sebag J. The Vitreous: Structure, Function and Pathology. New York: Springer-Verlag, 1989:47–55.
28. Osterlin SE. The synthesis of hyaluronic acid in the vitreous. III. Regeneration in the owl monkey. Exp Eye Res 1969;7:524–533.
29. Osterlin SE. The synthesis of hyaluronic acid in the vitreous. IV. In vivo metabolism in the owl monkey. Exp Eye Res 1969;8:521–534.
30. Berman ER, Gombos GM. Studies on the incorporation of U-14 C-glucose into vitreous polymers in vitro and in vivo. Invest Ophthalmol 1969;18:521–534.
31. Bleckmann H. Glycosaminoglycan metabolism of cultured fibroblasts from bovine vitreous. Graefes Arch Clin Exp Ophthalmol 1984;222:90 94.

32. Laurent UBG, Fraser JRE. Turnover of hyaluronate in aqueous humor and vitreous body of the rabbit. Exp Eye Res 1983;36:493–503.

33. Sebag J. Aging of the vitreous. Eye 1987;1:254–262.

34. Comper WD, Laurent TC. Physiological functions of connective tissue polysaccharides. Physiol Rev 1978;58:255–315.

35. Chakrabarti B, Park JW. Glycosaminoglycans: Structure and interaction. CRC Crit Rev Biochem Mol Biol 1980; 8:255–313.

36. Christiansson J. Changes in mucopolysaccharides during alloxan diabetes in the rabbit. Acta Ophthalmol 1958; 36:141–162.

37. Straatsma BR. Symposium: Surgery of the vitreous body. Trans Am Acad Ophthalmol Otolaryngol 1973;77:168–170.

38. Sebag J, Balazs EA. Morphology and ultrastructure of human vitreous fibers. Invest Ophthalmol Vis Sci 1989; 30:1867–1871.

39. Jacobson B. Degradation of glycosaminoglycans by extracts of calf vitreous hyalocytes. Exp Eye Res 1984; 39:373–385.

40. Balazs EA, Delinger JL. Aging Changes in the Vitreous. In Aging and Human Visual Function. New York: Liss, 1982;45–57.

41. Kinsey VE. Transfer of ascorbic acid and related compounds across the blood barrier. Am J Ophthalmol 1947;30:1262–1266.

42. Ringvold A. Aqueous humor and ultraviolet radiation. Acta Ophthalmol 1980;58:69–82.

43. Balazs EA. Studies of structure of vitreous body. Absorption of ultraviolet light. Am J Ophthalmol 1954; 38:21–28.

44. Ueno N, Sebag J, et al. Effects of visible-light irradiation on vitreous structure in the presence of a photosensitizer. Exp Eye Res 1987;44:863–870.

45. Balazs EA. Molecular Morphology of the Vitreous Body. In GK Smelser (ed), The Structure of the Eye. New York: Academic, 1961:293–310.

46. Steeten BA. Disorders of the Vitreous. In A Garner, GK Klintworth (eds), Pathobiology of Ocular Disease: A Dynamic Approach, Part B. New York: Dekker, 1982; 49:1381–1419.

47. Sebag J. Age-related differences in the human vitreo-retinal interface. Arch Ophthalmol 1991;109:966–971.

48. Fine BS, Tousimis AJ. The structure of the vitreous body and the suspensory ligaments of the lens. Arch Ophthalmol 1961;65:95–110.

49. Heegaard S, Jensen OA, et al. Structure of the vitreal face of the monkey optic disc (*Macaca mulatta*): SEM on frozen resin-cracked optic nerve heads supplemented by TEM and immunohistochemistry. Graefes Arch Clin Exp Ophthalmol 1988;226:377–383.

50. Sebag J, Balazs EA. Pathogenesis of CME: Anatomic consideration of vitreo-retinal adhesions. Surv Ophthalmol 1984;28:493–498.

51. Jaffe NS. Vitreous traction at the posterior pole of the fundus due to alterations in the vitreous posterior. Trans Am Acad Ophthalmol Otolaryngol 1967;71:642–652.

52. Jaffe NS. Macular retinopathy after separation of vitreoretinal adherence. Arch Ophthalmol 1967;78:585–591.

53. Schachat AP, Sommer A. Macular hemorrhages associated with posterior vitreous detachment. Am J Ophthalmol 1986;102:647–649.

54. Sebag J. Vitreo-retinal Interface and the Role of Vitreous in Macular Disease. In R Brancato, G Coscas, B Lumbroso (eds), Proceedings of the Retina Workshop. Amsterdam: Kugler & Ghedini, 1987:3–6.

55. Hogan MJ. The vitreous: Its structure in relation to the ciliary body and retina. Invest Ophthalmol 1963;2:418–445.

56. Reeser FH, Aabery T. Vitreous Humor. In PE Records (ed), Physiology of the Human Eye and Visual System. Hagerstown, MD: Harper & Row, 1979:1–31.

57. Foos RY. Vitreoretinal juncture: Topographical variations. Invest Ophthalmol 1972;11:801–808.

58. Foos RY. Anatomic and pathologic aspects of the vitreous body. Trans Am Acad Ophthalmol Otolaryngol 1973; 77:171–183.

59. Spencer LM, Straatsma RA, et al. Tractional degenerations of the peripheral retina. New Orleans Academy of Ophthalmology: Symposium of the Retina and Retinal Surgery. St. Louis: Mosby, 1969.

60. Foos RY. Vitreous Base, Retinal Tufts, and Retinal Tears: Pathogenic Relationships. In RC Pruett, CDJ Regan (eds), Retina Congress. New York: Appleton-Century-Croft, 1972:259–280.

61. Schepens CL. Retinal Detachment and Allied Diseases. Philadelphia: Saunders, 1983:186.

Chapter 3

Developmental Anomalies, Degeneration, and Diseases of the Peripheral Retina and Pars Plana

A number of degenerations of the peripheral retina are discussed in this chapter. Figure 3-1 illustrates several of the entities discussed.

Pars Plana Cysts and Epithelial Degeneration

Clinical Description

Pars plana cysts are clear cystoid spaces between the pigmented and nonpigmented epithelia. Most large cysts are oval, but smaller ones can be round, oblong, lobulated, oval, or irregularly shaped (Figures 3-2 and 3-3). They vary in size from one-fourth to three disc diameters and are usually located in the temporal side of the eye. Large cysts may occupy more than one bay and may extend from the ora serrata to the ciliary processes.

The cyst's inner walls may be flabby and poorly transparent, but most are distended and very transparent. Most pars plana cysts exhibit a smooth, taut, transparent surface that allows a view of the underlying pigment epithelium. The cysts are most often observed during binocular indirect ophthalmoscopy as a clear, blisterlike lesion just barely visible in the indirect condensing lens. The view of these cysts can be greatly enhanced by performing scleral depression. They look very much like a small retinoschisis of the pars plana, and similarly, they do not undulate with eye movements. Pars plana cysts may be solitary or occur in a row of multiple cysts abutting each other. Sometimes they have a light dusting of pigment on their inner walls. Pars plana cysts are present in 3–18% of all patients.[1–3]

Histopathology

Pars plana cysts are formed by a separation of the nonpigmented from the pigmented epithelium, which is analogous to a retinal detachment (Figure 3-4). The inner nonpigmented epithelium can be a single layer or consist of several cell layers.[2, 4] The inner layer may even produce extensions into the cystic cavity.[5] The cavities are filled with a fluid that presumably contains hyaluronic acid.

Clinical Significance

Most pars plana cysts are acquired; very few are congenital. They may be idiopathic or occur secondary to ocular disease. They are more commonly seen in eyes with retinal detachment, where they tend to be large. Their occurrence in eyes with retinal detachment may be the result of traction by the shrinking vitreous base.[6] The cysts may even communicate with the subretinal space in some cases. Pars plana cysts also frequently occur in eyes with posterior uveitis.

Pars plana cysts can be present in patients with multiple myeloma and seem to be filled with a para-aminosalicylic acid (PAS)-positive protein,

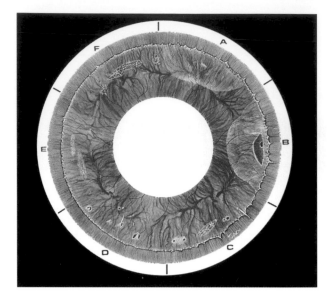

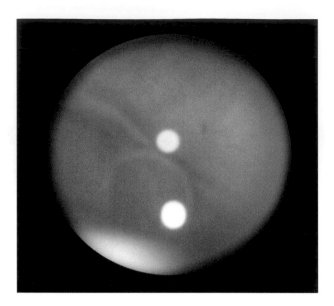

FIGURE 3-1
Peripheral retinal degenerations. Typical lattice degeneration is seen between 10:30 and 12 o'clock; the lattice at 5 o'clock has a hole within the lesion and a small tear at the nasal edge. The retinoschisis cavities are seen between 12 and 4 o'clock. The upper retinoschisis has snowflakes along its posterior margin and a thin pigmented demarcation line at its inferior nasal margin. The lower retinoschisis has an outer-layer tear with a rolled posterior edge and an inner-layer hole. Snail-track degeneration is found between 8:30 and 9:30. A meridional fold is seen at 4:30, with small localized retinal tears at the posterior and inferior margins. There are atrophic retinal holes at 4:30, and a small localized retinal detachment is associated with holes at 5:30. Horseshoe tears along with an operculated tear are seen between 6:30 and 8 o'clock. Note the pigment clump on the flap of the horseshoe tear at 6:30 and the vitreous strand on the flap of the tear at 7 o'clock. Peripheral cystoid degeneration is seen circumferentially next to the ora serrata. (Courtesy of MJ Garston, A Cavallerano. Degenerative changes associated with retinal detachment. Rev Optom1979;116:81–84.)

FIGURE 3-2
A pars plana cyst can be seen as a round transparent balloon (located between the light reflexes) on the inferior nasal pars plana. Also in view are the ora serrata and peripheral cystoid degeneration seen through an indirect condensing lens.

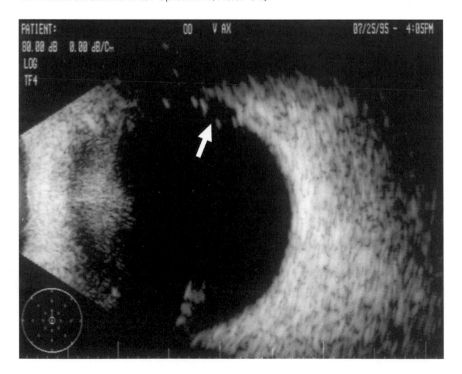

FIGURE 3-3
B-scan ultrasonogram of a large superior pars plana cyst (*arrow*).

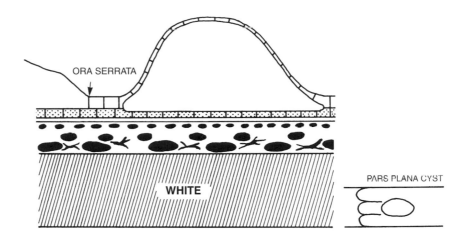

FIGURE 3-4
The pars plana cyst consists of a separation of the nonpigmented epithelium from the pigmented epithelium of the pars plana by a fluid-filled cavity.

which is the same myeloma protein (IgG) as is found in the patients' serum.[7] During fixation, the cysts of multiple myeloma become whitish, whereas other pars plana cysts remain clear.[8]

The nonpigmented epithelium may show hyaline or fatty degeneration with increasing age. Hyperplasia of the nonpigmented epithelium may cause pedunculated or senile wartlike growths to appear.[5] There can be erosion of the nonpigmented epithelium, causing a craterlike appearance to the pars plana (Figure 3-5). Tears of the nonpigmented epithelium also can occur. These are usually found along the anterior margin of the vitreous base and are generally associated with trauma.[6]

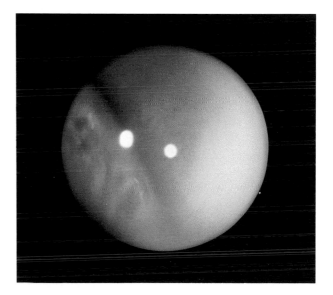

FIGURE 3-5
Degeneration of the superior temporal pars plana can be seen as areas of epithelial erosion, as viewed through an indirect condensing lens.

References

1. Allen RA, Miller DH, et al. Cysts of the posterior ciliary body (pars plana). Arch Ophthalmol 1961;66:302–313.
2. Okun E. Gross and microscopic pathology in autopsy eyes. IV. Pars plana cysts. Am J Ophthalmol 1961;51:1221–1228.
3. Grignolo A, Schepens CL, et al. Cysts of the pars plana ciliaris. Arch Ophthalmol 1957;58:530–543.
4. Gartner J. Fine structure of pars plana cysts. Am J Ophthalmol 1972;73:971–984.
5. Duke-Elder S, Perkins ES. Diseases of the Uveal Tract. In System of Ophthalmology. Vol. 9. London: Henry Kimpton, 1977:765–768.
6. Schepens CL. Retinal Detachment and Allied Diseases. Philadelphia: Saunders, 1983:163–187.
7. Bloch RS. Hematologic Disorders. In TD Duane, EA Jaeger (eds), Clinical Ophthalmology. Vol. 5. Philadelphia: Harper & Row, 1976:8.
8. Yanoff M, Fine BS. Ocular Pathology: A Text and Atlas (2nd ed). Philadelphia: Harper & Row, 1982:404.

Congenital Retinal Pigment Epithelium Hypertrophy

Clinical Description

The pigment epithelium of the retina and ciliary body is composed of a monolayer on cuboidal and columnar cells containing numerous pigment granules. These cells derive from the outer layer of the primitive optic cup and are located between the photoreceptors and the basal lamina (Bruch's membrane). Embryologically, the pigment epithelium has a different tissue origin than that of the choroidal melanocytes, which gives rise to different acquired disease manifestations. The pigment epithelial cells can undergo reactive proliferation and migration, but they do not have neoplastic capabilities.[1, 2] The choroidal melanocytes are branching, dendritic cells that are interspersed in the uveal space and are believed to originate from the neurocrest. They are capable of neoplastic transformation but are not inherently able to undergo reactive proliferation and migration.[3]

Congenital hypertrophy of the retinal pigment epithelium (RPE) may be either unifocal or multifocal. Unifocal congenital hypertrophy of the retinal pigment epithelium (CHRPE) results in pigmented, flat, round lesions with distinct margins (Figure 3-6).[4, 5] Areas of congenital hypertrophy range from light brown to jet black, depending on the amount of melanin in the epithelial cells.[5] Overlying retinal blood vessels appear normal. Areas of congenital hypertrophy are not to be confused with a choroidal nevus, which is usually flat, slate gray, and with indistinct margins. During scleral depression the pigmented lesion rolls evenly and without any apparent change in color. The lesions are almost always stable in size, but their color may change due to chorioretinal atrophy. On rare occasions, they have been shown to enlarge over many years.[6] A full or partial hypopigmented ring is sometimes seen around the lesions (Figure 3-7); this ring or halo is composed of epithelial cells devoid of melanin granules and is sometimes incorrectly diagnosed as a halo nevus (see Choroidal Nevus later in this chapter). Areas of pigment mottling and chorioretinal atrophy often occur; the areas of chorioretinal atrophy produce windowlike defects, called lacunae, that allow a clear view of the underlying choroid (Figure 3-8).[5, 7–9] One or many lacunae may be present within the boundary of the lesion (see Chorioretinal Atrophy later in this chapter). The prevalence of these lesions is quite common, although an estimated percentage for the general population has not been reported. The lacunae can enlarge over time.

FIGURE 3-6
Darkly pigmented congenital hypertrophy of the retinal pigment epithelium, with a clear halo around the lesion.

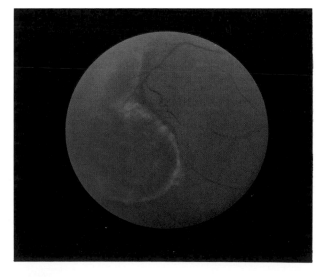

FIGURE 3-7
Congenital hypertrophy of the retinal pigment epithelium that is mildly pigmented with a classic halo and a large central lacuna.

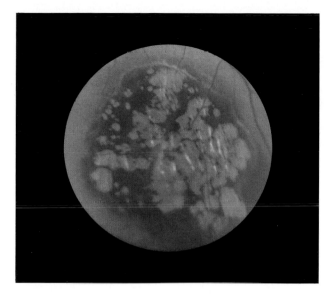

FIGURE 3-8
Retinal pigment epithelial hypertrophy with numerous lacunae (chorioretinal atrophy) and a slight surrounding clear halo.

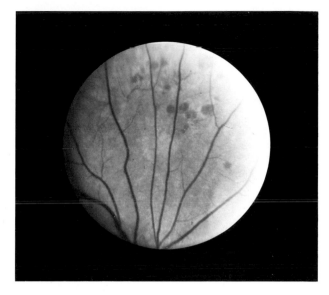
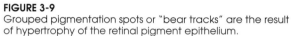

FIGURE 3-9
Grouped pigmentation spots or "bear tracks" are the result of hypertrophy of the retinal pigment epithelium.

A CHRPE can be found in any location in the retina, from adjacent to the ora serrata to a crescent around the optic disc, but about 70% occur in the temporal half of the fundus.[5] When a unifocal CHRPE is found in the region of the optic disc, often it partially surrounds the disc margin but abruptly ends at the edge of the disc. When it is found in the far periphery of the retina, it ends just before the ora serrata or immediately at the pars plana, never extending onto the pars plana.[3] CHRPEs can be scattered throughout the fundus, sometimes extending onto the disc without seeming to originate from the disc, as with a melanoma. Diameter usually varies from 2 to 6 mm,[7] but they have been known to range from a pinpoint to 14 disc diameters.[5, 10] Peripheral lesions tend to be larger than posterior lesions. A unifocal CHRPE is usually unilateral, but it does occur bilaterally in about 1–2% of the cases.[5] These lesions essentially never produce symptoms, and there is no predilection for gender or laterality. Although CHRPEs are probably more frequently discovered in whites, there seems to be no racial predisposition when studies are corrected for racial population densities.[3] The existence of CHRPE may be present as early as birth, but they have been found in infants as young as 3 months of age.[11]

Fluorescein angiography for a unifocal lesion that is uniformly pigmented shows hypofluorescence throughout the dye study. The fluorescein angiographic studies show blockage of the underlying choroidal fluorescence with normal fluorescence through the lacunae and depigmented area.[8] That the fluorescein study shows no leakage or staining suggests that the cellular integrity of the RPE is not compromised.[5] Lacunae are window defects that show early hyperfluorescence during the angiography that persists throughout the study. Like many other defects of the pigment epithelium, they may occasionally show an intense relative hyperfluorescence in the late phase of the angiogram due to stromal staining of the background sclera.[3]

A number of smaller lesions, usually numbering three to 30, ranging from 0.1 to 3.0 mm, and aggregated in a localized area of the fundus is known as multifocal CHRPE, grouped pigmentation spots, or bear tracks (Figure 3-9).[12] They are benign and stationary, and they are unilateral in about 85% of cases.[13] Generally, the larger lesions are located more peripherally. Visual field testing is characteristically normal. The clinical appearance has been associated with Coat's disease and enchondromatosis, but this may have been coincidental.[12] Occasionally, multifocal CHRPEs have been found in patients with neurofibromatosis.[3] Virtually the only differential diagnosis is sectorial retinitis pigmentosa.

Visual field defects have been associated with large unifocal CHRPEs that may be shallow and relative in young patients and absolute in older

Table 3-1. Congenital Retinal Pigment Epithelium (RPE) Hypertrophy vs. Acquired RPE Hyperplasia

Congenital RPE Hypertrophy	Acquired RPE Hyperplasia
Flat	Flat
Jet black to light black	Jet black to light black
Distinct margins	Distinct margins
May have chorioretinal atrophy (lacunae) within lesion	May have chorioretinal atrophy adjacent to lesion
May have clear halo	No halo
Typically round	Round to very irregular
May show scotoma consistent with size of lesion	Usually too small to produce detectable scotoma
No associated preceding event	May have history of trauma or inflammatory event
No vitreous traction	Vitreous traction may be present

Table 3-2. Congenital RPE Hypertrophy vs. Choroidal Nevus

Congenital RPE Hypertrophy	Choroidal Nevus
Flat	Flat to slightly elevated
Jet black to gray	Slate gray in color
Distinct margins	Indistinct margins
May show mottling due to RPE degeneration	May be mottled (drusen and RPE degeneration)
May have chorioretinal atrophy (lacunae) within lesion	No typical chorioretinal atrophy
May have a clear halo surrounding lesion	No halo
Typically round	Round to oval to irregular
Located in the pigment epithelium	Located in the choroid
May show scotoma on visual fields	Rarely displays a scotoma on visual fields
Blockage of underlying choroidal fluorescence during fluorescein angiography	Usually causes an area of hypofluorescence but sometimes hyperfluoresces during fluorescein angiography
Flat on ultrasonography	Usually flat but sometimes slightly elevated and sometimes demonstrates acoustic shadowing on ultrasonography

patients.[5, 8] The visual field defects are the result of degeneration of the photoreceptors in the lesion.[12, 14] Degeneration of the photoreceptors usually begins in the center of the lesion and spreads out. Ultrasonography is of little value because these lesions are usually flat. A ^{32}P test is not indicated but, if performed, would have a negative result.[5, 15]

The congenital lesions are benign but present a diagnostic challenge for the clinician (Tables 3-1 and 3-2). The differential diagnosis often includes choroidal nevus and choroidal melanoma. A malignant melanoma is almost always greater than 2 mm in thickness, whereas a CHRPE is flat. Choroidal nevi are rarely jet black and display indistinct margins, whereas CHRPE are often black with sharp borders. There have been cases of a unifocal CHRPE being misdiagnosed as a choroidal melanoma following enucleation and autopsy.[4, 14, 16] Other entities to include in the differential diagnosis are acquired hyperplasia of the RPE, old chorioretinal scar (e.g., old toxoplasmic retinochoroiditis), black sunburst from sickle cell retinopathy, and unknown pigmented lesions. All these acquired lesions usually display irregular pigmentation and margins, whereas CHRPEs have distinct and generally smooth borders.

Histopathology

In CHRPE, congenital hypertrophy (increased size of the cells) is present, and the cells contain large, oval, densely packed melanin granules (macromelanosomes) that obscure the nuclei (Figure 3-10)[4, 8, 9, 17–19]—thus, the lesions' typical darkly pigmented appearance. Although this is primarily a hypertrophy of the RPE, some cases have shown that hyperplasia may occur segmentally,[9, 18, 19] which may account for the rare instances of growth of these lesions.[9] Electron microscopy has shown the RPE cells to be twice their normal size. The normal RPE cells have small, rod-shaped, or elliptical pigment granules. There may be thickening of the basal lamina underneath the lesion, but the adjacent choroid is not affected, and the inner sensory retinal layers are usually normal.[3] The abnormal RPE is thought to lack the ability to phagocytose and digest photoreceptors' outer segments,[8, 9] which may explain

RETINAL PIGMENT EPITHELIUM HYPERPLASIA AND HYPERTROPHY

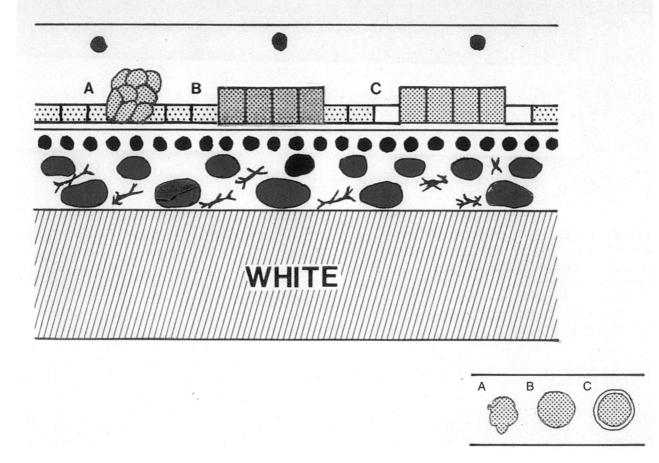

FIGURE 3-10
A. Acquired hyperplasia of the pigment epithelium, which has irregular margins. B. Congenital hypertrophy of the pigment epithelium with a uniform shape. C. Congenital hypertrophy of the pigment epithelium with a clear halo resulting from a relative absence of melanin in the pigment epithelium cells adjacent to the lesion. Lower right window view of the lesions A to C (from left to right) show acquired hyperplasia with irregular borders, congenital hypertrophy, and congenital hypertrophy with hypopigmented halo.

the histologic finding of degeneration of the overlying photoreceptors and that visual field defects can be plotted over these lesions.[4, 13, 16] Histologically, multifocal lesions are identical to unifocal lesions.[3] The lacunae seen in these lesions are the result of chorioretinal atrophy (Figure 3-11; see Chorioretinal Atrophy later in this chapter).

Clinical Significance

The prognosis is good because there have been no documented cases of CHRPE transforming into

malignant growth. If a CHRPE occurred in the fovea, the loss of photoreceptors could result in decreased vision, but this is an extremely rare event.[3] The CHRPE should be noted on the patient's chart along with its location and estimated size. It is often helpful to take a fundus photograph if the lesion is observable with the camera system. The lesion should be evaluated in 6–12 months to document stability.

Patients with familial adenomatous polyposis (FAP) and the related Gardner's syndrome may display CHRPE lesions.[7, 19–23] These CHRPE lesions may represent hamartomas and not just hypertrophy of the pigment epithelium.[24] The CHRPE of FAP

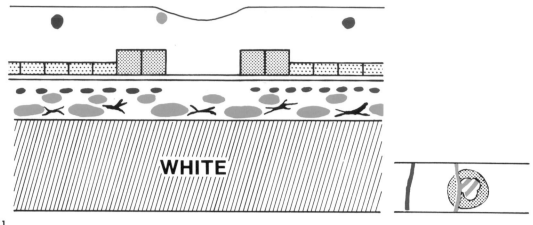

FIGURE 3-11
Chorioretinal atrophy has resulted in the formation of a lacuna within the lesion.

are often distinguishable from the typical retinal lesions by their bilaterality, family history, multiple lesions (>3), nonsectorial organization, and systemic associated abnormalities.[9, 10, 17] The retinal lesions associated with FAP represent defects in melanogenesis with both abnormal cellular hypertrophy and hyperplasia, which is more consistent with hamartoma of the retinal pigment.[19, 25] Therefore, the hypertrophy of the RPE of FAP histologically may be distinctly different from an isolated typical CHRPE. FAPs tend to have irregular borders with a tail of depigmentation on the margin of the lesion (Figure 3-12).[17] Whereas a typical unifocal lesion tends to be larger in the periphery, FAP-associated lesions tend to be smaller in the periphery and larger posterior to the equator.[9–11, 26] Usually, the FAP CHRPEs are considered benign and nonprogressive.[27] Grouped CHRPEs (multifocal) do not appear to be associated with FAP.[17] The cause of this retinal manifestation appears to be related to a widespread expression of an abnormal gene in the RPE cells. The functional abnormalities produced by these lesions seem to be localized to the epithelium and overlying photoreceptors.[28] Electro-oculographic studies have been reported to be normal in patients with FAP, and the normal recordings of the electro-oculographic studies and electroretinography (ERG) indicate no diffuse retinal disease.[8, 29] The visual acuity of two patients with FAP was decreased due to the rare presence of CHRPEs in the macula.[25] Other reported extracolonic ocular abnormalities are epidermal

cysts of the eyelids, exophthalmos secondary to orbital osteoma, and angioid streaks.[7, 30] These lesions are not necessarily a consistent finding, and CHRPE is the most common ocular finding associated with FAP. The absence of CHRPE does not exclude the diagnosis of FAP, but the presence of atypical CHRPE is considered a definite risk factor for the disease. Some families with FAP manifested CHRPE sporadically and displayed incomplete penetrance: Some family members had the retinal lesions and others did not.[26, 27]

The gene for FAP has been isolated to chromosome 5 and mapped to region 5q21–22 and it is known as the adenomatous polyposis tumor suppressor gene.[31–34] This gene is critical in the RPE proliferation and development.[24] Transmission is autosomal dominant. Even though genetic marking would be an excellent method to identify individuals with FAP, unfortunately only 33% of affected families can be accurately diagnosed with DNA testing due to the unavailability of family members and to new mutations of the DNA.[35] In patients without a family history (e.g., those who were adopted) and in cases of spontaneous mutation, the finding of multiple CHRPE lesions may be of particular benefit. The intestinal polyps of FAP usually develop between puberty and the fourth decade,[27] but in rare instances they have been found in 1-year-olds and elderly patients.[10] In the early stages of adenomatous polyp development, the patient is usually asymptomatic; however, when the symptoms of rectal bleeding, abdominal pain, mucus discharge, or diarrhea manifest, malignancy has developed in two-thirds of patients.[7, 10] Hundreds to thousands of intestinal polyps develop, and if the disease is left untreated, there is a 100% risk of the colorectal adenomatous condition becoming malignant.[10, 36] Colorectal carcinoma occurs in approximately 50% of the untreated cases by age 35 and in 100% by the fifth decade of life.[22] Prophylactic treatment is a colectomy,[37] and early diagnosis and intervention often prevents the occurrence of colorectal malignancy.

The first case of a transmission of CHRPE in a family with Gardner's syndrome was reported in 1980.[7] The expression of CHRPE has been reported to range from 58% to 100%.[10, 11, 23, 25, 26, 37–45] Patients with Gardner's syndrome may have CHRPE; however, both CHRPE and Gardner's syndrome may be seen in isolation with FAP. One study found that the finding of CHRPE in 25 families (of 75 patients, 32 had FAP) was 94% specific and 84% sensitive of patients at a high risk of FAP using the criteria that (1) the lesions were bilateral and (2) three or more lesions were larger than one-third of a disc diameter.[27] Patients with multiple CHRPE lesions should be asked about intestinal problems, and a referral to the patient's family practitioner is advisable.

FAP is an autosomal dominant condition characterized by multiple adenomatous polyps of the colon,[10, 26, 27] and when it is associated with extracolonic manifestation, it is known as Gardner's syndrome or Turcot's syndrome. Gardner's syndrome is characterized by osteomas, fibromas, lipomas, epidermal and sebaceous cysts, dermoid tumors, endocrine and hepatic tumors, and dental abnormalities. Some other extracolonic manifestations that are also thought to be associated with Gardner's syndrome are ampulla of Vater carcinoma, thyroid and skin cancer, and fibromas.[7, 27] Turcot's syndrome, which may show CHRPE, is characterized by multiple adenomatous polyps of the colon and neuroepithelial brain tumors, such as medulloblastomas and glioblastomas.[46] Many authorities believe that these two syndromes are a variable expression of the same genetic abnormality.[30, 37, 46] The extracolonic manifestations in both syndromes may not appear clinically before the polyps, and FAP may occur without any extracolonic signs.[10, 27, 37–39] CHRPE is also found in patients without any extracolonic manifestations. Patients with Gardner's syndrome may have CHRPE; however, both CHRPE and Gardner's syndrome may be seen in isolation with FAP. One study found that 55% of

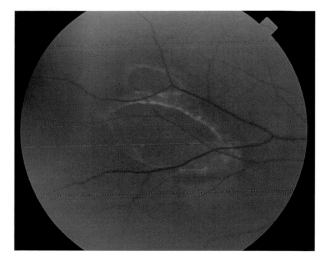

FIGURE 3-12
Congenital hypertrophy secondary to FAP tends to be irregular in shape.

patients with FAP and CHRPE (>4 retinal lesions) did not demonstrate the extracolonic lesions of Gardner's syndrome.[10] Another study found no statistical significance of CHRPE and other extracolonic manifestations of Gardner's syndrome in a study of 56 patients with FAP.[26]

An association between syringomyelia and CHRPE has also been reported.[4] One author found that patients with both unifocal and multiple CHRPE have been found to have a higher incidence of café-au-lait spots, suggesting a possible relationship to neurofibromatosis.[3]

References

1. Frayer WC. Reactivity of the retinal pigment epithelium. An experimental and histopathologic study. Trans Am Ophthalmol Soc 1966;64:587–643.
2. Hogan MJ, Zimmerman LE. Ophthalmic Pathology (2nd ed). Philadelphia: Saunders, 1962.
3. Shields JA. Diagnosis and Management of Intraocular Tumors. St. Louis: Mosby, 1983:122–143.
4. Kruz GH, Zimmerman LE. Vagaries of the retinal pigment epithelium. Int Ophthalmol Clin 1962;2:441–464.
5. Purcell JJ, Shields JA. Hypertrophy with hyperpigmentation of the retinal pigment epithelium. Arch Ophthalmol 1975;93:1122–1126.
6. Norris JL, Cleasby GW. An unusual case of congenital hypertrophy of the retinal pigment epithelium. Arch Ophthalmol 1976;94:1910–1911.
7. Blair NP, Trempe CL. Hypertrophy of the retinal pigment epithelium associated with Gardner's syndrome. Am J Ophthalmol 1980;90:661–667.

8. Buettner H. Congenital hypertrophy of the pigment epithelium. Am J Ophthalmol 1975;79:177–189.
9. Lloyd WC, Eagle RC, et al. Congenital hypertrophy of the retinal pigment epithelium: Electron microscopic and morphometric observations. Ophthalmology 1990;97:1052–1060.
10. Rominia A, Zakov AN, et al. Congenital hypertrophy of the retinal pigment epithelium in familial adenomatous polyposis. Ophthalmology 1989;96:879–884.
11. Traboulse EI, Krush AJ, et al. Prevalence and importance of pigmented ocular fundus lesions in Gardner's syndrome. N Engl J Med 1987;316:661–667.
12. Shields JA, Tso MO. Congenital grouped pigmentation of the retina. Arch Ophthalmol 1975;93:1153–1156.
13. Yanoff M, Fine BS. Ocular Pathology: A Text and Atlas (2nd ed). Philadelphia: Harper & Row, 1982:476–814.
14. Buettner H. Congenital hypertrophy of the pigment epithelium (RPE). Mod Probl Ophthalmol 1974;12:528–535.
15. Shields JA. Accuracy and limitations of the ^{32}P test in the diagnosis of ocular tumors. Ophthalmology 1978;85:950–966.
16. Reese AB, Jones IS. Benign melanomas of the retinal pigment epithelium. Am J Ophthalmol 1956;42:207–212.
17. Shields JA, Shields CL, et al. Lack of association among typical congenital hypertrophy of the retinal pigment epithelium, adenomatous polyposis, and Gardner syndrome. Ophthalmology 1992;99:1709–1713.
18. Chapion R, Daicker BC. Congenital hypertrophy of the pigment epithelium: Light microscopic and ultrastructural findings in young children. Retina 1989;9:44–48.
19. Kasner L, Traboulsi EI, et al. A histopathologic study of the pigmented fundus lesions in familial adenomatous polyposis. Retina 1992;12:35–42.
20. Gardner EJ. A genetic and clinical study of intestinal polyposis, a predisposing factor for carcinoma of the colon and rectum. Am J Hum Genet 1951;3:167–176.
21. Sheriff SM, Hegab S. A syndrome of multiple fundal anomalies in siblings with microcephaly without mental retardation. Ophthalmic Surgery 1988;19:353–355.
22. Lewis RA, Crowder WE, et al. The Gardner's syndrome: Significance of ocular features. Ophthalmology 1984;91:916–925.
23. Parisi ML. Congenital hypertrophy of the retinal pigment epithelium serves as a clinical marker in a family with familial adenomatous polyposis. J Am Optom Assoc 1995;66:106–112.
24. Marcus DM, Rustgi AK, Defoe D, et al. Retinal pigment epithelium abnormalities in mice with adenomatous polyposis coli gene disruption. Arch Ophthalmol 1997;115:645–650.
25. Romania A, Zakow ZN, et al. Retinal pigment epithelium lesions as a biomarker of disease in patients with familial adenomatous polyposis. A follow-up report. Ophthalmology 1992;99:911–913.
26. Heinemann MH, Baker RH, et al. Familial polyposis coli: The spectrum of ocular and other extracolonic manifestations. Graefes Arch Clin Exp Ophthalmol 1991;229:218–228.
27. Morton DG, Gibson J, et al. Role of congenital hypertrophy of the retinal pigment epithelium in the predictive diagnosis of familial adenomatous polyposis. Br J Surg 1992;79:689–693.
28. Santos A, Morales L, et al. Congenital hypertrophy of the retinal pigment epithelium associated with familial adenomatous polyposis. Retina 1994;14:6–9.
29. Stein EA, Brady KD. Ophthalmologic and electro-oculographic findings in Gardner's syndrome. Am J Ophthalmol 1988;106:326–331.
30. Martow J, Polmeno RC, et al. The importance of congenital hypertrophy of the retinal epithelium in familial adenomatous polyposis. Can J Ophthalmol 1990;25:290–292.
31. Solomon E, Voss R, et al. Chromosome 5 allele loss in human colorectal carcinomas. Nature 1987;328:616–619.
32. MacPherson AJS, Bjarnason I, et al. Discovery of the gene for familial adenomatous polyposis: May also increase our understanding of sporadic colorectal cancer. BMJ 1992;304:858–859.
33. Cottrell S, Bicknell D, et al. Molecular analysis of APC mutations in familial adenomatous polyposis and sporadic colon carcinomas. Lancet 1992;340:626–630.
34. Bodmer WF, Bailey CJ, Bodmer J, et al. Location of the gene for familial adenomatous polyposis on chromosome 5. Nature 1987;328:614–616.
35. MacDonald F, Morton DG, et al. Predictive diagnosis of familial adenomatous polyposis with linked DNA markers: Population based study. BMJ 1992;304:869–872.
36. Rustgi, AK, Marcus DM. Gastrointestinal and Nutritional Disorders. In DM Albert, FA Jakobiec (eds), Principles and Practice of Ophthalmology. Phildelphia: Saunders, 1994;5:2975–2985.
37. Moore AT, Maher ER, et al. Incidence and significance of congenital hypertrophy of the retinal epithelium (CHRPE) in familial adenomatous polyposis coli (FAPC). Ophthalmic Paediatr Genet 1992;13:67–71.
38. Berk T, Cohen Z, et al. Congenital hypertrophy of the retinal pigment epithelium serves as a clinical marker in a family with familial adenomatous polyposis. Dis Colon Rectum 1988;31:253–257.
39. Burn J, Chapman P, et al. The UK Northern Region genetic register for familial adenomatous polyposis coli: Use of age of onset, congenital hypertrophy of the retinal epithelium, and DNA markers in risk calculations. J Med Genet 1991;28:289–296.
40. Polkinghorne PJ, Ritchie S, et al. Pigmented lesions of the retinal epithelium and familial adenomatous polyposis. Eye 1990;4:216–221.
41. Diaz Llopis M, Menszo JL, et al. Congenital hypertrophy of the retinal epithelium and familial polyposis of the colon. Am J Ophthalmol 1987;103:235–236.
42. Lynch HT, Priluck I, et al. Congenital hypertrophy of the retinal epithelium in non-Gardner polyposis kindreds [letter]. Lancet 1987;2:333.
43. Luxenburg MN. Congenital hypertrophy of the retinal epithelium and familial adenomatous polyposis. Arch Ophthalmol 1988;106:412–413.
44. Iwana T, Mishima Y, et al. Association of congenital hypertrophy of the retinal epithelium with familial adenomatous polyposis. Br J Surg 1990;77:273–276.
45. Bertario L, Bandello F, et al. Congenital hypertrophy of the retinal pigment epithelium (CHRPE) as a clinical marker for familial adenomatous polyposis (FAP). Eur J Cancer Prev 1993;2:69–75.
46. Munden PM, Sobol WM, et al. Ocular findings in Turcot syndrome (glioma-polyposis). Ophthalmology 1991;98:111–114.

Acquired Hyperplasia of the Pigment Epithelium

Clinical Description

The retinal pigment epithelium (RPE) of the retina and ciliary body is composed of a monolayer on cuboidal and columnar cells containing numerous pigment granules. They derive from the outer layer of the primitive optic cup. These cells are located between the photoreceptors and the basal lamina (Bruch's membrane). Embryologically, the RPE has a different tissue origin than do choroidal melanocytes, which gives rise to different acquired disease manifestations. The RPE cells have the capability of undergoing reactive proliferation and migration, but they do not have neoplastic capabilities.[1, 2] The choroidal melanocytes are branching, dendritic cells interspersed throughout the uveal space and are believed to originate from the neurocrest. They do possess the ability of neoplastic transformation but do not have the inherent capability to undergo reactive proliferation and migration.[3]

Hyperplasia of the RPE is primarily caused by acquired lesions of the retina and underlying choroid. The acquired form is the result of some type of stimulus to the RPE and may denote a past episode of trauma (Figure 3-13) or postinflammatory or degenerative process that involves the retina or choroid (e.g., *Toxoplasmosis gondii*), but this condition has been seen in eyes with no pre-existing history of trauma or inflammation.[4, 5] Acquired hyperplasia of the RPE produce jet-black retinal lesions just like those seen in CHRPE, except that the lesions tend to be irregular in shape, may exhibit fibrosis or gliosis, and are not associated with depigmented rings. Acquired hyperplasia can be found in any region of the fundus and can vary in size from very tiny to many disc diameters. Acquired hyperplasia may show rapid progressive growth and often signs of resolution with time.[3]

Pigment clumping is a form of acquired hyperplasia of the RPE produced by isolated vitreous traction on the retina (Figure 3-14). The pigmentation slowly increases with time due to the continued traction by the vitreous in the involved area. Because of the time required to produce these lesions, they are most often found in adults. Pigment clumps are small areas of increased pigmentation of the retina, usually much less than one disc diameter in size (Figure 3-15). Condensed vitreous over the lesions can often be seen, particularly with scleral depression. CHRPEs usually do not have condensed vitreous over the area of involvement. Due to the intermittent episodes of vitreous traction in various directions, these clumps are usually round with irregular margins. The area of hyperplasia may invade the overlying sensory

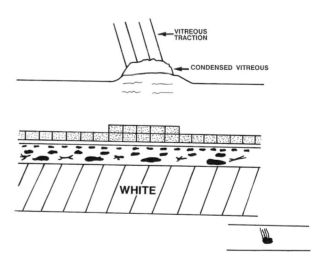

FIGURE 3-14
Diagram of retinal pigment clumping showing vitreous traction to area of condensed vitreous on the surface of the retina. The physical traction on the retina by the vitreous has caused the underlying pigment epithelial cells to undergo reactive hyperplasia and migration into the overlying sensory retina. Future posterior vitreal detachment may lead to excessive tractional force at this site of firm vitreoretinal adhesion and may lead to a retinal tear and possible detachment.

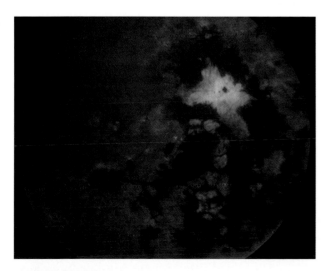

FIGURE 3-13
Previous severe blunt trauma from a brick falling on the eye resulted in peripheral retinal fibrosis and reactive pigment epithelial hyperplasia and migration.

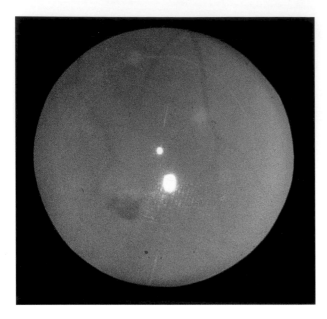

FIGURE 3-15
Pigment clump adjacent to the light reflexes as seen through an indirect condensing lens.

retina and result in a slight elevation of the involved area. These lesions are generally located in the equatorial region of the retina, rarely posterior to the equator. They seem to occur in all quadrants of the fundus without predilection for a particular one. It is likely that myopes and patients with vitreoretinal disorders are more likely to acquire pigment clumping due to the increase in vitreous degeneration and subsequent traction. Sometimes, a large pigment clump may look like a round atypical lattice degeneration lesion (see Table 3-10).

Another form of pigment clumping is known as clumped pigmentary retinal degeneration (CPRD), which is seen as numerous pigment spots scattered throughout the retinal midperiphery, of various size ranging from barely visible to 1 disc diameter. Pigment clumps are commonly found on routine eye examinations; the prevalence rate is probably close to that of peripheral pigmentary degeneration. These lesions can be found at any age but are more likely to be detected in older adults. The pathologic findings are those of abnormal RPE cells laden with melanin granules. There is loss of photoreceptors in areas of CPRD, which is the likely cause of functional deficit. The pigment spots do not usually show any "bone spicule" appearance. Studies show that the visual fields may be constricted, have elevated dark-adaptation thresholds, and reduced or delayed full-field ERGs. In more advanced cases the pigmentation can extend as far posterior as the tem-

poral arcades. The incidence of CRPD is reported to be about 0.5%.[6] People at risk are most likely those with myopia and other conditions causing vitreous degeneration. Some think that this condition may be inherited in a recessive mode.[6]

On fluorescein angiography, acquired hyperplasia of the RPE shows hypofluorescence throughout the dye study; areas of fibrosis and gliosis in the lesion display autofluorescence, progressive hyperfluorescence, and intense late staining.[3]

The differential diagnosis of acquired hyperplasia of the RPE includes CHRPE, choroidal nevus, malignant melanoma, and benign and malignant tumors of the RPE.

Histopathology

Acquired hyperplasia of the RPE results from the benign proliferation of RPE cells, and often these cells migrate anteriorly into the sensory retina. The pathology of this hyperplasia depends on the type of response producing the reaction and on whether the RPE undergoes metaplasia. The possible responses are (1) simple proliferation, (2) proliferation with the formation of cuticular masses, (3) proliferation with fibrous metaplasia, (4) proliferation with calcification, (5) proliferation with ossification, (6) migration, (7) proliferation in response to demand for phagocytes, and (8) pseudoepitheliomatous hyperplasia. Pigment clumps are acquired hyperplasia due to vitreous traction and, as such, demonstrate areas of condensed vitreous directly above the lesions. The reasons for the particular responses are poorly understood. Simple proliferation is a duplication of RPE cells uncomplicated by metaplasia or by the production of cuticular material. It is often found associated with retinal detachments and chorioretinal inflammation.[1]

Clinical Significance

Acquired hyperplasia of the RPE signifies that a stimulus to this layer was enough to cause a proliferation of the RPE cells. The most common types of stimulus are inflammation, trauma, and traction. The pigment epithelium needs time to respond in this proliferative process, which can vary depending on the strength of the stimulus. Following an episode of acute and intense stimulation, a reactive proliferation of RPE cells can be seen as a pigmented retinal lesion in 3–6 months. A longstanding, weak stimulus (e.g., mild vitreous traction) requires years to affect such a pigmented retinal lesion. Therefore, areas of retinal hyperplasia may indicate previous episodes of retinal or chorioretinal inflammation, previous episodes of ocular trauma, or sites of significant vitreous traction.

Pigment clumping occurs as a result of vitreous traction and therefore indicates an area of increased vitreoretinal adhesion.[7] Pigment clumping becomes important when the overlying vitreous traction increases dramatically at these spots of vitreoretinal adhesion, such as after ocular trauma or a posterior vitreous detachment (PVD). An increase in traction may result in photopsia or a retinal tear, which is most often noted after a PVD[8, 9]; therefore, pigment clumping is frequently seen next to operculated tears (sometimes on the operculum) or near the apex of a flap tear. The pigment is found next to the apex of the tear because that is the spot where the intense traction was initiated and thus began the tearing process. Because vitreous traction also causes other phenomena, pigment clumping may have a surrounding ring of white-without-pressure.[10] Pigment clumps in the equatorial region are more likely to produce a retinal break than those found close to the ora serrata.[10] During ophthalmoscopy, the viewer should always be observant of areas of pigment clumping because retinal tears are most likely to occur there. So even if no retinal breaks are found, the clinician should locate the areas of pigment clumping on the retinal drawing before sending the patient to the retinal specialist. Patients with pigment clumping should have yearly eye examinations and given the symptoms of a retinal tear and detachment.

The visual prognosis of patients with acquired hyperplasia of the RPE varies with the cause and the extent of the condition. If the area of involvement is the optic disc or fovea, a permanent decrease in vision may result. No cases of acquired hyperplasia have been documented to undergo a malignant transformation.[3]

References

1. Frayer WC. Reactivity of the retinal pigment epithelium. An experimental and histopathologic study. Trans Am Ophthalmol Soc 1966;64:587–643.
2. Hogan MJ, Zimmerman LE. Ophthalmic Pathology (2nd ed). Philadelphia: Saunders, 1962.
3. Shields JA. Diagnosis and Management of Intraocular Tumors. St. Louis: Mosby, 1983:122–143.
4. Spiers F, Jensen OA. Pseudo-epitheliomatous hyperplasia of the retinal pigment epithelium. Acta Ophthalmol 1963;41:722–727.
5. Stow MN. Hyperplasia of the pigment epithelium of the retina simulating a neoplasm. Trans Am Acad Ophthalmol Otolarygol 1949;53:674–677.
6. To KW, Adamian M, et al. Clinical and histopathologic findings in clumped pigmentary retinal degeneration. Arch Ophthalmol 1996;114:950–955.
7. Davis MD. Natural history of retinal breaks without detachment. Trans Am Ophthalmol Soc 1972;71:343–372.
8. Rutnin U, Schepens CL. Fundus appearance in normal eyes. IV. Retinal breaks and other findings. Am J Ophthalmol 1967;64:1063–1075.
9. Schepens CL. Retinal Detachment and Allied Diseases. Philadelphia: Saunders, 1983:164.
10. Dumas J, Schepens CL. Chorioretinal lesions predisposing to retinal breaks. Am J Ophthalmol 1966;61:620–630.

Choroidal Nevus

Clinical Description

A choroidal nevus appears as a pigmented area of the fundus, which can display a varied appearance. The shape of these lesions is generally round to oval but more irregular configurations may be seen. These lesions usually vary from 0.5 mm to 10.0 mm, with a majority being 1.5–5.0 mm in diameter.[1] In some cases, they cover half the fundus and, rarely, they can involve the entire fundus.[2] These lesions are usually flat but they can be elevated 1–2 diopters (this elevation is usually barely perceptible during ophthalmoscopy), and sometimes they are 2 mm or more.[3] Sometimes a choroidal nevus seems to be elevated because a retinal vessel traversing the lesion has an apparent elevation, but on close examination, it is found that the vessel just makes a turn over the area, and the bend in the path of the vessel gives the false impression of elevation. They are usually found as a single lesion but, occasionally, multiple nevi may be found in one eye. Also, they generally present as a unilateral entity, but bilateral presentations occur. Histologic studies have shown that 90% of choroidal nevi are found posterior to the equator.[3] There are no proven risk factors for these lesions, but they seem to be more common in lightly pigmented people.

The choroidal nevus is probably the most common intraocular tumor found in the ophthalmic practice.[1] The incidence of choroidal nevi is 1–2% in clinical studies and 6.5% in autopsy eyes.[4, 5] One study found the incidence of choroidal nevi in patients over 30 years of age to be 3.1%.[4] The time of onset of these lesions is uncertain, but it is an

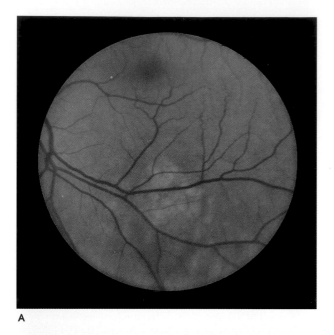

A

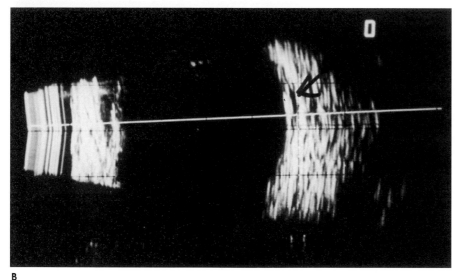

B

FIGURE 3-16
A. Choroidal nevus. Note the slate gray color, indistinct margins, and mottled appearance. B. Ultrasound showing some mild scleral shadowing (*arrow*).

extremely rare finding in infants and young children, becoming more common at about puberty.[6] It may well be that the potential cells are present in the choroid at birth but do not become very pigmented until puberty.[1]

Choroidal nevi appear slate gray (Figure 3-16A), which is the result of viewing them through the pigmented layer (the RPE). They have indistinct margins due to random reduction of choroidal melanocytes at the margins of the nevus. Also, viewing the edges of the nevus through the RPE tends to haze the margins. In contrast, congenital hypertrophy and acquired hyperplasia of the RPE produce pigmented lesions with rather sharp mar-

gins (see Table 3-2). Sometimes thin, flat nevi appear to be striated, which is due to the grouping of melanocytes in between choroidal vessels. Choroidal nevi can have a mottled coloration that is secondary to degeneration of the overlying RPE and formation of drusen. Drusen can be found in small or large lesions, and they may vary in number and location over months to years.[7] Choroidal nevi can also have orange pigment (lipofuscin) on the surface.[8] When the orange pigment is seen as tiny specks over the lesions, it usually is of little significance, but when the pigment spots are larger and confluent, an early malignant transformation may be indicated.[1] Amelanotic nevi are rare and are the result of melano-

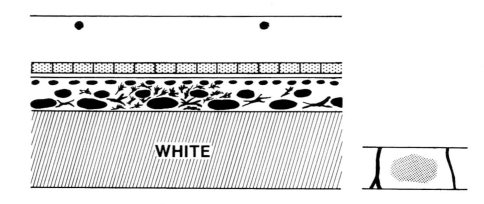

FIGURE 3-17
A choroidal nevus is composed of an aggregation of melanocytes within the choroid.

cytes that are not capable of producing melanin; sometimes only a portion of the nevus is partially nonpigmented.[9] A clinical variation of the choroidal nevus, a halo nevus, displays an irregular surrounding depigmented halo.

Because choroidal nevi are deep to the retina, they seem to disappear from view when using a red-free filter during ophthalmoscopy. Clinicopathologic studies have shown a loss of photoreceptors over a choroidal nevus,[3, 10, 11] and thus, it is not surprising to plot a visual defect over the nevus. But usually field defects are not produced by choroidal nevi; in one study of 42 choroidal nevi, 38% showed an associated scotoma.[12] Another study found a scotoma associated with these lesions in 85% of the cases.[13] However, such defects plotted over these lesions may appear identical to that caused by a melanoma.[14] Therefore, visual field testing is of little diagnostic value in these cases.

Usually, choroidal nevi show as an area of hypofluorescence during fluorescein angiography due to blockage of underlying choroidal fluorescence. Occasionally, however, large nevi that disrupt the RPE may hyperfluoresce and produce a pattern similar to a melanoma.[14] Ultrasonography can be used to help in determining the elevation of a choroidal nevus, but because most nevi have minimal elevation, this test is of little value. Ultrasonography can also be used to determine the presence of acoustic shadowing. Acoustic shadowing is an absence of reflected sound posterior to a retinal or choroidal lesion; it results from a mass of high acoustic density that does not allow the detection of reflected sound waves immediately behind it (Figure 3-16B). This phenomenon may be found with choroidal nevi, but it is not found with other pigmented fundus lesions, such as hypertrophy or hyperplasia of the RPE. The ^{32}P test is not usually indicated for obvious nevi but may be helpful with large lesions or those showing

some signs of growth and therefore suggesting a possible early melanoma.[14]

A clinical variant of the choroidal nevus is the choroidal "freckle," which differs from a nevus in that it always is flat and usually displays irregular or jagged margins. The freckle appears to be an increase in typical choroidal melanocytes, which do not replace the choroidal architecture, as is often true in nevi. Choroidal freckles are not believed to have the potential for malignant transformation.[1]

Differential diagnosis is limited, including small melanomas of the choroid, congenital hypertrophy and acquired hyperplasia of the RPE, subretinal hemorrhage, and combined hamartomas. Subretinal hemorrhages appear black when they occur under the pigment epithelium and thus are confused. Amelanotic nevi may resemble metastatic choroidal tumors, choroidal hemangiomas, and inflammatory lesions.[1]

Histopathology

A choroidal nevus is an accumulation of benign but atypical melanocytes (tumor) within the choroid (Figure 3-17). A nevus appears as flat lesions within the choroid, displaying variable degrees of pigmentation. They may have very distinct margins or blend imperceptibly into the adjacent choroid. A choroid nevus most commonly involves the outer choroid and generally spares the underlying choriocapillaris.[1] Cell types of this lesion are (1) a polygonal plump cell (a nevus made up exclusively of these cells is known as a melanocytoma), (2) an elongated spindle nevus cell, (3) plump fusiform and dendritic nevus cell, and (4) a balloon cell.[15] These cells are arranged in compact layers, and generally the thicker the nevus, the more darkly pigmented they appear. Many times there is loss of

Table 3-3. Choroidal Nevus vs. Malignant Choroidal Melanoma

Choroidal Nevus	Malignant Choroidal Melanoma
Flat to slightly elevated but remain below the basal lamina	Slightly elevated to dramatically elevated into the vitreous cavity and may perforate the basal lamina
Slate gray	Slate gray to grayish green to white (amelanotic) in color
Indistinct margins	Indistinct margins
May be mottled	Generally mottled
Lipofuscin rarely present	Lipofuscin is frequently present
Round to oval to irregular	Round to very irregular
May show scotoma consistent with size of lesion	Generally display a scotoma, which may be consistent with or larger than size of the lesion
Rarely associated with retinal detachment	Often have a secondary retinal detachment
Generally do not fluoresce during fluorescein angiography	Late hyperfluorescence on fluorescein angiography
Usually flat but sometimes slightly elevated and sometimes demonstrate acoustic shadowing on ultrasonography	Ultrasonography may show a slightly to dramatically elevated mass in the vitreous cavity, high reflective signal, and often prominent underlying acoustic scleral excavation
Negative ^{32}P test	Often show a positive ^{32}P test

photoreceptors in the retina above the lesions. The orange pigment over these lesions is characterized as clumps of macrophages laden with lipofuscin at the level of the disrupted RPE.[1] A halo nevus is a lesion showing choroidal balloon cell degeneration in the periphery.[16, 17]

Clinical Significance

The main clinical significance of a choroidal nevus lies in distinguishing it from a choroidal melanoma (Table 3-3).[18, 19, 20] Many authorities believe that choroidal nevi have the potential to transform into a melanoma. Therefore, suspicious nevi should be followed every 3–6 months to document stability of the lesion, and thereafter, yearly eye examinations are indicated. A suspicious nevus has been classified as one that is 3–5 mm in diameter and 1–2 mm thick.[1] Documentation should be made with fundus drawings or photographs. Small, flat, unsuspicious nevi have approximately a 5% chance of growing within 5 years; larger suspicious lesions (up to 2 mm in elevation) that have pigment epithelial alterations or subretinal fluid have a 15% chance of exhibiting growth.[14] Therefore, the larger the nevus, the greater the chance of becoming malignant, but the risk is very low,[1] occurring at the rate of 21 of 100,000 patients with nevi followed over a 10-year period,[5] and another reports that it occurs about 1 in 5,000 per year.[21] Any documented growth of a nevus should be suspected as a potentially malignant sign, especially if the lesion is greater than 5 mm in diameter and 2 mm in elevation, for nevi rarely attain a thickness greater than 2 mm.[3, 22] Certain findings suggest that a nevus is

more likely to grow on subsequent examinations but do not necessarily indicate malignancy: orange pigment on the tumor surface, fluorescence during fluorescein angiography, associated subretinal fluid, and a visual field defect.[22] One study found that lipofuscin occurred in 44 of 98 melanomas and only in five of 180 nevi (the five with lipofuscin later had documented growth and were reclassified as melanoma).[23] Probably the most reliable indication that a small nevus is becoming malignant is documented photographic growth: It is rare to find that a lesion is histologically benign after it displays documented growth.[24]

Choroidal nevi occasionally have a small serous retinal detachment adjacent to the lesion, especially if they are located in the macular area. Serous detachments are more commonly found with large nevi. They may result in blurred vision and visual distortion caused by a macular detachment similar to that seen in central serous chorioretinopathy, and these detachments are most frequently found because of complaints of blurred vision. A serous detachment does not necessarily indicate a malignant transformation: They have occurred in eyes with stationary, benign nevi.[22, 25, 26] Sometimes the serous detachment is located over the choroidal nevus and appears as a round, well-demarcated elevation. The persistence of subretinal fluid in the macular area may indicate the need for laser photocoagulation.[1]

Occasionally, a choroidal nevus may be associated with a subretinal neovascular membrane originating from the choriocapillaris; it is located between the RPE and the overlying lesion.[25] Retinal hemorrhages and exudates may be associated with the nevus; the existence of the neovascular membrane can be identified with fluorescein angiography.[1]

The follow-up of unsuspicious lesions is serial drawings or photography every year. Suspicious lesions should be followed more closely, at intervals of 3–6 months. Suspicious lesions may require baseline fluorescein angiography.[1]

References

1. Shields JA. Diagnosis and Management of Intraocular Tumors. St. Louis: Mosby, 1983:122–143.
2. Yanoff M, Fine BS. Ocular Pathology: A Text and Atlas (2nd ed). Philadelphia: Harper & Row, 1982:788.
3. Naumann GOH, Yanoff M, et al. Histogenesis of malignant melanomas of the uvea. I. Histopathologic characteristics of nevi of the choroid and ciliary body. Arch Ophthalmol 1966;76:784–796.
4. Ganley JP, Comstock GW. Benign nevi and malignant melanomas of the choroid. Am J Ophthalmol 1977; 76:19–25.
5. Hale PN, Allen RA, et al. Benign melanomas (nevi) of the choroid and ciliary body. Arch Ophthalmol 1965; 74:532–538.
6. Gass JDM. Problems in the differential diagnosis of choroidal nevi and malignant melanomas. The XXXIII Edward Jackson Memorial Lecture. Am J Ophthalmol 1977;83:299–323.
7. Pro M, Shields JA, et al. Serous detachment of the fovea associated with choroidal nevi. Arch Ophthalmol 1978; 96:1374–1377.
8. Shields JA, Rodrigues MM, et al. Lipofuscin pigment over benign and malignant choroidal tumors. Trans Am Acad Ophthalmol Otolaryngol 1976;81:871–881.
9. Brown GC, Shields JA, et al. Amelanotic choroidal nevi. Ophthalmology 1981;86:1116–1120.
10. Naumann GOH, Hellner K, et al. Pigmented nevi of the choroid. Clinical study of secondary changes in the overlying tissue. Trans Am Acad Ophthalmol 1971;75: 110–123.
11. Shields JA, Font RL. Melanocytoma of the choroid clinically simulating a choroidal melanoma. Arch Ophthalmol 1972;87:396–400.
12. Tamler E, Maumenee AE. Clinical study of choroidal nevi. Arch Ophthalmol 1959;62:196–202.
13. Flindall RJ, Drance SM. Visual field studies of benign choroidal melanomata. Arch Ophthalmol 1969;81: 41–44.
14. Shields JA. Tumors of the uveal tract. In TD Duane, EA Jaeger (eds), Clinical Ophthalmology. Vol. 4. Philadelphia: Harper & Row, 1989;26:2–3.
15. Naumann GOH, Yanoff M, et al. Histogenesis of malignant melanomas of the uvea. I. Histopathologic characteristics of nevi of the choroid and ciliary body. Arch Ophthalmol 1966;76:784–796.
16. Rodrigues MM, Shields JA. Malignant melanoma of the choroid with balloon cells. Can J Ophthalmol 1976; 11:208–216.
17. Shields JA, Annesley WH, et al. Nonfluorescent malignant melanoma of the choroid diagnosed with the ^{32}P test. Am J Ophthalmol 1975;79:634–664.
18. Gass JDM. Problems in the differential diagnosis of choroidal nevi and malignant melanomas. Am J Ophthalmol 1977;83:299–323.
19. Zimmerman LE. Problems in the diagnosis of malignant melanomas of the choroid and ciliary body. Am J Ophthalmol 1970;75:917–929.
20. Shields JA, McDonald PR. Improvements in the diagnosis of posterior uveal melanoma. Arch Ophthalmol 1974; 91:259–264.
21. Foss A. The problem of the suspecious naevus. Continuing Med Educ J Ophthalmol 1997;1:18.
22. Pro M, Shields JA, et al. Serous detachment of the fovea associated with presumed choroidal nevi. Arch Ophthalmol 1978;96:1374–1377.
23. Smith LT, Irvine AR. Diagnostic significance of orange accumulation over choroidal tumors. Am J Ophthalmol 1973;76:212–216.
22. MacIlwaine WA, Anderson B, et al. Enlargement of a histologically documented choroidal nevus. Am J Ophthalmol 1979;87:480–486.
23. Augsburger JJ, McCarthy EF, et al. Macular choroidal nevi. Int Ophthalmol 1981;21:99–106.
24. Slusher MM, Weaver RG. Presumed choroidal nevi and sensory retinal detachment. Br. J Ophthalmol 1977;61: 414–416.

Malignant Choroidal Melanoma

Clinical Description

Melanoma, although rare, is the most frequently occurring malignant intraocular tumor in the adult population.[1] Incidence in the white population over the age of 50 years is 21 per million per year[2]; another study found that they occur in about 1 in 150,000 white adults per year. The chance of developing bilateral melanomas of the choroid has been estimated to be around 1 in 50,000,000 patients in a lifetime.[1] The tumor is almost always benign in African-Americans and is less common in Asians and Hispanics. Also, Chinese and Hispanics tend to develop melanoma at an earlier age.[3] There has been speculation that darker-pigmented races have a natural immunity to developing such tumors, and it may be that the high concentration of melanocytes maintains the immune system's high surveillance for any abnormal pigment cells.

The appearance of a choroidal melanoma is highly variable, but it is usually a mottled, oval to round, elevated mass in the fundus and is often brown to greenish gray (see Figures 3-18A and 3-19A).[4, 5, 6] Sometimes the tumor may be a nodular

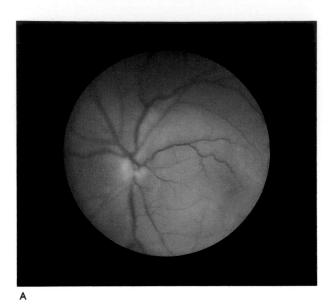

A

B

FIGURE 3-18
A. Juxtapapillary melanoma of the choroid. The circular hazy area in the inferior central portion of the tumor is a small serous retinal detachment. The golden orange spots on the surface of the tumor denote areas of concentrated lipofuscin. Tumor elevation is detected by observing the blood vessels traversing upward onto the tumor.
B. Histopathologic section of the eye showing juxtapapillary malignant melanoma that gives no sign of invading the optic nerve (*small arrow*). The dimensions of the tumor were 9 × 5 × 3 mm. Note the serous retinal detachment on the surface of the tumor, with fluid visible beneath the large arrow, underneath the detachment. Other sites of retinal detachment are the result of histologic preparation and thus display no evidence of serous fluid. The large arrow points to a retinal break that resulted from the histologic preparation.

mass that is bilobed or even multilobed.[7, 8] The mottled appearance is the result of drusen and degeneration of the RPE above the tumor. Orange stipples are often seen on the surface of this tumor (see Figure 3-18A) as the result of accumulation of lipofuscin (a wear-and-tear pigment released from the degenerating RPE cells).[9, 10] Choroidal nevi can also demonstrate mottling and sometimes orange stippling; therefore, these changes are not helpful in the differential diagnosis.[9] Large pigmented areas on these tumors, known as melanoma bodies, are pathognomonic of choroidal melanoma (see Table 3-3; see Figure 3-19A). Melanomas of the choroid are often asymptomatic but can cause blurred vision when fluid from the tumor extends into the macula or pain, which is likely secondary to a large tumor that produces glaucoma. Other less common symptoms are visual field defects, floaters, or photopsia, which are similar to that of a rhegmatogenous retinal detachment.

Tumor size can vary from a few millimeters in diameter (generally about 5–7 mm) to a lesion that

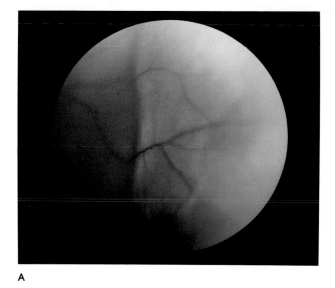

A

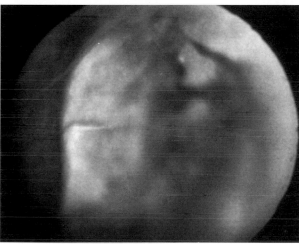

B

FIGURE 3-19
A. Choroidal melanoma located in the midperiphery. The hazy area adjacent to the tumor is a serous retinal detachment. The darkly pigmented spot on the surface is a melanoma body. Tumor elevation is detected by observing the blood vessels traversing upward onto the lesion. B. B-scan ultrasonogram of the melanoma showing elevation into the vitreous cavity (*white arrow*) and acoustic excavation of the underlying sclera (*black arrow*). C. Fluorescein angiography showing late hyperfluoresence.

C

occupies a majority of the fundus. Most malignant melanomas are 10–20 mm in diameter when initially discovered. The tumor may be flat and diffuse, but commonly it is elevated, from only a few millimeters to completely filling the vitreous cavity. Ultrasonography can be used to determine the size of an intraocular melanoma. The tumor is usually a rounded mass without lobular extensions when it is contained beneath the basal lamina (Bruch's membrane); however, it often takes on a so called collar button appearance after breaking through the basal lamina (Figures 3-20 and 3-21). The diffuse type of tumor tends to grow more within the boundary of the choroid and usually does not become very elevated and thus is less easy to detect on ophthalmoscopy or ultrasonography. The diffuse melanoma tends to show more malignant cytology and, commonly, to demonstrate extrascleral extension; therefore, this type has a worse prog-

nosis.[11] Diffuse melanomas have a greater tendency to invade the optic nerve; however, most melanomas show little tendency to invade the optic nerve.[12] Approximately 50% of uveal melanomas are found within 3 mm of the optic disc or fovea;[13] therefore, the number of peripheral tumors discovered is less frequent compared to those of the posterior pole.

Ultrasonography is helpful in diagnosing a melanoma. The A scan shows a high initial spike followed by low internal reflectivity. The B scan demonstrates a choroidal mass with a sharp anterior margin, choroidal or scleral excavation, acoustic hollowness, and orbital shadowing (see Figures 3-19B and 3-21). It may be difficult to differentiate a necrotic melanoma from a metastatic tumor or a choroidal hemorrhage.[14] An ultrasonogram is sometimes useful in diagnosing a melanoma in an eye with opaque media.[6, 15]

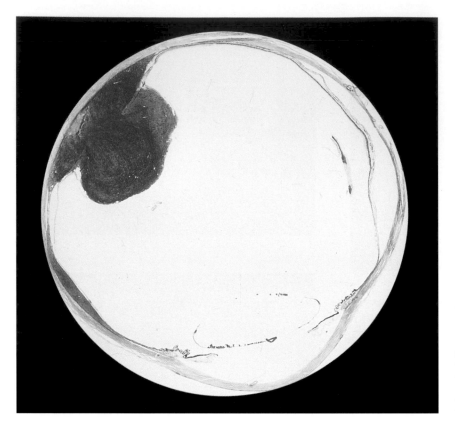

FIGURE 3-20
Histopathologic section of a malignant melanoma that has broken through the basal lamina and formed a mushroom-shaped elevated mass in the vitreous cavity. These findings indicate a more aggressive tumor and thus, worsens the prognosis. An extension of the tumor can be found more anteriorly within the choroid.

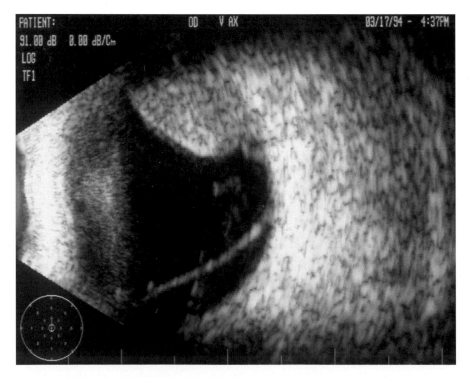

FIGURE 3-21
B-scan ultrasonogram of a superior collar-button malignant melanoma and an inferior secondary shifting retinal detachment.

Fluorescein angiography is also used in the diagnosis of an intraocular melanoma. Tumors usually show mottled hyperfluorescence in the arteriovenous stage and a prominent late hyperfluorescence (see Figure 3-19C), which is caused by leakage from the new blood vessels with poor endothelial junctions inside the tumor. New blood vessels occur as a response to the metabolic demands of the growing tumor. This test is most useful in differentiating a melanoma from a large nevus, choroidal hemangioma, or metastatic tumor.[14]

Visual fields are of little benefit due to the fact that similar defects can be plotted over other lesions of the fundus, such as metastatic tumors and other benign lesions that can simulate a melanoma.[14] The visual field changes are the direct result of degeneration of overlying photoreceptors.[12]

The ^{32}P test is valuable in differentiating a choroidal melanoma from a number of simulating benign lesions of the fundus.[16] The test cannot, however, differentiate a melanoma from a metastatic tumor because both produce a positive test result. In eyes with opaque media, the ultrasonogram and the ^{32}P test can be of marked importance in diagnosing an intraocular melanoma.[17] Immunologic tests are being developed to aid in the diagnosis of ocular melanomas and may become available soon.[18]

Recently, fine-needle aspiration biopsy (FNAB) has been used when the diagnosis cannot be confirmed by other tests.[19, 20] In FNAB, the needle is passed transvitreally through a pars plana entrance site into the suspected tumor. The test is useful in differentiating a metastatic tumor, hemangioma, or lymphoma from a melanoma. It is not so useful in differentiating a nevus or other spindle cell mass from a melanoma.[14] The FNAB has made the ^{32}P test less necessary in the differential diagnosis of a melanoma.

CT and MRI scans are mostly used to detect the elevation of the intraocular tumor (Figure 3-22B). At present these tests add little to the diagnostic information in most cases. CT scans are useful in determining extraocular extension of an intraocular melanoma and liver metastasis.[14]

Many melanomas have an associated secondary nonrhegmatogenous retinal detachment, which can shift. This type of retinal detachment is seen in about 2% of eyes with a choroidal melanoma.[21] The detachment can be small and localized to the surface of the tumor (see Figure 3-18) or extensive and some distance from the tumor. The secondary detachment is composed of a serous fluid that is somewhat viscous and tends to shift position due to gravity.[22, 23] Thus, the tumor may be located in the superior half of the ocular fundus, but the detachment is often located in the inferior dependent region when the patient is examined in the sitting position (see Figure 3-21). When the patient reclines, the detachment is relocated to the posterior pole of the fundus.

A serous detachment has a smooth surface, but a rhegmatogenous detachment has many folds. The serous detachment associated with a choroidal tumor typically extends from the mass and not from the ora serrata region, as is typically seen with a rhegmatogenous detachment. Often, loss of vision due to retinal detachment is the presenting symptom of a melanoma of the choroid. Sometimes the tumor is hidden by the retinal detachment, and shifting the patient's position during the examination may uncover its presence. Secondary detachments typically do not have retinal breaks, but if a break were to occur in a serous retinal detachment, the clinician might believe it is a primary rhegmatogenous retinal detachment. Rhegmatogenous retinal detachments associated with a melanoma are rare,[21, 24–29] occurring in less than 1% of eyes with a melanoma.[30] All these findings are not necessarily diagnostic, but they are certainly highly suggestive of a melanoma.[9] Sometimes the tumor can actually invade the sensory retina.[12] Even though photopsia is a common symptom of a rhegmatogenous detachment, it is sometimes noticed in patients with a malignant melanoma.[31]

The rate of growth of a choroidal melanoma is typically slow, and over extended periods of time it may show no growth; however, in some cases, rapid growth was observed in only 60 days.[32] One study found that out of 116 patients with a uveal melanoma, 69 patients with 64 small tumors and 5 with medium-size tumors demonstrated no growth over a 5-year period. None of these patients showed signs of metastasis. Of the remaining tumors, 47 medium and five large tumors did show growth during this period of observation. The study found that only 7% of the small tumors that exhibited growth caused metastatic death. This study demonstrated that there was no increase in the mortality rate of patients followed with small tumors before enucleation.[33] The appearance of drusen on the surface of the tumor and the absence of drusen in the fellow eye is a sign of slow growth; the presence of subretinal fluid and the lack of drusen on the surface of the tumor may indicate rapid growth.[1]

Other ocular complications associated with an intraocular melanoma include corneal edema, rubeosis iridis, secondary cataract, vitreous hemorrhage, vitreous seeding (see Figure 3-22A), uveitis,

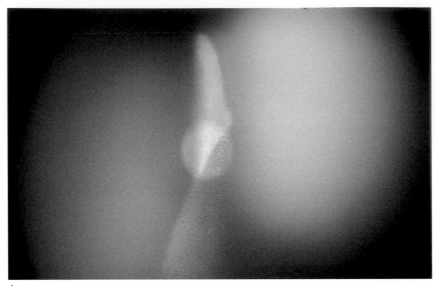

A

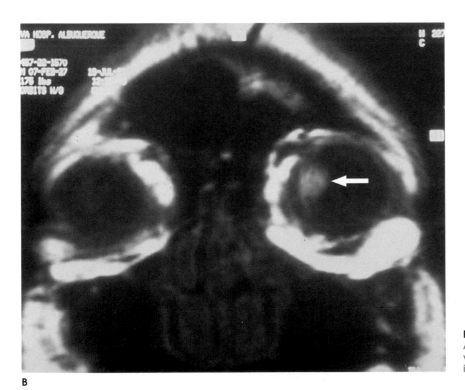

B

FIGURE 3-22
A. Ciliary body melanoma displaying vitreous seeding. B. MRI of the same ciliary body melanoma (*arrow*).

glaucoma, and, rarely, choroidal neovascular membrane.[6, 14, 34, 35] Intravitreal seeding of malignant cells is a rather uncommonly reported event.[33–39] Even cystoid macular edema may result from a peripheral tumor, although the mechanism for this is uncertain. In some cases, a melanoma remains quiet for years and only becomes known after associated problems occur in the involved eye, such as glaucoma, corneal edema, or cataract. A vitreous hemorrhage most likely originates from a ruptured blood vessel or necrosis of the tumor. Another interesting retinal change associated with choroidal melanomas is chorioretinal atrophy in the form of paving-stone degeneration. These lesions of chorioretinal atrophy are typically 1–2 mm in diameter and are seen in the retina just peripheral to the mass. This condition is believed to result from regional deprivation of blood circulation.[12]

Several studies have found that an unsuspected melanoma was found in 10% of enucleated eyes.[40, 41] Many unsuspected melanomas are discovered at autopsy after removal of blind, painful eyes. Other studies have found that up to 21% of eyes with unsuspected uveal melanomas have opaque media at the time of surgical enucleation.[40, 42, 43] The most common reasons for opaque ocular media are corneal edema, hyphema, cataract, and vitreous hemorrhage. Sometimes a uveal melanoma is misdiagnosed as a choroidal detachment after cataract surgery.[12] Any eye with opaque media should have an ultrasonogram (especially if the opacification is unexplained) to rule out an intraocular melanoma or some other intraocular mass.

Lesions that most are most commonly mistaken for a melanoma (pseudomelanomas) are choroidal nevus, lesions of the RPE, rhegmatogenous retinal detachment, disciform macular degeneration, metastatic tumors to the choroid, and choroidal hemangioma.[44, 45] In the past, many eyes were mistakenly enucleated for pseudomelanoma,[13, 46] but this has mostly ceased in recent years.[45, 47]

Melanomas of the ciliary body are more difficult to detect because they are hidden behind the iris, usually becoming visible only after they grow to a large size, when they can be seen just over the iris margin. Ciliary body melanomas may show various degrees of pigmentation and growth patterns (see Figure 3-22A).[21, 48, 49] An initial sign of a ciliary body melanoma is dilated episcleral vessels (sentinel vessels) in the same quadrant. The tumor may erode through the thin iris root and then be seen in the anterior chamber, and it can even erode through emissary channels in the sclera and appear as a pigmented area of the sclera. In the anterior chamber, the tumor can infiltrate the trabecular meshwork, which may result in a severe secondary glaucoma. Ciliary body melanomas can occasionally extend around the ciliary body for 360 degrees (a ring melanoma), which has worse prognosis than a typical ciliary body melanoma. Extrascleral extension worsens the prognosis. As the tumor enlarges, it can cause secondary astigmatism, localized cataract, subluxated lens, hyphema, rubeosis iridis, glaucoma, and retinal detachment.[12] Any patient with unexplained unilateral lenticular astigmatism should be examined for a possible ciliary body melanoma.

Fluorescein angiography for ciliary body melanomas is difficult but visual fluoroscopy is possible to perform with the binocular indirect ophthalmoscope. Transillumination is useful in examining a ciliary body melanoma because it allows an external view of the mass. This technique can be used to determine the size and location of the tumor, which is important in deciding if an iridocyclectomy or enucleation should be performed and for positioning the irradiation scleral plaque.[14] Ultrasonography can be helpful in studying larger tumors of the ciliary body but is not very helpful in examining small tumors. The ^{32}P test seems to be highly reliable in the diagnosis of ciliary body melanomas.[16]

Histopathology

Gross uveal melanomas can have placoid, oval, mushroom, or diffuse growth patterns.[14] The tumor is composed of malignant melanocytes, which are either spindle-shaped or epithelioid. Other cell types (based on Callender's classification) are fascicular, mixed, and necrotic. If the cell type cannot be determined due to tumor necrosis, it is known as necrotic. The tumor may not be homogeneous in cell type, and a center of epithelioid cells may be surrounded by spindle cells (mixed cell type). The epithelioid cell is associated with a much higher degree of malignancy and, thus, a higher frequency of patient fatality. The lipofuscin found associated with the tumor is located in clumps of macrophages at the level of the RPE.[12]

Clinical Significance

The significance of a melanoma of the choroid is its potential for fatal consequences. The primary intraocular tumor usually spreads by way of the circulatory system to the liver. The patient dies secondary to liver failure. The other two most common sites of metastasis are the lungs and brain. A metastatic workup (consisting of liver function studies; liver, lung, and brain scans; and chest x-ray) is necessary for all patients diagnosed with an intraocular melanoma.

The prognosis of a melanoma is based on a number of factors, the most important of which is the cell type, spindle cell (A and B) being the least malignant (14% 5-year mortality rate with spindle B) and epithelioid being the most malignant (69% 5-year mortality).[14, 50] In general, the 5-year survival rate is between 20% and 50% depending on the prognostic factors found concerning the tumor.[14] Other considerations are the size of the tumor, especially the greatest diameter, and patients with large tumors have a worse prognosis. The incidence of metastasis in small melanomas is very low, and one study showed the risk of metastasis from a series of 1,329 tumors less than 3 mm in thickness was 3%.[51] Diffuse tumors have a very poor prognosis because they are large and usually contain epithelioid cells.[52] Prognosis may also be influenced by the degree of mitotic activity displayed by the tumor on histopathology examination. The presence of extrascleral extension worsens the prognosis, for tumors with more malignant cell types are often associated with extrascleral extension.[36, 53] Due to the tissue attempting to nourish the rapidly growing tumor, deficient metabolism is fairly common in melanomas, and thus, there is some degree of spontaneous necrosis in 35–79% of these lesions.[54, 55] Also, spontaneous tumor necrosis in choroidal tumors often leads to a large hemorrhage that may invade the vitreous.[4]

The treatment of intraocular melanoma is very controversial. The conventional treatment for intraocular choroidal melanoma has been enucleation, especially for large tumors (>13 mm in base diameter and >8 mm in thickness) and for some smaller tumors located near the optic disc or macula.[14, 18] Enucleation is advisable in these cases because the amount of radiation needed to treat large tumors can cause serious complications. Many feel that enucleation is the treatment of choice in most cases.[56] The prognosis after enucleation of large tumors is poor, with a 30% mortality rate in 5 years and 50% in 10 years after surgery from metastatic disease.[1] After analyses of melanoma data, however, it is apparent that enucleation may not prevent death from metastasis and may in fact contribute to increased mortality by spread of the tumor at the time of surgery.[57, 58] Therefore, many suggest a gentle handling (no-touch; minimal manipulation techniques) of the globe during enucleation in a theoretical effort to reduce metastasis.[59] It has been found that for patients over 65 years of age, enucleation has resulted in a decrease in the probability of mortality compared to patients with similar medical history who did not have a choroidal melanoma.[1] After the discovery of systemic metastasis is made, the survival rate is only about 2–4 months.[59]

Due to the concern that enucleation may lead to metastasis, authorities have increasingly relied on specialized modalities of irradiation for melanomas (especially for small or medium-size tumors), including charged-particle irradiation with proton beams or helium nuclei.[19, 45, 60–65] The overall 5-year probability of tumor control after proton beam irradiation is 97%.[66] Radioactive episcleral plaques sutured under the base of the melanoma have also proved successful.[67–69] The plaques are calculated to deliver 10,000 R to the apex of the tumor (ultrasonography is used to determine the height of the tumor so it can be used to calculate the proper dosage). The response to such treatment often requires several weeks to months. Usually this type of therapy is used for tumors demonstrating growth because small, stable lesions show little effect from radiotherapy.[14] Pre-enucleation with radiation has been done in the hope that it would reduce the mortality rate from this malignancy, but, unfortunately, studies have shown little benefit.[19, 70, 71] The morbidity and mortality rates for patients receiving proton beam radiation is about the same as that for enucleation.[72] Because about 50% of uveal melanomas are within 3 mm of the optic disc and fovea, the use of either treatment mode is limited due to the development of radiation maculopathy and optic neuropathy in 41% of cases.[73–76] Another study found a 55% incidence of visual deterioration after plaque treatment of tumors located within 3 disc diameters of the optic disc.[77] Studies have shown that 5 years after plaque treatment, there are late radiation complications in approximately 50% of eyes.[78, 79]

Another treatment modality used is hyperthermia, which enhances the therapeutic gain of radiation.[80–82] The goal of such treatment is to increase the temperature of the tumor to 42–44°C, which augments the effects of radiation. Hyperthermia can be induced with microwaves,[83–86] localized current field,[87, 88] ultrasound,[71, 89, 90] ferromagnetic thermoseeds,[91] and transpupillary thermotherapy.[13] Transpupillary thermotherapy along with radiation plaque treatment allows for maximum therapeutic effects at the top and the bottom of the tumor and therefore can be used to treat tumors higher than 5 mm, whereas radiation plaque is limited to tumors no higher than 5 mm.[13] Also, this treatment modality is useful in the treatment of tumors near the optic disc and macula due to the low lateral spread of heat into adjacent tissues.

Less common forms of treatment include photocoagulation,[90–95] cryotherapy, diathermy, and chemotherapy. Photocoagulation requires multiple treatments due to the rather superficial necrosis accomplished by this method[96–98]; results were not acceptable, with 19% of the treated tumors displaying regrowth and 42–50% of eyes requiring later enucleation.[99, 100] Photocoagulation is now used only to supplement radiation treatment when tumor regression is not deemed sufficient.[101–106] Penetration of the tumor by photocoagulation has been enhanced by the intravenous use of indocyanine green.[107] Today, neither diathermy nor cryotherapy are used due to post-treatment complications.

Sclerochorioretinal resection (full-thickness eye wall resection) is used to treat choroidal melanomas, especially if they are located anteriorly, but this surgical approach is difficult and controversial.[108] More recently, partial lamellar sclerouvectomy (removal of the tumor with an attempt to preserve the outer sclera, retina, and vitreous) seems to have advantages over full-thickness eye wall resection.[109, 110] The indications for eye wall resection are for tumors confined to the ciliary body or located anterior in the choroid (not more than 4 mm posterior to the equator).[14] Exenteration or a modified exenteration is not often used and is indicated only for intraocular melanomas with massive extrascleral extension.[40, 111] The treatment for small ciliary body melanomas, especially in older patients, is periodic observation; for more suspicious tumors, treatment is iridocyclectomy.[14] No matter which treatment mode is used, the prognosis does not seem to be altered.[112]

Any suspected tumor of the ocular fundus should be followed with serial fundus drawings or photographs to document changes in its physical characteristics. Observation (with photography, ultrasonography, and other ancillary tests) is sometimes justified for a small or slow-growing melanoma in older patients.[13] Follow-up may consist of periodic observation at intervals, such as 3, 6, and 12 months, depending on the clinical findings. A documented change in size necessitates referral to a retinal specialist. Yearly metastatic evaluation of patients with known melanomas has been recommended because of the tendency for metastases to show up months to years after treatment or enucleation. It is quite possible that subclinical metastasis to the liver has occurred before treatment of an intraocular melanoma.[56, 113, 114] Once metastasis has occurred, the disease becomes uniformly fatal, and even the use of chemotherapy for liver metastasis can prolong the survival rate for only a few months.[115]

References

1. Shields JA. Intraocular Tumors. Philadelphia: Saunders, 1992.
2. Yanoff M, Fine BS. Ocular Pathology: A Text and Atlas (2nd ed). Philadelphia: Harper & Row, 1982:788,826,831.
3. Hudson HL, Vallure S, et al. Choroidal melanomas in Hispanic patients. Am J Ophthalmol 1994;118:57–62.
4. Reese AB. Tumors of the Eye. Hagerstown, MD: Harper & Row, 1976:173–238.
5. Gass JDM. Differential Diagnosis of Intraocular Tumors. A Stereoscopic Presentation. St. Louis: Mosby, 1974.
6. Jacobiec FA. Ocular and Adnexal Tumors. Birmingham, AL: Aesculapius, 1978.
7. Augsburger JJ, Shields JA, et al. Diffuse primary choroidal melanoma after prior cutaneous melanoma. Arch Ophthalmol 1980;98:1261–1264.
8. Shields JA, Leonard BC, et al. Multilobed uveal melanoma masquerading as a postoperative choroidal detachment. Br J Ophthalmol 1976;60:386–389.
9. Shields JA, Rodrigues MM, et al. Lipofuscin pigment over benign and malignant choroidal tumors. Trans Am Acad Ophthalmol Otolaryngol 1976;81:871–881.
10. Font RL, Zimmerman LE, et al. The nature of the orange pigment over a choroidal melanoma: Histochemical and electron microscopic observations. Arch Ophthalmol 1974;91:359–362.
11. Font RL, Spaulding AG, et al. Diffuse malignant melanomas of the uveal tract. Trans Am Acad Ophthalmol Otolaryngol 1968;72:877–895.
12. Shields JA. Intraocular Tumors. Philadelphia: Saunders, 1983:144–170.
13. Oosterhuis JA, Hanneke G, et al. Transpupillary thermotherapy in choroidal melanomas. Arch Ophthalmol 1995;113:315–321.
14. Shields JA. Tumors of the Uveal Tract. In TD Duane, EA Jaeger (eds), Clinical Ophthalmology. Vol. 4. Philadelphia: Harper & Row, 1989;67:2–3.
15. Shields JA, McDonald PR, et al. Ultrasonography and ^{32}P test in the diagnosis of malignant melanomas in eyes with hazy media. Trans Am Ophthalmol Soc 1976;74:262–281.
16. Shields JA. Accuracy and limitations of the ^{32}P test in the diagnosis of ocular tumors: An analysis of 500 cases. Ophthalmology 1978;85:950–966.
17. Shields JA, McDonald PR, et al. The diagnosis of uveal malignant melanomas in eyes with opaque media. Am J Ophthalmol 1977;83:95–105.
18. Shields JA. Current approaches to the diagnosis and management of choroidal melanomas. Surv Ophthalmol 1977;21:443–463.
19. Augsburger JJ, Shields JA. Fine-needle aspiration biopsy of solid intraocular tumors: Indications, instrumentation, and techniques. Ophthalmic Surg 1984;15:34–40.
20. Augsburger JJ, Shields JA, et al. Fine-needle aspiration biopsy in the diagnosis of intraocular cancer: Cytologic-histologic correlations. Ophthalmology 1985;92:39–49.
21. Boniuk M, Zimmerman LE. Occurrence and behavior of choroidal melanomas in eyes subjected to operations for retinal detachment. Trans Am Acad Ophthalmol Otolaryngol 1962;66:642–657.
22. Pischel DK. Retinal Detachment: A Manual (2nd ed). Am Acad Ophthalmol Otolaryngol 1965:80–81.
23. Schepens CL. Retinal Detachment and Allied Diseases. Philadelphia: Harper & Row, 1983:224–225,705–730.
24. McGraw JL. Malignant melanoma associated with retinal hole. Arch Ophthalmol 1951;46:666–667.
25. Boniuk M, Zimmerman LE. Problems in differentiating idiopathic serous detachments from solid retinal detachments. Int Ophthalmol Clin 1962;2:411–430.
26. Manschot WA. Retinal hole in a case of choroidal melanoma. Arch Ophthalmol 1965;73:666–668.
27. Berson E, Bigger JF, Smith ME. Malignant melanoma, retinal hole, and retinal detachment. Arch Ophthalmol 1967;77:223–225.
28. Bedford MA, Chignell AH. U-shaped retinal tear associated with a presumed malignant melanoma of the choroid. Br J Ophthalmol 1970;54:200–202.
29. Robertson DM, Curtin VT. Rhegmatogenous retinal detachment and choroidal melanoma. Am J Ophthalmol 1971;72:351–355.

30. Shields JA, Shields CL. Differential Diagnosis of Posterior Uveal Melanoma. In Intraocular Tumors: A Text and Atlas. Philadelphia: Saunders, 1992:150.

31. Gass JDM. Problems in the differential diagnosis of choroidal nevi and malignant melanomas. Am J Ophthalmol 1977;83:299–323.

32. Fineberg TR, Fineberg E, et al. Extremely rapid growth of a primary choroidal melanoma. Arch Ophthalmol 1983;101:1375–1377.

33. Gass JDM. Observation of suspected choroidal and ciliary body melanomas for the evidence of growth prior to enucleation. Presented to the Annual Meeting of the American Academy of Ophthalmology, Nov. 5–9, 1979.

34. Eagle RC Jr., Shields JA. Pseudoretinitis pigmentosa secondary to preretinal malignant melanoma cells. Retina 1982;2:51–55.

35. Halverson KD, Ruder AJ, et al. Intraocular melanoma. Clin Eye Vision Care 1994;6:146–148.

36. Traboulsi EI, Jalkh AE, Frangieh GT, et al. Vitreous histopathology of primary choroidal malignant melanoma. Ann Ophthalmol 1987;19:45–47.

37. Dunn WU, Lambert HM, Kincaid MC, et al. Choroidal malignant melanoma with early vitreous seeding. Retina 1988;8:188–192.

38. El Baba F, Hagler WS, De La Cruz, et al. Choroidal melanoma with pigment dispersion in vitreous and melanomalytic glaucoma. Ophthalmology 1988;95:370–377.

39. Robertson DM, Campbell RJ. Intravitreal invasion of malignant cells from choroidal melanoma after brachytherapy. Arch Ophthalmol 1997;115:793–795.

40. Zimmerman LE. Problems in the diagnosis of malignant melanomas of the choroid and ciliary body. Am J Ophthalmol 1973;75:917–929.

41. Shields JA, Augsburger JJ. Cataract extraction and intraocular lenses in patients with malignant melanoma of the ciliary body and choroid. Ophthalmology 1985;92:823–826.

42. Makley TA, Teed RW. Unsuspected intraocular malignant melanomas. Arch Ophthalmol 1958;60:475–478.

43. Shields JA, Zimmerman LE. Lesions simulating malignant melanomas of the posterior uvea. Arch Ophthalmol 1973;89:466–471.

44. Shields JA. Diagnosis and Management of Intraocular Tumors. St. Louis: Mosby, 1983.

45. Shields JA, Augsburger JJ, et al. The differential diagnosis of posterior uveal melanoma. Ophthalmology 1980;87:543–548.

46. Ferry AP. Lesions mistaken for malignant melanoma of the posterior uvea. Arch Ophthalmol 1964;72:463–469.

47. Shields JA, McDonald PR. Improvements in the diagnosis of posterior uveal melanomas. Trans Am Ophthalmol Soc 1973;71:193–211.

48. Shields JA, Federman JL. Malignant Melanoma of the Uveal Tract. In WH Clark, LI Goldman, MJ Mastrangelo (eds), Human Malignant Melanoma. New York: Grune & Stratton, 1979.

49. Shields JA, Young SE. Malignant tumors of the uveal tract. Curr Probl Cancer 1980;5:1–35.

50. McLean IW, Foster WD, et al. Prognostic factors in small malignant melanomas of the choroid and ciliary body. Arch Ophthalmol 1977;94:48–58.

51. Shields CL, Shields JA, Kiratli H, et al. Risk factors for growth and metastasis of small choroidal melanocytic lesions. Ophthalmology 1995;201:1351–1361.

52. Font RL, Spaulding AG, et al. Diffuse malignant melanoma of the uveal tract: A clinico-pathologic report of 54 cases. Trans Am Acad Ophthalmol 1968;72:877–895.

53. Starr HJ, Zimmerman LE. Extrascleral extension and orbital recurrence of malignant melanomas of the choroid and ciliary body. Int Ophthalmol Clin 1962;2:369–385.

54. Reese AB, Archila EA, et al. Necrosis of malignant melanoma of the choroid. Am J Ophthalmol 1970;69:91–104.

55. Samuels B. Anatomic and clinical manifestations of necrosis in 84 cases of choroidal sarcoma. Arch Ophthalmol 1934;11:988–1027.

56. Manschot WA, van Piperzell HA. Choroidal melanoma: Enucleation or observation? A new approach. Arch Ophthalmol 1980;98:71–77.

57. Zimmerman LE, McLean IW. An evaluation of enucleation in the management of uveal melanoma. Am J Ophthalmol 1979;87:741–760.

58. Zimmerman LE, McLean IW. Metastatic disease from untreated uveal melanoma. Am J Ophthalmol 1979;88:524–534.

59. Wilson RS, Fraunfelder FT. "No-touch" cryosurgical enucleation: A minimal trauma technique for eyes harboring intraocular malignancy. Ophthalmology 1978;85:1170–1175.

60. Young LHY, Egan KM, et al. Familial uveal melanoma. Am J Ophthalmol 1994;117:516–520.

61. Gragoudas ES, Goitein M, et al. Proton beam irradiation of uveal melanoma. Arch Ophthalmol 1982;100:928–934.

62. Char DH, Phillips TD. The potential for adjunct radiation radiotherapy in choroidal melanoma. Arch Ophthalmol 1982;100:247–248.

63. Char DH, Castro JR. Helium ion therapy for choroidal melanoma. Arch Ophthalmol 1982;100:935–938.

64. Gragoudas ES, Seddon J, et al. Current results of proton beam radiation of melanomas. Ophthalmology 1985;92:284–291.

65. Char DH, Saunders W, et al. Helium ion therapy for choroidal melanoma. Ophthalmology 1983;90:1219–1225.

66. Gragoudas ES, Egan KM, Seddon JM, et al. Intraocular recurrence after proton beam irradiation. Ophthalmology 1992;99:760–766.

67. Shields JA, Augsburger JJ, et al. Cobalt plaque therapy of posterior uveal melanomas. Ophthalmology 1988;89:1201–1207.

68. Shields JA, Augsburger JJ, et al. Selection of Radioactive Plaques for Treatment of Posterior Uveal Melanoma. In ES Gragoudas, L Zagrofos, et al. (eds), Transactions of the Second International Congress on Intraocular Tumors.

69. Packer S, Rotman M, et al. Irradiation of choroidal melanoma with iodine 125 ophthalmic plaque. Arch Ophthalmol 1980;98:1453–1457.

70. Char DH, Phillips TL, et al. Pre-Enucleation Irradiation of Uveal Melanoma. In PK Lommatzsch, L Aografos, ES Gragoudas (eds), Proceedings of the Second International Meeting on the Diagnosis and Treatment of Intraocular Tumors. Berlin: Akademie-Verlag, 1990.

71. Augsburger JJ, Corallo D, et al. Pre-Enucleation Irradiation of Uveal Melanoma. In PK Lommatzsch, L Aografos, ES Gragoudas (eds), Proceedings of the Second International Meeting on the Diagnosis and Treatment of Intraocular Tumors. Berlin: Akademie-Verlag, 1990.

72. Seddon JM, Gragoudas ES, et al. Relative survival rates after alternative therapies of uveal melanoma. Ophthalmology 1990;97:769–777.

73. Coleman DJ, Lizzi FL, et al. Ultrasonic hyperthermia and radiation in the management of intraocular malignant melanoma. Am J Ophthalmol 1986;101:635–642.

74. Char DH, Castro JR, et al. Uveal melanoma radiation. [125]I brachytherapy versus helium ion irradiation. Ophthalmology 1989;96:1708–1715.
75. Brown GC, Shields JA, et al. Radiation optic neuropathy. Ophthalmology 1982;89:1489–1493.
76. Brown GC, Shields JA, et al. Radiation retinopathy. Ophthalmology 1982;89:1494–1501.
77. Garretson BR, Robertson DM, et al. Choroidal melanoma treatment with iodine 125 brachytherapy. Arch Ophthalmol 1987;105:1394–1397.
78. Halk BG, Jereb EB, et al. Ophthalmic Radiotherapy. In N Lliff (ed), Complications in Ophthalmic Therapy. New York: Churchill Livingstone, 1983:449–485.
79. Lommatzsch PK, Kirsch IH. 106Ru/106Rh plaque radiotherapy for malignant melanomas of the choroid. Doc Ophthalmol 1988;68:225–238.
80. Kim JH, Hahn EW, et al. Combination hyperthermia and radiation therapy for cutaneous malignant melanoma. Cancer 1978;41:2143–2148.
81. Overgaard J, Overgaard M. Hyperthermia as an adjuvant to radiotherapy in the treatment of malignant melanoma. Int J Hyperthermia 1987;3:483–501.
82. Emami B, Perez CA, et al. Thermoradiotherapy of malignant melanoma. Int J Hyperthermia 1988;4:373–381.
83. Lagendijk JJW. Microwave applicator for hyperthermic treatment of retinoblastoma. Natl Cancer Inst Monogr 1982;61:469–471.
84. Riedel KG. Hypertherme therapieverfahren in erganzung zur stahlenbehandlung maligner intraokularer tumoren. Klin Monatsbl Augenheilkd 1988;193:131–137.
85. Swift PS, Stauffer PR, et al. Microwave hyperthermia for choroidal melanoma in rabbits. Ophthalmol Vis Sci 1990;31:1754–1760.
86. Finger PT. Microwave plaque thermoradiotherapy for choroidal melanoma. Br J Ophthalmol 1992;76:358–364.
87. Liggett PE, Prince KJ, et al. Localized current field hyperthermia. Effect on normal ocular tissue. Int J Hyperthermia 1990;6:517–527.
88. Petrovich Z, Astrahan MA, et al. Episcleral plaque thermoradiotherapy in patients with choroidal melanoma. Int J Radiat Oncol Biol Phys 1992;23:599–603.
89. Coleman DJ, Silverman RH, et al. Histopathologic effects of ultrasonically induced hyperthermia in intraocular malignant melanoma. Ophthalmology 1986;101:635–642.
90. Braakman R, van der Valk, et al. The effects of ultrasonically induced hyperthermia on experimental tumors in the rabbit eye. Invest Ophthalmol Vis Sci 1989;30:835–844.
91. Mieler WF, Jaffe GJ, et al. Ferromagnetic hyperthermia and iodine 125 brachytherapy in the treatment of choroidal melanoma in a rabbit model. Arch Ophthalmol 1989;107:1524–1528.
92. Minckler D, Thompson FB. Photocoagulation of malignant melanoma. Arch Ophthalmol 1979;97:120–123.
93. Shields JA. The expanding role of laser photocoagulation for intraocular tumors. Retina 1994;14:310–322.
94. Meyer-Schwickerath G, Bornfeld N. Photocoagulation of Choroidal Melanomas. Thirty Years Experience. In PK Lommatzsch, FC Blodi (eds), Intraocular Tumors. Berlin: Akademie-Verlag, 1983:269–276.
95. Francois J. Treatment of malignant choroidal melanomas by photocoagulation. Ophthalmologica 1982;184:121–130.
96. Makley TA, Havener WH, et al. Light coagulation of intraocular tumors. Am J Ophthalmol 1965;60:1082–1089.
97. Hepler RS, Allen RA, et al. Photocoagulation of choroidal melanoma: Early and late histopathologic consequences. Arch Ophthalmol 1968;79:177–181.
98. Apple DJ, Goldberg MF, et al. Argon laser photocoagulation of choroidal malignant melanoma: Tissue effects after a single treatment. Arch Ophthalmol 1973;90:97–101.
99. Meyer-Schwickerath G. Photocoagulation of choroidal melanomas. Doc Ophthalmol 1980;50:57–61.
100. DeLaey JJ, Hanssens M, et al. Photocoagulation of malignant melanomas of the choroid. A reappraisal. Bull Soc Belge Ophtalmol 1986;213:9–18.
101. Boniuk M, Cohen JS. Combined use of radiation plaques and photocoagulation in the treatment of choroidal melanomas. In FA Jakobiec (ed), Ocular and Adnexal Tumors. Birmingham, AL: Aesculapius, 1978:80–85.
102. Aygulska-Mach H, Maciejewski Z, et al. Conservative Treatment of Choroidal Melanomas. Combined Use of Cobalt Plaques and Photocoagulation. In PK Lommatzsch, FC Blodi (eds), Intraocular Tumors. Berlin: Akademie-Verlag, 1983:269–276.
103. Moura RA, McPherson AR, et al. Malignant melanoma of the choroid: Treatment with episcleral [198]Au plaque and xenon-arc photocoagulation. Ann Ophthalmol 1985;17:114–125.
104. Lee KY, Sabetes FN, et al. Combined Iodine-125 Plaque Irradiation and Laser Photocoagulation in the Treatment of Choroidal Malignant Melanoma. In N Bornfeld, ES Gragoudas, W Hopping, et al. (eds), Tumors of the Eye. Amsterdam: Kupler, 1991:441–447.
105. Foulds WS, Damato BE. Low energy long-exposure laser therapy in the management of choroidal melanoma. Graefes Arch Clin Exp Ophthalmol 1986;224:26–31.
106. Augsburger JJ, Kleineidam M, et al. Combined iodine-125 plaque irradiation and indirect ophthalmoscope laser therapy of choroidal malignant melanomas: Comparison with iodine-125 and cobalt-60 plaque therapy alone. Graefes Arch Clin Exp Ophthalmol 1993;231:500–507.
107. Chong LP, Ozler SA, et al. Indocyanine green-enhanced diode laser treatment of melanoma in a rabbit model. Retina 1993;13:251–259.
108. Peyman GA, Juarez CP, et al. Ten years experience with eye wall resection of uveal malignant melanomas. Ophthalmology 1984;91:1720–1724.
109. Shields JA, Shields CL. Lamellar sclerouvectomy for posterior uveal melanomas. Ophthalmic Surg 1988;19:774–780.
110. Shields JA, Shields CL, et al. Partial lamellar sclerouvectomy for ciliary body and choroidal tumors. Ophthalmology 1991;98:971–983.
111. Shields JA, Shields CL. Massive orbital extension of posterior uveal melanomas. Ophthal Plast Reconstr Surg 1991;7:238–251.
112. Augsburger JJ, Gamel JW, et al. Enucleation vs. cobalt plaque radiotherapy for malignant melanomas of the choroid and ciliary body. Arch Ophthalmol 1986;104:655–661.
113. Zimmerman LE, McLean IW. An evaluation of enucleation in the management of uveal melanoma. Am J Ophthalmol 1979;87:741–760.
114. Shields JA. Counseling the patient with a posterior uveal melanoma. Am J Ophthalmol 1988;106:88–91.
115. Mavligit GM, Charnsangavej C, et al. Regression of ocular melanoma metastatic to the liver after hepatic arterial chemoembolization with cisplatin and polyvinyl sponge. JAMA 1988;260:974–976.

Peripheral Tapetochoroidal Degeneration

Clinical Description

Typical peripheral tapetochoroidal degeneration (also known as peripheral senile pigmentary degeneration) gives a pigmented, granular appearance to the peripheral retina and is usually found between the ora serrata and the equator. Degeneration of the peripheral pigment epithelium releases pigment granules into the overlying sensory retina, thus producing areas of hyperpigmentation and hypopigmentation as a scattered circumferential band. The anterior border is irregular and difficult to see, but the posterior border is smooth and well defined.[1] When the pigmentation takes on the appearance of a fine network of criss-crossing pigmented lines, it is called reticular pigmentary degeneration (Figure 3-23). Peripheral retinal drusen are sometimes associated with this entity. During scleral depression, the areas of pigmentary degeneration appear flat, and the involved tissues may take on a whiter appearance due to the mild associated retinal degeneration.

This degenerative condition is usually seen after the fifth decade of life, and it slowly increases in prominence with age. No symptoms are associated with this condition. It does not cause defects on visual fields or dark-adaptation studies. The incidence is 20% of the population over 40 years of age and is bilateral in all cases.[2] Axial myopia has a higher frequency (16.9%) of this condition as compared to the general population of all ages.[3]

Histopathology

The RPE displays some cells with loss of pigment granules and others with an increase in pigment granules (Figure 3-24). Pigment released from degenerating RPE cells is scattered through the retinal tissue. There is also some loss of photoreceptors, thickening of the basal lamina, and sclerosis of the choriocapillaris. Macrophages may engulf the melanin granules and carry them to the retinal venules, where they may deposit the granules along the venules (pigment cuffing) during diapedesis (Figures 3-24 and 3-25).

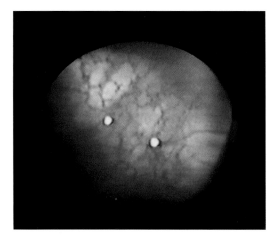

FIGURE 3-23
Reticular senile peripheral retinal pigmentary degeneration seen through the indirect condensing lens. Note criss-crossing pattern to the lines of pigmentation.

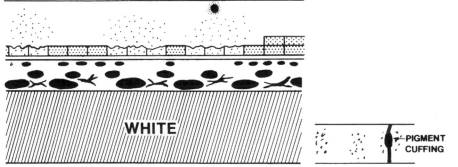

FIGURE 3-24
Degeneration of the choriocapillaris and pigment epithelium leads to dispersion of pigment granules in the sensory retina. Macrophages may engulf the melanin granules and carry them into the retina, where they may deposit the granules along venules (pigment cuffing) during diapedesis.

Clinical Significance

Peripheral tapetochoroidal degeneration is a benign involutionary process without symptoms and does not require treatment. It should be drawn on the patient's chart for future reference. Confusion may exist over the possibility of retinitis pigmentosa; the pigmentation in this condition usually has a bone spicule appearance, but sometimes it may be granular. Other signs necessary to diagnose retinitis pigmentosa are midperipheral location in the fundus, a waxy yellow pallor to the disc, visual field defects, attenuated vessels, night blindness, an abnormal electroretinogram, and younger age group (Table 3-4).

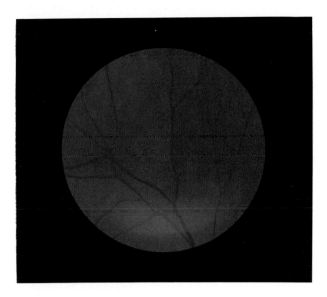

FIGURE 3-25
Two areas of pigment cuffing along retinal venules.

Table 3-4. Peripheral Tapetochoroidal Pigmentary Degeneration vs. Retinitis Pigmentosa

Peripheral Tapetochoroidal Pigmentary Degeneration	Retinitis Pigmentosa
Small, irregularly shaped, pigmented areas	Small, "bone spicule," pigmented areas
Not extensively found along retinal vessels	Typically found along venules
Generally found in the far periphery	Generally found in the midperiphery
No night blindness	Night blindness
Retinal vessels may show age-related arteriosclerosis	Marked vessel attenuation
No associated optic disc pallor	Disc pallor common
Normal electroretinogram	Abnormal electroretinogram
No associated decrease in visual acuity	May show a decrease in visual acuity late in the disease process
No scotoma	Ring scotoma

References

1. Foos RY, Spencer LM, et al. Trophic Degeneration of the Peripheral Retina. In New Orleans Academy of Ophthalmology: Symposium on Retina and Retinal Surgery. St. Louis: Mosby, 1969.

2. Glasgow BJ, Foos RY, et al. Degenerative Diseases of the Peripheral Retina. In TD Duane, EA Jaeger (eds), Clinical Ophthalmology. Vol. 3. Philadelphia: Harper & Row, 1993;26:1–29.

3. Pierro L, Camesasca FI, et al. Peripheral retinal changes and axial myopia. Retina 1992;12:12–17.

Peripheral Chorioretinal Degeneration

Clinical Description

Peripheral chorioretinal degeneration is a whitish smooth area adjacent to the ora serrata (Figure 3-26). The posterior edge merges discretely into the normal retina without producing an obvious demarcation line. The RPE under the chorioretinal degeneration is hyperpigmented.

This degeneration usually does not extend more than two disc diameters from the ora serrata. Blood vessels that pass through an area of chorioretinal degeneration may become sclerotic and may be surrounded by pigment. The more advanced areas of degeneration occur closer to the ora serrata, perhaps as the result of irritation of the peripheral retina by traction forces on the vitreous base.[1]

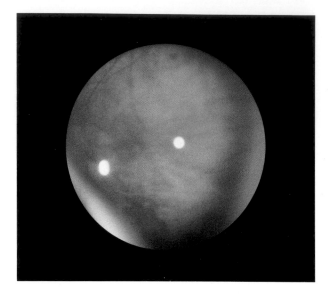

FIGURE 3-26
Peripheral chorioretinal degeneration is seen as a whitish band just posterior to the ora serrata. View is of the nasal ora serrata through the indirect condensing lens with scleral depression.

Peripheral chorioretinal degeneration is found in about two-thirds of the population to some degree. It generally begins in the fourth decade of life and increases with age.[2] There appears to be no predilection either for sex or for location in the peripheral fundus.

Histopathology

Chorioretinal degeneration is highlighted by decreased profusion of the peripheral retinal and choroidal blood vessels (Figure 3-27). This is probably the result of arteriosclerosis. There is degeneration and shrinkage of the retinal tissue and subsequent glial proliferation. The atrophic retina adheres tightly to the underlying choroid. Because this is a fairly mild degenerative process, there is gliotic repair and reactive pigment proliferation. If the process is severe, repair is not possible, and chorioretinal atrophy results.[2]

Clinical Significance

Peripheral chorioretinal degeneration and peripheral cystoid degeneration commonly occur in the same region of the fundus and have many of the same degenerative characteristics. These two conditions seem to inhibit each other because chorioretinal degeneration is frequently found posterior to cystoid degeneration and acts as a natural barrier to the posterior progression of cystoid degeneration.[2] Peripheral chorioretinal degeneration appears to be benign and does not seem to play a role in the production of retinal breaks.

References

1. Goldbaum MH. Retinal Examination and Surgery. In GA Peyman, DR Sanders, MF Goldberg (eds), Principles and Practice of Ophthalmology. Vol. 2. Philadelphia: Saunders, 1980;15:1029.
2. Schepens CL. Retinal Detachment and Allied Diseases. Philadelphia: Saunders, 1983:145–154.

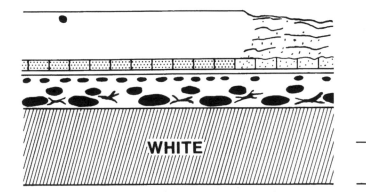

FIGURE 3-27
Peripheral chorioretinal degeneration. Note the loss of the choriocapillaris and the retinal degeneration located posterior to the ora serrata.

Peripheral Retinal Hemorrhage

Clinical Description

A bleed from a retinal artery or vein results in a retinal hemorrhage. Peripheral retinal hemorrhages appear as red spots that are usually less than 1 disc diameter in size (frequently 0.125–0.250 mm). Hemorrhages located in the peripheral retina are of various shapes, but most are irregularly round or oval (Figure 3-28). Flame-shaped hemorrhages are found in the superficial retinal layers and derive their shape from their characteristic orientation in the nerve fiber layer. Most peripheral hemorrhages are blot- and dot-shaped and are found in the middle layers of the retina. Small peripheral hemorrhages tend to be absorbed rather quickly, but at times they can take several months to absorb.

Histopathology

The vessel wall displays a rupture, and the surrounding retina has a pool of extravasated blood. Most of these hemorrhages result from a bleed in the deep capillary bed of the retina. They may be the result of a localized degeneration in the vessel wall or an increase invenous pressure. It is far more common to have a bleed in the venous system than in the arterial system of the retina. Hemorrhages in the inner layers of the sensory retina spread out in a flame shape, and those in the middle layers have a dot or blot appearance (Figure 3-29).

Clinical Significance

Peripheral retinal hemorrhages can be secondary to any type of hemorrhagic retinopathy. Patients with known vascular diseases and other blood disorders, such as diabetes mellitus, systemic hypertension, anemia,[1, 2] anticardiolipin antibody disease,[3, 4] thrombocytopenia and other platelet disorders,[5, 6] polycythemia,[7] and leukemia (29%)[8] may have peripheral hemorrhages. Peripheral hemorrhages commonly occur in venous stasis conditions and are sometimes seen in patients with chronic obstructive pulmonary disease[9, 10] or in patients on anticoagu-

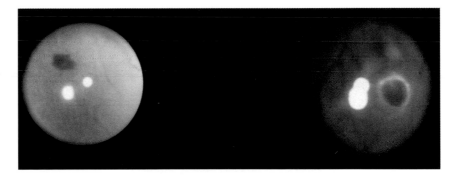

FIGURE 3-28
A peripheral retinal hemorrhage on the left and an operculated tear on the right seen through the indirect condensing lens. Note that there is no degenerated or detached retinal tissue around the hemorrhage as is seen with retinal break. The operculum from the retinal tear can be seen floating above the tear. The white ring around the tear indicates an old localized retinal detachment.

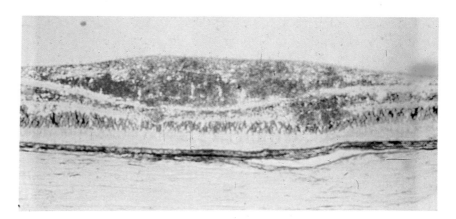

FIGURE 3-29
Histologic section of retinal tissue with hemorrhages. Note large superficial hemorrhage, which would have a flame- or splinter-shaped configuration when viewed during ophthalmoscopy. Deeper hemorrhages in the outer plexiform layer would look like dots or blots during ophthalmoscopy.

Table 3-5. Retinal Hemorrhage vs. Retinal Hole

Retinal Hemorrhage	Round Retinal Hole
Flat	Edges may be raised and an elevated surrounding retinal detachment may be present
Pinpoint to many disc diameters in size	Usually ⅛ disc diameter to almost a disc diameter in size
Red	Red when seen in attached retina
Red color remains during scleral depression	Red color may blanch on scleral depression
Margins may be distinct or slightly hazy	Distinct margins
Round to oval to irregular	Usually round but sometimes oval
Rarely encircled by a white collar of edema	May be encircled by a white collar of retinal degeneration or localized detachment
May show scotoma if large and located posteriorly	Generally too small to produce a scotoma unless it is a large break or surrounded by a detachment and is located posteriorly
Generally located from the posterior pole, but may be round anywhere in the retina	Most often found between the equator and the posterior margin of the vitreous base

lant therapy. Finally, they are often idiopathic or secondary to old age. Some of the age-related peripheral hemorrhages are secondary to posterior vitreous detachments.

A retinal hemorrhage that is mostly round can be mistaken for a retinal hole. Unlike a hemorrhage, retinal holes are almost always symmetrically round. The overlying retina is usually flat with hemorrhages, the exception being large hemorrhages, which may show mild elevation. On scleral depression, hemorrhages roll smoothly and do not exhibit an edge, as a hole does (see Figures 5-2, 5-4, and 5-5). Retinal holes may change slightly in color when being rolled but hemorrhages do not (Table 3-5). Retinal hemorrhages are usually multiple, whereas retinal holes are usually solitary lesions. A discussion of the differential diagnosis of a small round retinal hemorrhage and a retinal hole can be found in Chapter 5.

Peripheral hemorrhages usually resolve without any sequelae, and it may be impossible to detect their previous retinal location. If peripheral hemorrhages occur without a known etiology, a follow-up examination in a few months is indicated to see if there is an increase in hemorrhaging and to see if further changes in the involved area leads to a diagnosis for the underlying cause of the bleeding. These patients should be referred to their primary care physician to rule out underlying systemic diseases. The peripheral hemorrhages should be drawn on the patient's chart or photodocumented if observable with the camera system.

References

1. Rubenstein RA, Yanoff M, et al. Thrombocytopenia, anemia and retinal hemorrhages. Am J Ophthalmol 1968;65:435–439.
2. Merin S, Freund M. Retinopathy in severe anemia. Am J Ophthalmol 1968;66:1102–1106.
3. Levine SR, Croffs JW, et al. Visual symptoms associated with the presence of lupus anticoagulant. Ophthalmology 1988;95:686–692.
4. Kleiner RC, Najarian LV, et al. Vaso-occlusive retinopathy associated with antiphospholipoid antibodies (lupus anticoagulant retinopathy). Ophthalmology 1989;96:896–901.
5. Stefani FH, Brandt F, et al. Periarteritis nodosa and thrombotic thrombocytopenic purpura with serous retinal detachment in siblings. Br J Ophthalmol 1978;62:402–407.
6. Lambert SR, High KA, et al. Serous retinal detachments in thrombotic thrombocytopenia purpura. Arch Ophthalmol 1985;103:1172–1174.
7. Rothstein T. Bilateral central retinal vein closure as the initial manifestation of polycythemia. Am J Ophthalmol 1972;74:256–260.
8. Williams GA. Ocular Manifestation of Hematologic Diseases. In TD Duane, EA Jaeger (eds), Clinical Ophthalmology. Vol. 5. Philadelphia: Harper & Row, 1991; 23:1–12.
9. Spalter HF, Bruce GM. Ocular changes in pulmonary insufficiency. Trans Am Acad Ophthalmol Otolaryngol 1964;68:661–676.
10. Gottlieb F, Harris D, et al. The peripheral eyeground in chronic respiratory disease. Arch Ophthalmol 1969;82:611–619.

Peripheral Retinal Neovascularization

Clinical Description

Peripheral retinal neovascularization occurs in a number of ocular disease conditions and from iatrogenic causes. A study of 100 consecutive patients' (156) eyes with peripheral proliferative retinopathies found the following underlying reasons for the proliferative diseases: sickle cell hemoglobinopathies (49%), branch retinal vein occlusions (20%), diabetes mellitus (9%), sarcoid (4%), intravenous drug abuse (4%), ocular ischemic syndrome (1%), pars planitis (1%), Coat's disease (1%), retinitis pigmentosa or retinal detachment (1%), and no obvious cause (10%).[1] Chronic leukemia has also been reported to cause peripheral neovascularization as well as neovascularization of the disc.[2] Neovascularization of the near retinal periphery is most commonly seen in proliferative diabetic retinopathy (Figure 3-30). Optic disc neovascularization is a sign of diffuse retinal ischemia, and neovascularization elsewhere is more closely related to localized retinal ischemia.[3]

In the far periphery of the retina, the most common cause of neovascularization appears to be related to sickle cell retinopathy.[4] It characteristically displays a proliferative vascular formation known as a sea fan, which resembles the marine invertebrate *Gorgonia flabellum*. Fibrosis and intraretinal and preretinal hemorrhages are often associated with sea fans. Sometimes a vitreous detachment may elevate the sea fan into the vitreous cavity. Sea fans are seen in 59–72% of patients with the sickle cell form of the disease,[5, 6] in 33% of patients with sickle cell thalassemia,[7] and uncommonly in patients with the other hemoglobinopathies (10%).[5] Sea fans are most frequently located in the superior temporal quadrant and, in descending order of frequency, the inferior temporal, superior nasal, and inferior nasal quadrants.[8] They may grow in a circumferential pattern, and rarely do they come close to the posterior pole. Other retinal findings include salmon patches and black sunbursts.

Retrolental fibroplasia can also produce neovascularization of the far retinal periphery. Less commonly it occurs during the recovery phase of branch vein occlusions[9] and after incisions into the vitreous through the pars plana and peripheral retina during retinal and vitreous surgery.[10]

Histopathology

Trypsin-digest studies of sickle cell retinopathy show arteriolar occlusions, peripheral zones of infarcted capillaries, arteriovenous anastomoses, capillary budding microaneurysmal formations, vessel enlargement, and neovascular tissue. Sometimes, vitreous traction bands are attached to the neovascular tissue.[8] The neovascular tissue demonstrates marked endothelial proliferation arising from residual vascular complexes immediately adjacent to areas of retinal capillary closure.

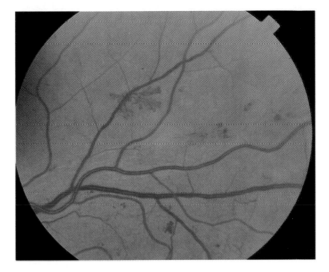

FIGURE 3-30
Neovascularization in the midperiphery due to proliferative diabetic retinopathy.

Clinical Significance

Hemorrhaging is the all too common consequence of neovascularization anywhere in the eye. Vitreous hemorrhage is a fairly common event in peripheral retinal neovascularization and was present in 23% of patients with sickle cell disease and 3% of patients with the SS trait.[7]

After a vitreous hemorrhage there is vitreous degeneration and scarring, which frequently leads to increased vitreous traction on the retina. The traction may result in a retinal break and subsequent rhegmatogenous retinal detachment.[11] Sometimes severe vitreous traction may produce a purely tractional retinal detachment.

Treatment for peripheral neovascularization of the retina consists of one or a combination of the following modalities: photocoagulation, diathermy, and transconjunctival cryotherapy.[12–14]

References

1. Brown GC, Brown RH, et al. Peripheral proliferative retinopathies. Int Ophthalmol 1987;11:41–50.
2. Kincaid MC, Green WR. Ocular and orbital involvement in leukemia. Surv Ophthalmol 1983;27:211–232.
3. Kincaid MC, Cunningham RD. Retinopathy of Blood Dyscrasias. In W Tasman, EA Jaeger (eds), Clinical Ophthalmology. Vol. 3. Philadelphia: Harper & Row, 1993;17:4.
4. Romayananda N, Goldberg MF, et al. Histopathology of

sickle cell retinopathy. Trans Am Acad Ophthalmol 1973;77:652–676.

5. Welsh RB, Goldberg MF. Sickle-cell hemoglobin and its relation to fundus abnormalities. Arch Ophthalmol 1966;75:353–362.

6. Goldberg MF. Natural history of untreated proliferative sickle cell retinopathy. Am J Ophthalmol 1971;71:649–665.

7. Goldberg MF, Charache S, et al. Ophthalmologic manifestations of sickle cell thalassemia. Arch Intern Med 1971;128:33–39.

8. Goldberg MF. Sickle cell retinopathy. In TD Duane, EA Jaeger (eds), Clinical Ophthalmology. Vol. 3. Philadelphia: Harper & Row, 1979;17:1–45.

9. Jaeger EA. Venous Obstructive Disease of the Retina. In TD Duane, EA Jaeger (eds), Clinical Ophthalmology. Vol. 3. Philadelphia: Harper & Row, 1979;15:1–21.

10. Schepens CL. Retinal Detachment and Allied Diseases. Philadelphia: Saunders, 1983:1042.

11. Goldberg MF. Retinal detachment associated with proliferative retinopathies. Isr J Med Sci 1972;8:1447–1461.

12. Hannon J. Vitreous hemorrhage associated with sickle cell-hemoglobin C disease. Am J Ophthalmol 1956;42:707–711.

13. Goldberg MF. Treatment of proliferative sickle retinopathy. Trans Am Acad Ophthalmol Otolaryngol 1971;75:532–556.

14. Goldberg MF, Acacio I. Argon laser photocoagulation of proliferative sickle retinopathy. Arch Ophthalmol 1973;90:35–44.

Peripheral Retinal Drusen

Clinical Description

Retinal drusen are white to yellowish, round, dome-shaped areas deep in the retina (Figure 3-31). They can vary in size and shape, but they are usually small and round. They have a glistening crystalline quality from which they derive their German name *drusen*, meaning "stone nodule." When they occur in the midperiphery of the fundus, they are called equatorial drusen. Equatorial drusen have a greater tendency to collect hyperpigmented clumps; these are called pigment-ringed drusen. Drusen may appear white when they have become calcified. Drusen can coalesce to form larger, irregularly shaped drusen bodies.

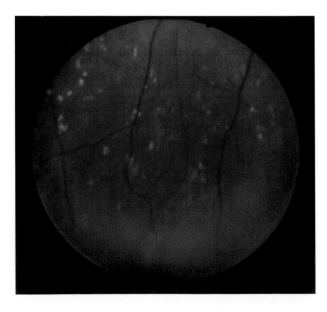

FIGURE 3-31
Peripheral retinal drusen are seen as tiny, clear to yellowish areas.

During ophthalmoscopy, indirect illumination of a drusen causes it to glow more brightly than the surrounding retina because there is less pigment epithelium covering it (Figure 3-32). This same phenomenon produces a window defect during fluorescein angiography that results in early hyperfluorescent spots during the choroidal flush and a gradual diminution as the concentration of fluorescein in the choroid decreases.

Histopathology

Drusen are focal, irregular, homogeneous, mound-like extensions of the basal lamina (Bruch's membrane) (see Figure 3-32). They are most likely the deposit of a hyaline material (an acid mucopolysaccharide) from degenerated pigment epithelial cells onto the cuticular portion of the basal lamina (Bruch's membrane). Because drusen commonly occur with increasing age, natural degeneration of the choroidal vessels and pigment epithelium is probably responsible for most of them. The pigment epithelium appears degenerated and stretched thin over the drusen. Drusen can undergo further degeneration and the hyaline material may be replaced with dystrophic calcium, thus giving them a white appearance.[1]

Clinical Significance

Peripheral retinal drusen are generally considered a benign degeneration that increases with age and produces little consequence in most cases. Rarely, they are involved in the formation of a peripheral

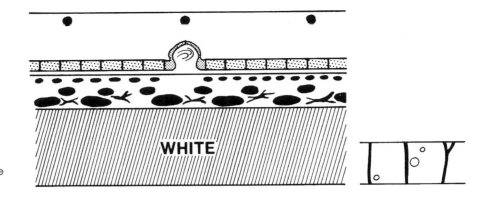

FIGURE 3-32
The drusen have elevated and thinned the pigment epithelium, which makes them appear rather transparent when seen through the retina.

subretinal neovascular membrane.[2] They can be associated with a number of ocular and systemic diseases such as dysproteinemia, chronic leukemia, pseudoxanthoma elasticum, scleroderma, Rendu-Osler-Weber syndrome, and many other conditions.[3] It is not uncommon to find drusen overlying choroidal tumors, such as malignant melanoma. They are seen in Doyne's honeycomb choroiditis, also known as dominant and familial drusen.

References

1. Cavender JC, Ai E. Hereditary Macular Dystrophies. In TD Duane, EA Jaeger (eds), Clinical Ophthalmology. Vol. 3. Philadelphia: Harper & Row, 1982;9:18–19.
2. Gass JDM. Drusen and disciform macular detachment and degeneration. Arch Ophthalmol 1973;90:206–217.
3. Duke-Elder S, Perkins ES. Diseases of the Uveal Tract. In System of Ophthalmology. Vol. 10. London: Henry Kimpton, 1977;5:536.

Retinal Tufts

Clinical Description

Retinal tufts, also known as granular tissue, are grayish to white lesions in the postbasal peripheral retina that have a dull, irregular appearance (Figure 3-33). They are usually very small, ranging from a few microns to approximately 3 mm, and have a great variety of shapes. Zonular traction tufts vary from barely raised to markedly elevated. Retinal tufts and tags are much easier to see during scleral depression.

These lesions may be solitary or occur in clusters (Figure 3-34). They are generally located between the equator and the ora serrata, commonly in the nasal half of the fundus.[1] The usual location is just posterior to the ora serrata within the vitreous base. These lesions tend to occur bilaterally.[2, 3] Vitreous traction is usually present and is frequently attached to the apex of the tuft.[4, 5] Vitreous traction may pull small pieces of the tuft into the vitreous, resulting in small vitreous floaters. Longstanding traction can result in hyperplasia of the adjacent pigment epithelium, called pigment clumping. These lesions remain stationary in size and do not increase in number with age, suggesting that they are developmental in origin.[6] Retinal tufts usually

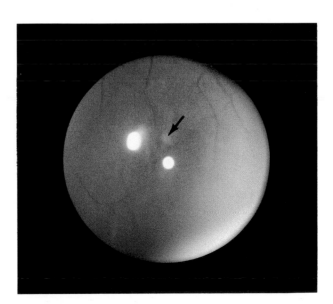

FIGURE 3-33
Peripheral retinal tuft (*arrow*) seen through the indirect condensing lens.

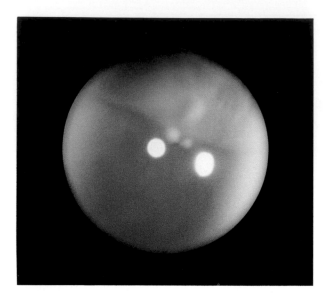

FIGURE 3-34
Three peripheral retinal tufts seen in the indirect condensing lens with scleral depression.

tinuous vitreous traction. Retinal or granular tags consist of degenerated tissue that has been thinned and elongated by vitreous traction. They tend to be very small and sometimes are just barely visible during indirect ophthalmoscopy. They usually appear as tiny white posts protruding from the retinal surface into the vitreous (see Figures 2-4 and 3-40). These lesions are sometimes associated with other peripheral degenerative anomalies, such as meridional folds. Vitreous traction can cause these tags to avulse from the retinal surface, resulting in a vitreous floater or retinal break. A noncystic retinal tuft is a noncystic retinal degeneration composed of degenerated retinal tissue and proliferated glial cells. They are most often located in the vitreous base and can be found in any quadrant of the fundus. Noncystic tufts tend to be small (<0.1 mm in diameter) and irregularly shaped and may have pointed projections on their surface due to vitreous traction. They are present in 72% of the adult population, occurring bilaterally in half the cases, and thus are present in 59% of adult eyes.[7]

A cystic retinal tuft is the result of cystic retinal degeneration, in which a number of microcystic spaces are found within the lesion (Figure 3-35). Cystic tufts are congenital development abnormalities (having been seen in newborns).[8] Foos[9] suggests that these tufts originate in the primitive peripheral retina and consist of glial cell proliferation. These tend to be larger than noncystic tufts

do not produce symptoms, but occasionally they may cause photopsia due to significant vitreous traction, especially during the formation of a posterior vitreous detachment.

Retinal tufts vary in appearance and are usually stable in size and shape over time. Occasionally, the size and shape can vary slightly due to con-

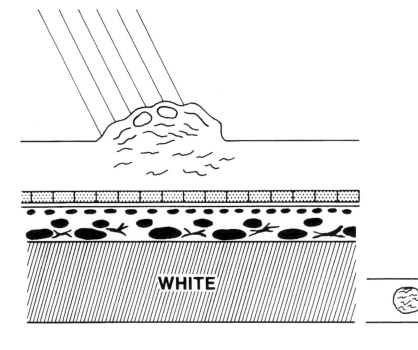

WHITE

FIGURE 3-35
Cystic retinal tuft with vitreous traction.

(0.1–1.0 mm) and have a more honeycombed appearance. Cystic tufts tend to be spherical with a flat bottom and have the clinical appearance of a small wet cotton ball on the surface of the retina. The retina surrounding the tuft often shows degeneration.[10, 11] Because vitreous traction may be associated with these tufts, it is not unusual to find pigment at the base of a tuft. Cystic tufts can be located within or posterior to the vitreous base, but 78% occur in the equatorial zone. They can be found in any quadrant of the retina and are most often unilateral and occur singularly (80%). They are found in 5% of the adult population, are bilateral in only 6% of cases, and thus are detected in 2.5% of adult eyes.[7] Others have reported that they occur in 5–59% of eyes that have undergone autopsy.[8]

A zonular traction tuft is produced by the tractional force of a zonule. The developing inner layer of the optic cup may produce zonules posterior to the ora serrata,[7] and as the globe grows, a zonule attached to the peripheral retina may pull retinal tissue forward into a traction tuft. The appearance is like that of gliotic strand being pulled anteriorly into the vitreous, making a sharp angle with the retina (Figure 3-36). The length of these tufts varies greatly, probably as a result of the difference in tractional forces. They have a triangular base that thins to a fairly sharp point at the apex, and they are usually attached to the retina less than 0.5 mm posterior to the ora serrata and rarely attached posterior to the vitreous base (Figure 3-37). These lesions

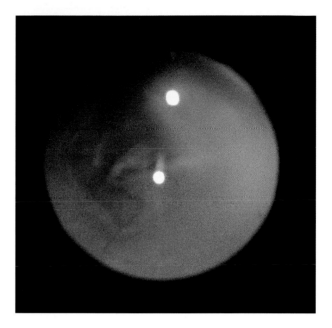

FIGURE 3-36
Zonular traction tuft seen through the indirect condensing lens. The retina is to the left and the pars plana is to the right. Note that the traction tuft is traveling down to the retina from left to right. The tuft has produced a retinal tear at the posterior margin of its anchorage to the retina (reddish mouth appearance).

occur in 15% of the population and are present bilaterally in 15% of cases and thus are evident in 9% of all eyes.[3,7] They are commonly found in the nasal half of the fundus.[4]

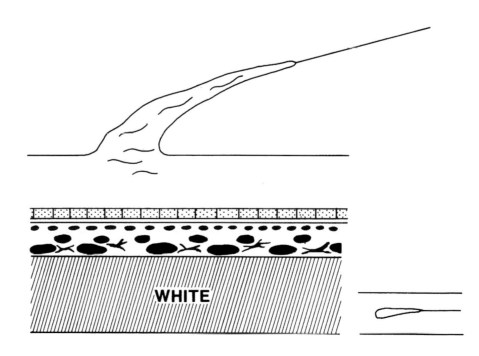

FIGURE 3-37
Traction zonule in the vitreous is pulling the retinal tuft in an anterior direction.

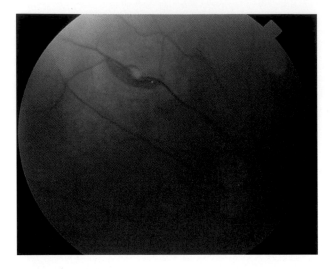

FIGURE 3-38
A tuft in the equatorial region of the retina has resulted in a bi-flap retinal tear and has pulled a vessel up into the vitreous. Due to the observation of considerable traction on the tear by watching the flaps move from side to side during eye movements, retinopexy was performed.

Histopathology

Retinal tufts and tags are composed of degenerated retinal tissue and proliferated glial cells. Retinal disorganization seems to involve the entire sensory retina, and there can be an associated disruption of the pigment epithelium. Frequently, microcystic degeneration occurs, and vitreous traction is almost always present (see Figure 3-35).

Clinical Significance

Vitreous traction is mainly responsible for the formation of the retinal breaks associated with retinal tufts. The continuous tractional forces can cause both retinal holes and tears. Retinal tufts are most likely to produce operculated or flap tears when strong vitreous traction is applied (Figure 3-38).[10–12] These breaks can occur on any side of a retinal tag, a noncystic tuft, or a cystic tuft. Zonular traction tufts tend to form retinal breaks on the posterior edge of the base and only accounted for 0.11% of retinal tears in autopsied eyes; because these lesions are intrabasal (within the vitreous base) they rarely cause a retinal detachment.[7] Cystic retinal tufts may account for 10% of rhegmatogenous retinal detach-ments, but only 0.28% of cystic tufts produce a retinal detachment.[12] Atrophic holes adjacent to a cystic tuft rarely result in a retinal detachment (risk of 0.3%).[3, 4, 9, 13–15] Retinal tufts without breaks should be watched every 1–2 years and their location drawn on the patient's chart. Those with breaks should be watched more frequently, depending on the clinical circumstances. Retinal tufts are infrequently associated with retinal detachments. Treatment is rarely indicated and consists of either cryopexy or photocoagulation.

References

1. Teng CC, Katzin HM. An anatomic study of the periphery of the retina. Part 1. Nonpigmented epithelial cell proliferation and hole formation. Am J Ophthalmol 1951; 34:1237–1248.
2. Spencer LM, Foos RY. Paravascular vitreoretinal attachments. Arch Ophthalmol 1970;84:557–564.
3. Spencer LM, Straatsma BR, et al. Tractional Degenerations of the Peripheral Retina. In New Orleans Academy of Ophthalmology: Symposium on Retina and Retinal Surgery. St. Louis: Mosby, 1969:103–127.
4. Byer NE. Cystic retinal tufts and their relationship to retinal detachment. Arch Ophthalmol 1981;99:1788–1790.
5. Foos RY. Vitreous Base, Retinal Tufts and Retinal Tears: Pathological Relationships. In RC Pruett (ed), Retina Congress. New York: Appleton-Century-Crofts, 1974:259.
6. Schepens CL. Retinal Detachment and Allied Diseases. Philadelphia: Saunders, 1983:139–140.
7. Glasgow BJ, Foos RY, et al. Degenerative Diseases of the Peripheral Retina. In TD Duane, EA Jaeger (eds), Clinical Ophthalmology. Vol. 3. Philadelphia: Harper & Row, 1993;26:1–29.
8. Dunker S, Glinz J, Faulborn J. Morphologic studies of the peripheral vitreoretinal interface in humans reveal structures implicated in the pathogenesis of retinal tears. Retina 1997;17:124–130.
9. Foos RY. Zonular traction tufts of the peripheral retina in cadaver eyes. Arch Ophthalmol 1969;82:620–632.
10. Bec P, Ravault M, Arne JL, et al. La peripherie du fond d'oeil. Paris: Masson, 1980.
11. Foos RY, Allen RA. Retinal tears and lesser lesions of the peripheral retina in cadaver eyes. Am J Ophthalmol 1967;64:643–655.
12. Byer NE. Discussion of "Vitreous in lattice degeneration of retina." Ophthalmology 1984;91:457.
13. Schepens CL, Bahn GC. Examination of the ora serrata: Its importance in retinal detachments. Arch Ophthalmol 1950;44:677–690.
14. Foos RY. Postoral peripheral retinal tears. Ann Ophthalmol 1974;6:679–687.
15. Murakami-Nagasako F, Ohba N. Phakic retinal detachment associated with cystic retinal tuft. Graefes Arch Clin Exp Ophthalmol 1982;219:188–192.

Meridional Fold and Complex

Clinical Description

A meridional fold is a spindle-shaped roll of redundant retinal tissue that is elevated into the vitreous (Figures 3-39 and 3-40; see also Figure 3-1). It is an asymptomatic developmental anomaly produced by a stretching of the retina in an anteroposterior direction and is thought of as an exaggerated ora tooth. They are a developmental variation of the peripheral retina, like enclosed ora bays and peripheral retinal excavations. Developmental variations of the peripheral retina are found in approximately 20% of all eyes and share common features, including presence at birth, tendency for symmetry in both eyes, persistence throughout life, and association with other developmental anomalies.[1] These acquired lesions can increase in size with age. Meridional folds usually originate in an ora tooth (81%), but they can develop in the middle of the posterior edge of an ora bay (19%).[2] The length of folds can vary from 0.5 disc diameter to 4 disc diameters and extend posteriorly for 0.6–6.0 mm.[3] Vitreous bands originate from the posterior end of a meridional fold and traverse in both anterior and posterior directions. Occasionally, a zonule may be attached to the apex of a meridional fold.[4]

During ophthalmoscopy, the clinician usually only sees the posterior end of the fold that appears as a white spot or streak at the edge of the condensing lens, but scleral depression allows for a full view of the fold. On scleral depression, the fold appears as a slightly raised white ridge with an irregular surface. The fold can be seen to begin just posterior to the ora and usually extends anteriorly between two ora bays as a large ora tooth, but sometimes the fold terminates anteriorly at the middle of an ora bay. Often a small white floater may be seen above the fold, which is a piece of the fold pulled off into the vitreous due to vitreous traction.

Meridional folds occur in about 26% of the population, are bilateral in 55% of cases, and thus are present in 20% of all eyes.[3] They more commonly affect males.[3] The number of folds per eye varies from one to ten. Although some state that there is usually only fold one per eye,[5] it has been my experience to find more than one fold in close proximity to each other in most eyes. Multiple folds are found in only 27% of affected eyes.[4] Folds are most frequently found in the superonasal quadrant and are more frequently superior and nasal than inferior and temporal.[3] Cystoid degeneration is often found adjacent to the folds.

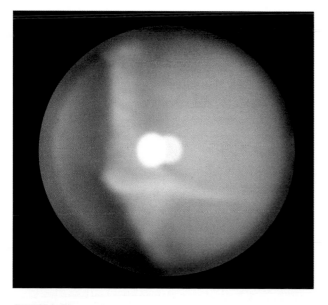

FIGURE 3-39
A meridional fold in an ora tooth between two ora bays on the nasal ora serrata seen through the indirect condensing lens during scleral depression.

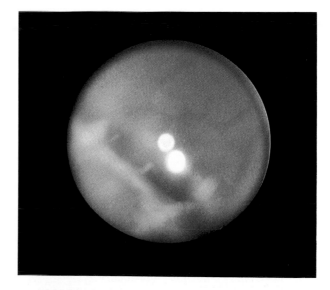

FIGURE 3-40
Two adjacent meridional folds, each in an ora tooth and with two retinal tags (noncystic retinal tufts) between them. They are seen on the superior nasal ora serrata through the indirect condensing lens with scleral depression.

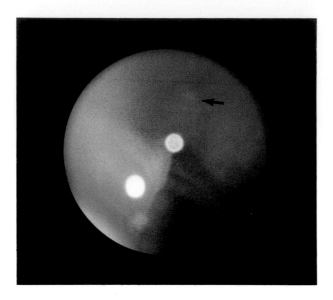

FIGURE 3-41
A meridional complex is a fold extending anteriorly all the way to a large ciliary process, and posterior to the meridional fold is a tiny area of retinal excavation (*arrow*). The lesion is located in the nasal fundus and seen through the indirect condensing lens with scleral depression.

A meridional complex is composed of an enlarged dentate and ciliary process associated with a meridional fold (Figure 3-41). They are more commonly found in the superior nasal quadrant of the retina. A peripheral retinal excavation can be located posterior to the complex. Meridional complexes are found in 16% of the population, are bilateral in 58%

of cases, and thus are present in 12% of all eyes. They are multiple in 45% of affected eyes.[3]

Histopathology

Meridional folds are thickened folds of retinal tissue (Figure 3-42). The surface can display proliferation of glial cells, and beneath the surface there are often microcystoid changes. Underneath the degenerative inner retinal tissue are the outer retinal layers, which are essentially intact.

Clinical Significance

In general, meridional folds and complexes seldom cause significant retinal problems.[4, 6] Vitreous traction on meridional folds and complexes may result in the formation of retinal breaks.[1] Retinal breaks and excavations can be found just posterior to a meridional fold (Figure 3-43). Retinal breaks are more likely to occur if a posterior vitreous detachment is present. Meridional folds located in the temporal fundus or that extend posterior to the ora serrata are more likely to develop retinal breaks. These breaks may be located anywhere along the edge of the fold but are more frequently found at the posterior margin. Breaks associated with meridional folds or the vitreous base are usually located in the upper half of the fundus, with the upper nasal quadrant being affected most frequently.[7] Me-

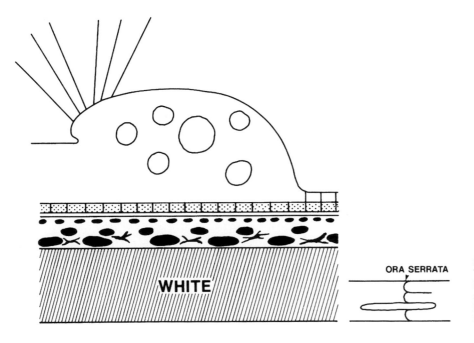

ORA SERRATA

FIGURE 3-42
The meridional fold is located in both the retina and pars plana, shows cystoid degeneration, and has vitreous traction on the posterior portion of the fold.

ridional folds are not a common cause of retinal detachment,[4, 6] which is probably due to the fact that these lesions are found in the region of the vitreous base. Even though meridional folds do not increase the risk of developing a retinal detachment, a retinal tear in an eye with a detachment may be found at the posterior edge of a fold.[4, 8, 9]

Periodic examinations should be performed with indirect ophthalmoscopy with and without scleral depression and a three-mirror contact lens to determine the existence of retinal breaks associated with meridional folds or complexes. The lesions should be drawn on the patient's chart for future reference. The patient should be followed on a routine basis every 1–2 years, and if an associated retinal tear is present, the patient should be given the symptoms of a retinal detachment. Because of the anterior location of these lesions, cryopexy is the preferred treatment for an associated retinal break.

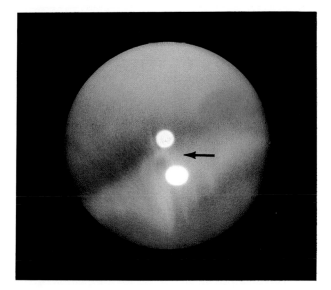

FIGURE 3-43
There is a small hole at the posterior end of a meridional fold (arrow), and signs of a vitreous traction. The location is the superior nasal ora serrata, seen through the indirect condensing lens with scleral depression.

References

1. Spencer LM, Foos RY, et al. Meridional folds and meridional complexes of the peripheral retina. Trans Am Ophthalmol Otolaryngol 1969;73:204.
2. Rutnin U, Schepens CL. Fundus appearance in normal eyes. II. The standard peripheral fundus and developmental variation. Am J Ophthalmol 1967;64:840–852.
3. Glasgow BJ, Foos RY, et al. Degenerative Diseases of the Peripheral Retina. In TD Duane, EA Jaeger (eds), Clinical Ophthalmology. Vol. 3. Philadelphia: Harper & Row, 1993;26:1–29.
4. Spencer LM, Foos RY, et al. Meridional folds, meridional complexes and associated abnormalities of the peripheral retina. Am J Ophthalmol 1970;70:697–718.
5. Schepens CL. Retinal Detachment and Allied Diseases. Philadelphia: Saunders, 1983:139.
6. Straatsma BR, Landers MB, et al. The ora serrata in the adult human eye. Arch Ophthalmol 1968;80:3–20.
7. Pischel DK. Retinal Detachment: A Manual (2nd ed). Am Acad Ophthalmol Otolaryngol 1965;72.
8. Spencer LM, Foos RY, et al. Enclosed bays of the ora serrata: Relationships to retinal tears. Arch Ophthalmol 1970;83:421–425.
9. Rutnin U, Schepens CL. Fundus appearance in normal eyes. IV. Retinal breaks and other findings. Am J Ophthalmol 1967;64:1063–1078.

Enclosed Ora Bay

Clinical Description

An enclosed ora bay, also known as a ring tooth or hole-in-a-tooth,[1] results from the enclosing of an island of pars plana epithelium by peripheral retina at the ora serrata. They are a developmental variation of the peripheral retina, like peripheral retinal excavations and meridional folds. Developmental variations of the peripheral retina are found in approximately 20% of all eyes and share common features, such as presence at birth, tendency to occur symmetrically in both eyes, persistence throughout life, and association with other developmental anomalies.[2] The ora bay can be partially or totally enclosed. A partially enclosed ora bay or open ring is produced when two adjacent teeth come close to each other but never unite (Figure 3-44A). A totally enclosed ora bay can be produced by two slender adjacent teeth uniting at their anterior apices (ring tooth) or, if two adjacent teeth merge to form one large tooth, a hole-in-a-tooth (Figures 3-44B and 3-45).

Enclosed ora bays are brownish depressions, frequently displaying cystoid degeneration, surrounded by normal-appearing retina. Enclosed ora bays occur in about 3–4% of all eyes and 6% of all

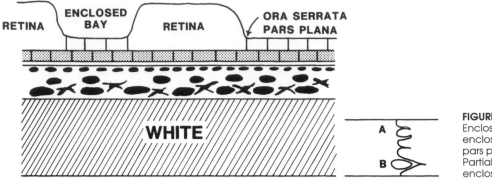

FIGURE 3-44
Enclosed ora bay. Note that the enclosed bay is isolated from the pars plana by peripheral retina. A. Partially enclosed bay. B. Totally enclosed bay.

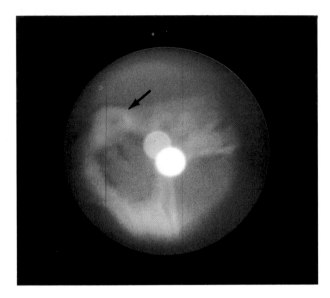

FIGURE 3-45
Completely enclosed ora bay is isolated from the pars plana by two large ora teeth that unite anterior to the enclosed bay. Note the small retinal erosion at the posterior edge of the enclosed bay (*arrow*). View is through the indirect condensing lens with scleral depression.

patients, and they are bilateral in 8% of affected individuals.[3–5] A ring tooth is found in 2% of eyes.[5] In two studies, 73% of enclosed bays were associated with a meridional complex in the same clock position, and sometimes a bay was part of a complex; also, 20% of enclosed bays had a meridional fold immediately anterior or posterior to them. They are usually located near the horizontal meridian and occur equally between the nasal and temporal halves of the fundus.[5, 6]

Histopathology

An enclosed ora bay is composed of a thin layer of pars plana surrounded by sensory retina (see Figure 3-44).

Clinical Significance

An enclosed ora bay may be mistaken for a retinal hole; however, careful examination with indirect ophthalmoscopy with or without scleral depression, a 90-diopter condensing lens, or a three-mirror contact lens reveals the brownish color of the pars plana island and that the suspected hole is anterior to the ora serrata. A retinal erosion or full-thickness break may be found immediately posterior to an enclosed bay (see Figure 3-45). Strong vitreous traction may be present at the edges of enclosed ora bays. Retinal breaks may occur in one of six enclosed ora bays at the posterior edge. These were found in 16.7% of all eyes, and all were associated with a posterior vitreous detachment.[5]

References

1. Schepens CL. Retinal Detachment and Allied Diseases. Philadelphia: Saunders, 1983;8:137–138.
2. Spencer LM, Foos RY, et al. Meridional folds and meridional complexes of the peripheral retina. Trans Am Ophthalmol Otolaryngol 1969;73:204.
3. Glasgow BJ, Foos RY, et al. Degenerative Diseases of the Peripheral Retina. In TD Duane, EA Jaeger (eds), Clinical Ophthalmology. Vol. 3. Philadelphia: Harper & Row, 1993;26:1–29.
4. Rutnin U, Schepens CL. Fundus appearance in normal eyes. IV. Retinal breaks and other findings. Am J Ophthalmol 1967;64:1063–1078.
5. Spencer LM, Foos RY, et al. Enclosed ora bays of the ora serrata: relationship to retinal tears. Arch Ophthalmol 1970;83:421–425.
6. Spencer LM, Foos RY, et al. Meridional folds, meridional complexes, and associated abnormalities of the peripheral retina. Am J Ophthalmol 1970;70:697–714.

Pearls of the Ora Serrata

Clinical Description

Pearls of the ora serrata are bright, glistening white spheroids near or on the dentate processes (Figure 3-46). They are usually single and are located between the base and the tip of the dentate process. In the early stage of development, they appear as dark brown, round bodies in an ora tooth due to the covering of the pigment epithelium. Later, they become highly visible when the pigment epithelium over the pearl becomes thinned or absent.

Ora pearls occur in any quadrant of the fundus, and approximately 20% of 700 consecutive studied autopsied eyes had a recognizable pearl. If both eyes were examined, there was a remarkable degree of bilaterality and symmetry to the distribution of pearls.[1]

Histopathology

The pearls are drusenlike structures that are analogous to a giant drusen of the retina. They occur between the pigment epithelium and the basal lamina (Bruch's membrane) (Figure 3-47). Histologically, they stain as acid carbonate.[1]

Clinical Significance

Pearls of the ora serrata are a benign finding.[2]

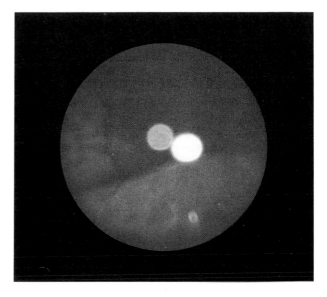

FIGURE 3-46
A small ora pearl can be seen on the ora serrata through the indirect condensing lens.

References

1. Lonn LI, Smith TR. Ora serrata pearls: Clinical and histological correlation. Arch Ophthalmol 1967;77:809–813.
2. Goldbaum MH. Retinal Examination and Surgery. In GA Peyman, DR Sanders (eds), Principles and Practice of Ophthalmology. Vol. 2. Philadelphia: Saunders, 1980; 15:1032.

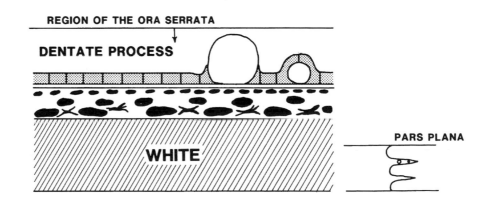

FIGURE 3-47
Two ora pearls in a dentate process. The smaller pearl is covered with pigment epithelium and appears dark. The larger pearl has broken through the pigment epithelium and thus displays its crystalline properties.

Chorioretinal Atrophy (Paving-Stone Degeneration)

Clinical Description

Chorioretinal atrophy usually appears as round, depigmented areas in the retina in which a clear view of the medium- and large-sized vessels of the choroid are seen against the white background of the sclera. Chorioretinal atrophy is believed to be the result of the occlusion of a single lobule of choroidal circulation that produces a focal postischemic atrophy of the pigment epithelium and outer layers of the sensory retina. They usually vary from 0.1 to 1.5 mm but occasionally are many disc diameters in size. Pigment can be found at the edges, on incomplete septa, or in the centers of these lesions.[1] Small lesions may coalesce into large areas with convex scalloped margins and incomplete septa. Single lesions are called chorioretinal atrophy, but when the lesions are aligned in a row parallel to the ora serrata, the condition is known as paving-stone or cobblestone degeneration (Figures 3-48 and 3-49; see also Figure 2-4). During scleral depression, chorioretinal atrophy appears flat and the overall appearance does not change.

Paving-stone degeneration is present in 22–27% of adults,[2, 3] and its prevalence increases markedly with age, from 10% in persons in their twenties to more than 30% of those greater than 70 years of age.[1, 4] There is a higher incidence of chorioretinal atrophy in myopes where it has been reported to have an incidence of 27.1%[3] and at 40% in myopic individuals over 40 years of age.[5] There seems to be a preference for the inferior region of the fundus, and more than half of these lesions are located between the 5 and 7 o'clock positions.[1] They are bilateral in 38.0–41.4% of eyes[6, 7] and in 57% of myopic eyes.[5] The majority are found just posterior to the ora serrata; rarely, paving-stone degeneration can occur as far posterior as the equator. It can, however, occasionally be seen in the posterior pole and pars plana. Paving-stone degeneration is also found anterior to peripheral intraocular tumors, such as choroidal malignant melanoma and nevi, and metastatic choroidal tumors. It is believed that the association of this entity and intraocular tumors has to do with peripheral choroidal insufficiency induced by the space-occupying masses.[8] Chorioretinal degeneration and atrophy can affect the same areas of the peripheral retina.

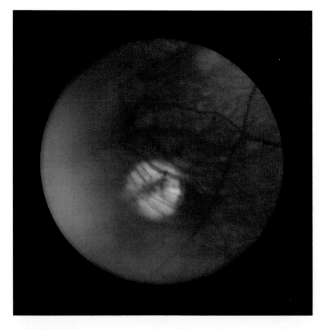

FIGURE 3-48
Chorioretinal atrophy in the inferior fundus. Note that the large and medium-sized choroidal vessels are seen more easily through the lesion and that there is pigment on the edges and in the center of the lesion.

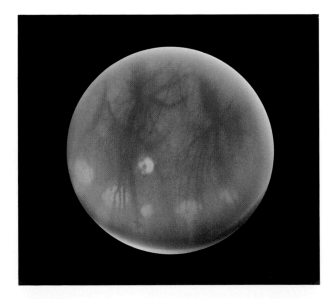

FIGURE 3-49
Paving-stone degeneration in the inferior fundus. Note that the large and medium-sized choroidal vessels are seen more easily through the lesions and that there is pigment on the edges and in the center of the lesions.

FIGURE 3-50
The chorioretinal atrophy shows a loss of the choriocapillaris and the outer five layers of the retina, resulting in loss of tissue and small depression of the retina. Loss of pigment epithelium and choriocapillaris allows a clear "window view" of the choroid and sclera. There can be pigment epithelial hyperplasia at the edges of the lesion and pigment migration from the degenerated pigment epithelium into the sensory retina.

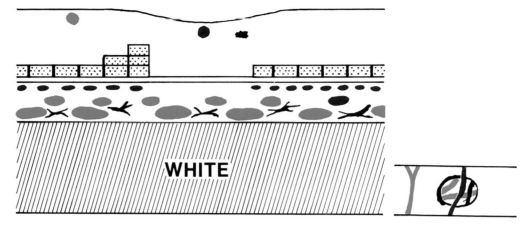

Histopathology

The pathology appears to result from the closure of small areas of the choriocapillaris, which produces subsequent atrophy of the overlying pigment epithelium and outer layers of the sensory retina (Figure 3-50). There is loss of photoreceptors and the external limiting membrane. All these retinal layers are nourished by the choriocapillaris. The inner layers of the retina are essentially intact because the retinal circulation supplies these layers. Thus, there is a clear windowlike view of the choroid and sclera through the intact inner retinal layers. The inner surface of these lesions is slightly depressed as a result of tissue loss in the choroid and retina, but this depression is not detectable on routine ophthalmoscopy. The pigmented borders and septa are the result of the proliferation of pigment epithelial cells at the edges of the lesions. Other pigmented areas may be the result of pigment migration from the degenerated pigment epithelial cells that were within the boundaries of the chorioretinal atrophy. The remaining inner retinal layers become tightly adherent to the basal lamina (Bruch's membrane), which may show damage in its inner layers. Histopathologically, the areas of chorioretinal atrophy look similar to the scars produced by retinal cryopexy.[9]

Clinical Significance

Because the inner retinal layers are spared in the degenerative process, there are no breaks through which fluid can penetrate into the subretinal region to produce a retinal detachment. Therefore, these lesions do not predispose to retinal detachment. If a retinal detachment involves an area of chorioretinal atrophy, however, the tight adherence to the basal lamina may produce an additional tear in the retina at the edge of the lesion. These breaks are often small and irregular in shape, and close examination may be necessary to detect them. Sometimes, small round chorioretinal atrophy lesions are mistaken for retinal holes because they are round with sharp margins (Table 3-6). This is especially true if a choroidal vessel is immediately beneath the lesion and gives it a

Table 3-6. Chorioretinal Atrophy vs. Retinal Hole

Chorioretinal Atrophy	Retinal Hole
Flat	Edges may be raised and an elevated surrounding retinal detachment may be present
⅛ disc diameter to greater than 1 disc diameter	Usually ⅛ disc diameter to almost 1 disc diameter
White to yellow white with a "window view" of the large or medium size choroidal vessel directly underneath	Choroid and sclera but sometimes red when seen through a small lesion in attached retina
Distinct margins	Distinct margins
Round to oval to scalloped	Usually round but sometimes oval
No white surrounding collar	No white surrounding collar
Scotoma consistent with the size of the lesion is found posteriorly	Generally too small to produce a scotoma unless it is a large break or surrounded by a detachment and is located posteriorly
Generally located close to ora serrata but occasionally found in the posterior region	Most often found between the equator and the posterior margin of the vitreous base

red color, as is found in a retinal hole. Occasionally, an advancing retinal detachment has been halted along a line of paving-stone degeneration.[9]

References

1. O'Malley PF, Allen RA, et al. Paving-stone degeneration of the retina. Arch Ophthalmol 1965;73:169–182.
2. Straatsma BR, Foos RY, et al. Degenerative Diseases of the Peripheral Retina. In TD Duane, EA Jaeger (eds), Clinical Ophthalmology. Vol. 3. Philadelphia: Harper & Row, 1980;26:13–15.
3. Pierro L, Camesasca FI, et al. Peripheral retinal changes and axial myopia. Retina 1992;12:12–17.
4. Rutnin U, Schepens CL. Fundus appearance in normal eyes. II. The standard peripheral fundus and developmental variations. Am J Ophthalmol 1967;64:840–852.
5. Karlin BD, Curtin BJ. Peripheral chorioretinal lesions and axial length of the myopic eye. Am J Ophthalmol 1976;81:625–635.
6. Yanoff M, Fine BS. Ocular Pathology: A Text and Atlas (2nd ed). Philadelphia: Harper & Row, 1982:513.
7. Rutnin U, Schepens CL. Fundus appearance in normal eyes. III. Peripheral degenerations. Am J Ophthalmol 1967;64:1040–1062.
8. Brown GC, Shields JA. Choroidal melanomas and paving stone degeneration. Ann Ophthalmol 1983;15:705–708.
9. Folberg R, Bernardino VB Jr. Pathologic Correlates in Ophthalmoscopy. In TD Duane, EA Jaeger (eds), Clinical Ophthalmology. Vol. 3. Philadelphia: Harper & Row, 1980;26:8–10.

White-with-Pressure and White-Without-Pressure

Clinical Description

White-with-pressure is an optical phenomenon in which the fundus changes from its usually orange-red color to a translucent white or grayish-white on scleral depression (Figure 3-51). White-without-pressure, first described by Charles Schepens[1] in 1952, has the same appearance without the physical application of scleral indention (Figure 3-52; see also Figure 2-4); however, scleral depression can enhance the whitish appearance and better delineate the borders of the lesion. This condition can occur in a small isolated area or be seen as a circumferential band that travels the entire perimeter of the retina. The circumferential band can have smooth or scalloped margins. The area of white-with- or -without-pressure can be migratory in nature, and therefore its shape can be different on subsequent examinations.[2] The posterior margin tends to be very sharp, and the anterior margin gently fades into the peripheral retina. It is not unusual to see just posterior to an area of white-without-pressure a small zone where the retina appears to be darker red (Figure 3-53) and gives the false impression of a linear retinal tear. The etiology of this dark zone is presumed to be the same as that of white-without-pressure. This condition is generally found from the ora serrata to approximately three disc diameters posteriorly; however, it can occur as far posterior as the equator and, rarely, as far as the temporal arcades.

White-with- or -without-pressure is presumed to be an optical phenomenon associated with the vitreoretinal interface. It is believed that continued mild vitreal traction is responsible for changes in the transparency of this interface. These areas of vit-

reoretinal adhesion may be portions of the vitreous base that are located further posterior than usual. The whitish appearance may be due to collagenic formations in the peripheral retina or to the way that the ophthalmoscope light reflects off tangential bundles of dense vitreous collagen.[3, 4] There have been reports in the literature of mild retinal degeneration with loss of retinal transparency found in an area of white-without-pressure.[5] These degenerative findings may be the result of this condition occurring over prolonged periods. Loss of transparency may be fairly mild initially and may only be detected on scleral depression.

Vitreous changes that may be associated with this condition are a posterior vitreous detachment with collapse or extensive liquefaction of the middle and posterior vitreous body (see Chapter 4). In either case, tractional forces are produced on the peripheral retina with subsequent degeneration.

White-with- or -without-pressure is found to some extent in more than 30% of normal eyes, with a strong tendency toward bilaterality. Individuals under 20 years of age have only a 5% occurrence, whereas those over 70 years of age have approximately a 66% frequency.[6] A study of myopes found a prevalence of 0% in myopic eyes with the shortest axial length and 54% in eyes with axial lengths greater than 33 mm.[7] In patients of all ages, it is most frequently found in myopic patients at 22.8%.[8] In the elderly, it is probably related to the increased vitreous degeneration.[9] White-without-pressure has also been reported to occur more frequently in African-Americans,[9] but this may be due to the increased contrast of this phenomenon against a dark fundus background. It generally occurs in the

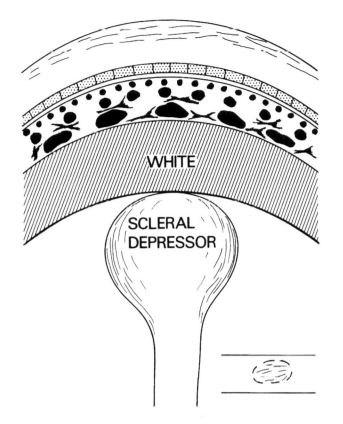

FIGURE 3-51
White-with-pressure is produced by pushing an area of mild retinal degeneration into the vitreous cavity with a scleral depressor.

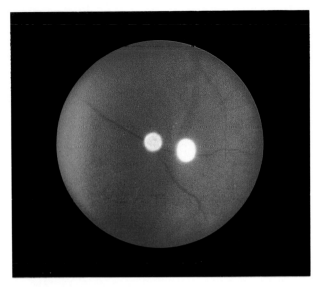

FIGURE 3-52
An area of white-without-pressure can be seen as a whitish patch peripheral in the fundus with a sharp demarcation line. The area is the temporal fundus as seen through the indirect condensing lens.

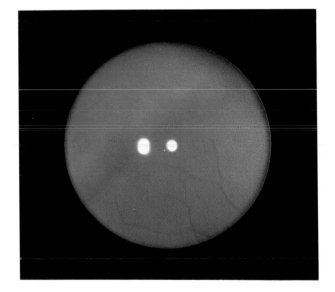

FIGURE 3-53
A small band of darker red retina is seen immediately posterior to an area of white without pressure. The area is the nasal fundus through the indirect condensing lens.

superior or temporal regions of the fundus, and it is not uncommon to see this condition on the posterior edge of lattice degeneration (Figure 3-54) and on the edge of a posterior staphyloma.

White-with- or -without-pressure can have an island of normal-appearing retina within its borders (Figure 3-55). This is sometimes mistaken for a retinal tear (pseudo–retinal tear) surrounded by a retinal detachment (Table 3-7). It can be differentiated from a true retinal break and detachment with the use of scleral depression, a three-mirror contact lens, or a 90-diopter precorneal lens examination. With this procedure, the observer can see the absence of retinal elevation or torn edges of the suspected tear.

The phenomenon of white-with-pressure can be used to enhance the detection of retinal degeneration (with or without retinal breaks) during scleral depression. Degeneration of the sensory retina almost always produces a whitish discoloration, and scleral depression can enhance this whitish appearance. Sometimes in very mild cases of degeneration it does not appear whitish until the sclera is depressed. When a retinal break is not very

evident on ophthalmoscopy, its appearance can be enhanced with scleral depression. Retinal breaks tend to be located in areas of retinal degeneration and, if the degeneration is mild, white-with-pres-

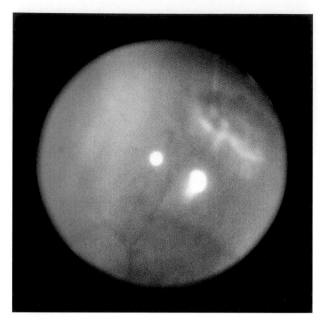

FIGURE 3-54
(*From top to bottom*) Lattice degeneration with a break along the anterior border, white-without-pressure, and normal peripheral retina. The view is through the indirect condensing lens and shows the superior retina.

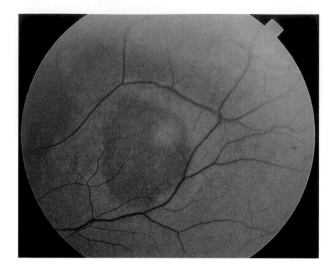

FIGURE 3-55
An island of normal-appearing retina is surrounded by white-without-pressure, which is known as a pseudo–retinal break. Small, round, whitish area in the center of the figure is an artifact.

sure may help locate such areas during scleral depression (Figure 3-56). Scleral depression is recommended in areas of the fundus where vitreous floaters are found, to determine whether they originated from a barely visible retinal break. A pseudo-white-with-pressure can be seen in infants or in persons with darkly pigmented fundi; it has a watered-silk appearance.

Sometimes white-without-pressure is confused with a retinoschisis or a retinal detachment because of the broad area of involvement, whitish appearance, and mild loss of choroidal detail. In consider-

ing the differential diagnosis of a retinoschisis, this confusion can be corrected by noting that the suspicious area is not elevated (with or without scleral depression). Regarding a retinal detachment, white-without-pressure does not have retinal folds, does not undulate on eye movement, and is not elevated on scleral depression. Another important clue to differentiate the phenomenon from either a retinoschisis or retinal detachment is that the posterior margin of white-without-pressure is concave in relation to the posterior pole and that a retinoschisis or detachment is almost always convex in relation to the posterior pole due to expansion of the detachment or retinoschisis from the periphery (Table 3-8).

Table 3-7. Pseudo–Retinal Break vs. Retinal Break

Pseudo–Retinal Break	Retinal Break
Flat (even on depression)	Edges may be raised and an elevated surrounding retinal detachment may be present
Irregular margins	Margins are usually smooth and regularly shaped but may sometimes be tattered
Area of darker color than the surrounding fundus	Red when seen in attached retina
Often in an area of white-without-pressure	White-without-pressure is not commonly associated with retinal breaks
Generally not perfectly round or horseshoe shaped	Generally round or horseshoe shaped

Histopathology

White-with- or -without-pressure gives a thinned and atrophic appearance to the retina (Figure 3-57). In one histologic study, the inner limiting membrane was disrupted or absent, the neural elements were disorganized, and the pigment epithelium was disrupted with evidence of pigment proliferation and migration. There was also a layer of fluid between the pigment epithelium and the sensory retina.[5] Loss of retinal transparency may be due to the following retinal changes: fluid accumulation above the pigment epithelium, intraretinal edema, degenerated retinal tissue, or fibrous condensation of the vitreous cortex.[10] Vitreous strands are seen attached to the areas displaying this condition.

Clinical Significance

White-with- or -without-pressure is accompanied by a high frequency of extensive vitreous degeneration and posterior vitreous detachment, and the clinician should be aware of such changes in these patients. It generally does not require treatment because its propensity to produce a retinal break is not great.[11] This condition should be followed on a periodic basis because it has been associated with both horseshoe tears and giant retinal tears at its posterior margin.[4] These tears seem to occur more frequently if the posterior margin of the area is irregular and scalloped or if there is extensive vitreous degeneration and traction in the involved area. In eyes in which an area of white-with- or -without-pressure seems to be at

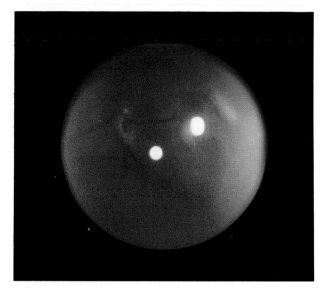

FIGURE 3-56
Scleral depression of the retinal break demonstrates the white-with-pressure phenomenon, which is seen as a white halo around the hole. View is through the indirect condensing lens.

great risk of developing a retinal break, prophylactic treatment with photocoagulation or cryoapplication may be used.

Because white-without-pressure is seldom associated with a retinal tear or detachment, the prognosis is good. Follow-up examinations should be performed every 1–2 years. The patient should be advised of the symptoms of a retinal tear or detachment and told to return immediately for a dilated retinal examination if any of the symptoms occur.

Table 3-8. White-Without-Pressure vs. Retinal Detachment

White-Without-Pressure	Retinal Detachment
Flat (even on depression)	Slightly elevated to bullous, which may be enhanced on scleral depression
White	Recent detachments are white
Usually fairly distinct margins	Often indistinct margins in fresh cases and distinct in long-standing cases
Margins are frequently irregular	Margins are generally smooth and curvilinear
No retinal folds	Retinal folds
No undulation on eye movements	Recent detachments undulate on eye movements
Occasionally retinal breaks may be present	Generally have retinal breaks present
Shape is almost always concave or rather straight to the posterior pole	Shape is almost always convex to the posterior pole
Often mildly obscure underlying choroidal detail	Obscure underlying choroidal detail
No visual field loss	Relative scotoma with sloping margins
No elevation on ultrasonography	Slight to bullous elevation on ultrasonography

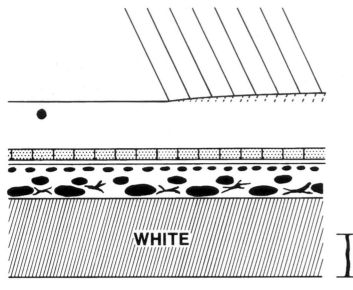

WHITE

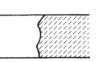

FIGURE 3-57
White-without-pressure. Vitreous traction has produced an optical disturbance and mild superficial retinal degeneration at the vitreo-retinal interface.

References

1. Schepens CL. Subclinical retinal detachments. Arch Ophthalmol 1952;47:593–606.
2. Nagpal KC, Huamonte F, et al. Migratory white-without-pressure retinal lesions. Arch Ophthalmol 1976;94:576–579.
3. Daicker B. Sind die symptome "Weiss mit Druck" und "Weiss ohne Druck" durch die peripherie netzshaut-sklerose bedingt? Mod Probl Ophthalmol 1975;15:82–90.
4. Green WR. Vitreoretinal juncture. In SJ Ryan (ed), Retinal Disease. St. Louis: Mosby, 1989:13–69.
5. Watzke RC. The ophthalmoscopic sign "white with pressure": a clinicopathic correlation. Arch Ophthalmol 1961;65:812–823.
6. Schepens CL. Retinal Detachment and Allied Diseases. Philadelphia: Saunders, 1983:156–158.
7. Karlin BD, Curtin BJ. Peripheral chorioretinal lesions and axial length of the myopic eye. Am J Ophthalmol 1976;81:625–635.
8. Pierro I, Camesaca FI, et al. Peripheral retinal changes and axial myopia. Retina 1992;12:12–17.
9. Folberg R, Bernardina VB Jr. Pathologic Correlates in Ophthalmoscopy. In TD Duane, EA Jaeger (eds), Clinical Ophthalmology, Vol. 3. Philadelphia: Harper & Row, 1985;7:1–25.
10. Tolentino FI, Schepens CL, et al. Vitreoretinal Disorders: Diagnosis and Management. Philadelphia: Saunders; 1976:339.
11. Byer NE. The Peripheral Retina in Profile: A Stereoscopic Atlas. Torrance, CA: Criterion Press, 1982.

Peripheral Cystoid Degeneration

Clinical Description

Peripheral cystoid degeneration appears as translucent grayish or red dots in an area with grayish white margins. It is composed of a band of intraretinal cystoid cavities that are usually found about one-half a disc diameter from the ora serrata (see Figures 2-4 and 3-1), but they can extend as far posteriorly as the equator. The involved retina has up to three times its normal thickness. The surface of the retina has small white depressions that are the ends of the pillars between the intervening round domes, which are the inner walls of the cystoid spaces. During ophthalmoscopy, peripheral cystoid degeneration has a rather honeycomb appearance, which is more obvious on scleral depression. Scleral depression also makes the area whiter. The cystoid spaces appear reddish due to the increased visibility of the choroidal reflex during ophthalmoscopy.[1] Dentate processes are commonly involved in cystoid degeneration. With age, the involved area often becomes whitish.

Peripheral cystoid degeneration occurs more frequently in the temporal half of the retina than in the nasal half, and more frequently in the superior than the inferior half.[2–4] It seems to begin next to the ora serrata and slowly spreads posteriorly. There can be changes in the vitreous above cystoid degeneration consisting of vitreous strands and grayish opacities that sometimes resemble snowflakes.

There are two types of peripheral cystoid degeneration, typical and reticular. Typical cystoid degeneration appears as dark reddish dots caused by the retinal thinning in the cystoid spaces, which may coalesce to form interlacing tunnels (Figure 3-58). The intraretinal pillars and intervening domes (the cystoid spaces) cause retinal depression stippling.[5] This condition starts at the ora serrata, particularly at the base of dentate processes, and extends both circumferentially and posteriorly.[6] This form occurs bilaterally, is seen in all patients more than 8 years old, and increases with age.[3] It has been found in infants as young as 1 year of age. One theory posits that peripheral cystoid degeneration is caused by the traction and movement of the ora serrata during accommodation.[7]

Reticular cystoid degeneration appears as a finely stippled surface with a linear reticular pattern that corresponds to sclerotic retinal vessels. The involved areas may be single or multiple, are irregularly shaped, and have sharp angular margins. The posterior limit of these patches is often marked by retinal blood vessels.[8] Reticular cystoid degeneration is located posterior to and continuous with typical cystoid degeneration. Spaces develop in the nerve fiber layer that are divided by delicate retinal pillars.[6] Reticular peripheral cystoid degeneration is most easily seen with a biomicroscope using a contact lens or a precorneal lens.

Reticular cystoid degeneration is found in 18% of the adult population and is bilateral in 41% of the patients, and thus is seen in 13% of all adult eyes.[6] This condition occurs in persons in every decade of life and does not seem to be related to the aging process of the peripheral retina.

Histopathology

Typical cystoid degeneration begins as cystoid spaces in the outer plexiform and adjacent nuclear layers of the retina (Figures 3-59 and 3-60).[9] With time, these cavities can extend from the inner to the outer limiting membrane. Cystoid cavities are separated by pillars composed of compressed Müller cells and photoreceptor axons. The cavities contain hyaluronic acid, which may represent degenerative neural tissue. The pillars may break, thus producing larger cystoid cavities, and a massive rupturing of these pillars may be the mechanism by which a retinoschisis forms. Peripheral cystoid degeneration always occurs anterior to retinoschises. The pigment epithelium under cystoid degeneration does not show signs of involvement.[10]

Reticular cystoid degeneration begins as small cystoid spaces in the nerve fiber layer of the retina.

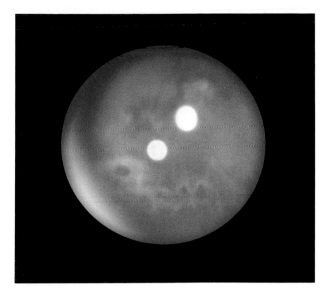

FIGURE 3-58
Peripheral cystoid degeneration has produced a red retinal hole with a small, localized surrounding retinal detachment, as seen through the indirect condensing lens during scleral depression. The whitish lesion above the hole is a cryopexy scar from a previously treated retinal hole.

With time, these cavities can extend from the inner limiting membrane to the outer plexiform layer. These smaller cystoid spaces in the inner layers of the retina are responsible for the finely stippled surface. These cavities are also filled with hyaluronic acid.[11]

Clinical Significance

Retinal holes can develop in peripheral cystoid degeneration, usually as the result of a rupture of the inner wall of a cystoid cavity (see Figure 3-58). The inner wall of the cavity is thinner than the outer wall, making it more susceptible to rupturing. The outer wall usually remains intact, and thus liquefied vitreous is able to fill only the cavity itself. Therefore, retinal holes in cystoid degeneration generally do not require treatment because they usually do not produce a retinal detachment. If there is a rupture in both the outer and inner walls of the cystoid cavity, a retinal detachment can occur. There have been a few reports of a retinal detachment caused by a hole in cystoid degeneration.

The other clinically significant aspect of peripheral cystoid degeneration is its possible implication in the formation of a retinoschisis (see Retinoschisis). Peripheral cystoid degeneration should be noted on the patient's chart and re-examined periodically.

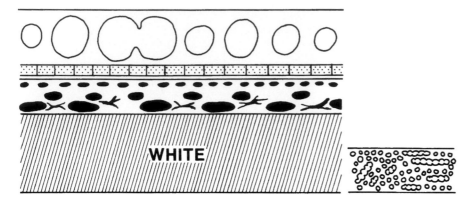

FIGURE 3-59
Peripheral cystoid degeneration. The cystoid process starts in the inner retinal layers and enlarges circumferentially. The pillars between the cystoid spaces may break.

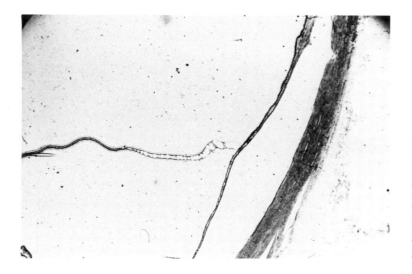

FIGURE 3-60
Histology section shows peripheral cystoid degeneration in an artifactually separated retina. The peripheral cystoid spaces are large, and many of the interseptal pillars have broken, which may be the mechanism in the formation of a retinoschisis. The remnants of the pillars can be seen on the inner and outer walls; those on the inner wall may be responsible for the snowflakes on a retinoschisis. The inner and outer retinal walls become thin as degeneration progresses.

References

1. Hines JL, Jones WL. Peripheral microcystoid retinal degeneration and retinoschisis. J Am Optom Assoc 1982;53:541–545.
2. Straatsma BR, Foos RY. Typical and reticular degenerative retinoschisis. Am J Ophthalmol 1973;75:551–575.
3. O'Malley PF, Allen RA. Peripheral cystoid degeneration of the retina: incidence and distribution in 1,000 autopsy eyes. Arch Ophthalmol 1967;77:769–776.
4. Foos RY, Spencer LM, et al. Tropic Degeneration of the Retina. In New Orleans Academy of Ophthalmology: Symposium on Retina and Retina Surgery. St. Louis: Mosby, 1969.
5. Rutnin U, Schepens CL. Fundus appearance in normal eyes. III. Peripheral degenerations. Am J Ophthalmol 1967;64:1040–1062.
6. Glasgow BJ, Foos RY, et al. Degenerative Diseases of the Peripheral Retina. In TD Duane, EA Jaeger (eds), Clinical Ophthalmology, Vol. 3. Philadelphia: Harper & Row, 1993;26:1–29.
7. Teng CC, Katzen HM. An anatomic study of the periphery of the retina. II. Peripheral cystoid degeneration of the retina: Formation of cysts and holes. Am J Ophthalmol 1953;36:29–39.
8. Foos RY, Freeman SS. Reticular cystoid degeneration of the peripheral retina. Am J Ophthalmol 1973;69:392–403.
9. Gottinger W. Senile Retinoschisis. Stuttgart, Germany: Georg Thieme, 1978.
10. Foos RY. Senile retinoschisis: Relationship to cystoid degeneration. Trans Am Acad Ophthalmol Otolaryngol 1970;74:33–51.
11. Yanoff M, Fine BS. Ocular Pathology: A Text and Atlas (2nd ed). Philadelphia: Harper & Row, 1982:504–505.

Retinoschisis

Clinical Description

Retinoschisis was first reported by Bartels and given the name retinoschisis by Wilczek in the 1800s.[1-3] "Cystoid degeneration of the retina," "retinocoele," and "retinal cyst" are terms formerly used to describe this entity.[4, 5] Retinoschisis results from the splitting of the sensory retina into two layers, which often results in an elevated bullous lesion (like a blister of the retina). Therefore, it has been defined as a splitting of the retina that is large enough to be a clinically visible cavity.[6] Histopathologically, it is defined as an intraretinal cavity that is at least 2 mm (1.3 disc diameters) in size.[7] It may be congenital or acquired, and although the physical appearance is essentially the same, the pathogenesis of the two forms is different.

Retinoschises due to heredity and degeneration are a primary pathologic entity and therefore are found in 100% of these patients. The secondary forms, however, are very uncommon and are associated with various pathologic entities, such as vitreoretinal traction, cystic degeneration, intraretinal hemorrhage, exudation, and inflammation. The secondary retinoschises produced by vitreoretinal traction include proliferative diabetic retinopathy, retinopathy of prematurity, and sickle-cell retinopathy.[8,9] Other entities causing cystic spaces that may coalesce into a retinoschisis cavity are malignant melanoma, choroidal hemangioma, and combined hamartoma of the retinal and pigment epithelium.[10, 11] Massive intraretinal hemorrhaging can physically split the retina in a retinoschisis; this can be found in such conditions as battered baby syndrome, neonatal hemorrhage, central retinal vein occlusion, aplastic anemia, and blunt trauma.[10, 12, 13] Massive exudation can also cause a splitting of the retina, which may be seen in Coat's disease.[10] Inflammatory conditions rarely produce a retinoschisis and have been reported in cases of pars planitis, chronic iridocyclitis, and uveitis.[10, 14]

Acquired retinoschisis, also known as adult or senile degenerative retinoschisis, is a separation of the sensory retina at the outer plexiform and inner nuclear layers. Acquired degenerative retinoschisis is divided into typical or reticular forms, depending on the histologic response. The typical degenerative form has a flat appearance, and the reticular form shows obvious elevation.[4] It is most often found in the temporal half of the fundus, especially the infe-rior temporal region (70%), and about 25% in the superior temporal quadrant[15-18]; however, it may not have a greater frequency for either quadrant.[19] Typical degenerative retinoschisis is seen clinically as a round or oval splitting of the sensory retina. In typical cases, the retinal vessels are located in the outer layer, which has a moderately irregular appearance. The typical degenerative retinoschises are bilateral and fairly symmetric in about 33–80% of adult patients[17, 18, 20]; therefore, the discovery of a retinoschisis in one eye may be accompanied by the finding of one in the fellow eye. One of the clinical clues to differentiate it from a retinal detachment is that a detachment is usually unilateral and a retinoschisis is usually bilateral. When examining the fellow eye for a possible retinoschisis, it is wise to perform scleral depression in the temporal region because a shallow retinoschisis may not be easily seen without depression. Typical degenerative retinoschisis is seen in about 1–4% of persons, and because they are bilateral 33% of the time, they are seen in 0.7% of adult eyes.[15, 20] An autopsy study of eyes with no history of disease found that nearly 1% had senile retinoschisis with outer layer breaks.[21] It is commonly found in those 38 years of age or older and is rare under the age of 20 years.[4, 18, 22] Retinoschisis seems to occur more frequently in females and more often in hyperopes.[23] The typical form is only rarely associated with breaks in either layer, which do not extend posteriorly to threaten the macula, therefore, treatment is usually not indicated.

Reticular retinoschisis has a more bullous architecture and is associated with a prominent reticular cystoid degeneration. Reticular form appears round or oval and displays an extremely thin and pitted outer layer. The degenerative changes in the reticular form are more advanced than that found in the typical form. The retinal vessels on the surface of the inner layer give the lesion the reticular appearance when seen with magnification. Round or oval breaks are often found in the outer layer; these may be single or multiple, usually large, and having rolled edges. Breaks are more likely to be found near the posterior or anterior margins of the lesion. Reticular degenerative retinoschises are found in 1.6% of adult patients, are bilateral in 15% of these cases, and therefore are seen in 0.95% of adult eyes.[20]

Advanced retinoschisis is found in approximately 7% of persons over 40 years of age.[24] The condition tends to be bilateral (82.1%)[18] and sym-

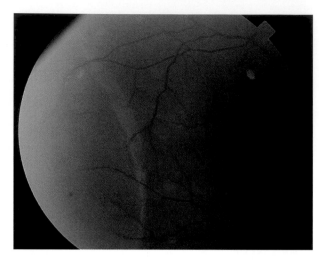

FIGURE 3-61
Bullous retinoschisis of the inferior temporal fundus. Blood vessels travel upward in the inner layer of the schisis; note the slightly pigmented demarcation line. The macula can be seen nasal to the retinoschisis.

metric. It usually is not thought to be inherited, but some authors believe that advanced retinoschisis may be transmitted by an autosomal recessive or incomplete dominant trait.[25]

Retinoschisis is typically seen as an elevated bullous lesion in the peripheral fundus (Figure 3-61; see also Figures 3-1 and 3-70A). A retinoschisis has a smooth, taut surface that does not undulate on eye movements, as commonly occurs with retinal detachments (Table 3-9). On scleral depression, the roll can be seen to move right under the inner layer, and it appears to fill most of the retinoschisis cavity. As the scleral roll fills the retinoschisis cavity, the inner layer appears to be stretched, resembling the stretched upper surface of a balloon after pressure of a hand on the bottom of the balloon. The retinoschisis does not enlarge or form breaks during depression but remains taut and smooth. In contrast, the depression of a fresh retinal detachment causes it to move and change shape easily.

Some retinoschises are shallow and share the characteristics of shallow retinal detachments, including loss of underlying choroidal detail, greater difficulty of visualization during ophthalmoscopy, and the casting of a shadow of a vessel in the inner layer onto the underlying outer layer and choroid. The loss of choroidal detail is probably the most effective means of detecting a shallow retinoschisis (Figure 3-62). Ultrasonography is also effective in determining the existence of a shallow retinoschisis (Figure 3-63). Frequently, retinoschises localized in the posterior retina are shallower. A

shallow retinoschisis has a particularly interesting appearance on scleral depression due to placing the inner and outer layers on a cross-sectional view. Scleral depression allows for a side-section view of the inner layer and the underlying cavity, giving the appearance of a "fog bank" over the roll (Figure 3-64). This phenomenon is also seen on depression of a shallow retinal detachment.

The inner layer of the retinoschisis is very thin and can be essentially transparent to fairly translucent during ophthalmoscopy. The outer layer covers the choroid with a faint haze, but otherwise it does not show any particular difference from the general fundus appearance. Because the inner layer is very thin, ultrasonography displays a very attenuated membrane in the vitreous cavity (Figure 3-65). A fresh retinal detachment is thicker than a retinoschisis and therefore is more prominent on ultrasonography. This is demonstrated both by the prominence of the tissue layer in the vitreous cavity during B-scan and by the height of the A-scan peak of the tissue during ultrasonography. Therefore, the prominence or echo signal height during ultrasonography can be used to differentiate between a retinoschisis and a fresh retinal detachment. Many times the detection of a retinoschisis depends on the observation of blood vessels traversing upward into the vitreous cavity in the inner layer of the lesion (see Figures 3-61 and 3-70A).[26] Sometimes, retinal vessels can be found in the outer layer of the retinoschisis, and they may be stretched between the two layers. Such a vessel may rupture and fill the retinoschisis cavity with a layered hemorrhage.[24] Frequently, occluded, white, sclerotic vessels are present in the inner layer, which helps to differentiate a retinoschisis from a detachment. White sclerotic vessels are not frequently found on a fresh retinal detachment but can be found on a long-standing detachment.

Tiny snowflakes can be present on the surface of 70% of lesions.[18] They are either the result of condensation of the vitreous onto the inner layer, remnants of glial pillars attached to the inner wall, or the footplates of Müller cells (Figure 3-66).[27] Snowflakes are usually found on the posterior portion of the retinoschisis, on or just internal to the inner layer. Sometimes a retinoschisis is detected only after the discovery of snowflakes that seem to be floating in the vitreous over the peripheral retina.

Both the inner and outer layers of a retinoschisis may have a honeycomb or beaten-metal appearance, especially when viewed with a three-mirror contact lens or with a precorneal fundus lens during biomicroscopy. It is much more common to see this

Table 3-9. Retinoschisis vs. Retinal Detachment

Retinoschisis	Retinal Detachment
Usually bullous but may be shallow	Usually bullous but may be shallow
Usually very transparent	Whitish in recent detachments but may become semitransparent in long-standing detachments
Sharp margins that may be difficult to detect	Margins are often indistinct and even more difficult to determine in shallow detachments
Usually semicircular with the base at the ora serrata	Large peripheral detachments involving a quadrant are usually semicircular, with the base toward the ora serrata; larger ones can have many semicircular bullous areas, but small localized detachments around breaks are almost always circular
Surface is generally smooth and taut (looks like a retinal blister)	Surface can have many tiny folds and some large folds
No movement on eye movements	Undulations of the detached retina on eye movements; however, usually long-standing detachments do not move
Inner- and outer-layer breaks may be present and look atrophic	Retinal breaks are usually present
Some loss of underlying choroidal detail	Usually greater loss of underlying choroidal detail
Rarely demonstrate a pigmented demarcation line, which is often thin and discontinuous (broken line)	Pigmented demarcation lines are more frequently present in long-standing cases
Enlarge very slowly	May enlarge slowly (faster than a retinoschisis) or quickly, in just a few days
Tiny, snowflakelike deposits may be found on the surface of the inner layer	Surface may have pigmented spots, small hemorrhages, and whitish subretinal precipitates
White sclerotic vessels may be seen in the inner layer	On recent detachments the vessels are usually not sclerotic unless associated with lattice degeneration; however, long-standing detachments may have white sclerotic vessels
Argon laser photocoagulation often produces a white burn in the outer layer but this is not a reliable test for definitive diagnosis	Argon laser photocoagulation of the lesion usually does not produce a white burn spot
Infrequently invade within the posterior pole, especially within the temporal arcades	Often invade the posterior pole
Produce an absolute scotoma with sharp margins on visual fields if the advancing border progresses posterior to the equator	Produce a relative scotoma with sloping margins
Generally are symptomatic unless they encroach on the temporal arcades or produce a vitreous bleed	Often are symptomatic with symptoms of photopsia, sudden onset of tiny black floaters, curtain or veil encroaching on visual field, and loss of central visual acuity; however, detachments may be present before symptoms occur
Remains taut and smooth during scleral depression	Easily moves and changes shape with or without scleral depression, unless it is long-standing, then it remains fairly stable
Thin inner layer produces a reduced acoustic signal height on ultrasonography	Obvious vitreous membrane with folds and significant acoustic height (greater than retinoschisis) seen on ultrasonography
Generally not treated unless there is encroachment on the temporal arcades or if both inner- and outer-layer breaks present	Generally treated unless the detachment is small and deemed by the examiner not to be a significant threat to the patient's vision

in the inner layer, and it signifies long-standing retinal degeneration. This honeycomb appearance can also be detected in long-standing retinal detachments. Long-standing retinal detachments can be mistaken as a retinoschisis due to the honeycomb appearance, thinning, and increased transparency of such lesions that is the result of atrophy of the detached tissue.

Rarely, pigmented or white demarcation lines occur along the posterior margin of a retinoschisis (see Figure 3-1); however, such lines are much more frequently associated with retinal detachments. Pigmented demarcation lines have been seen associated with outer layer breaks and secondary retinal detachments in retinoschises.[28] Multiple pigmented demarcation lines in the inner layer from a slowly advancing retinoschisis are very uncommon (see the section on Demarcation Lines).

Sometimes a small retinal hemorrhage can be found at the posterior margin of a retinoschisis; it is

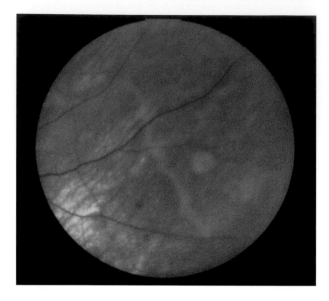

FIGURE 3-62
A large, shallow retinoschisis is seen in the temporal, midperipheral retina. Note the serrated posterior margin, the loss of choroidal detail underneath the lesion, and the smooth, taut surface.

probably the result of the angulation (kinking) on the retinal vessels as they travel up onto the inner layer or it may be secondary to vitreous traction. The hemorrhaging can be so extensive as to fill the vitreous cavity. A rare finding is a number of small retinal hemorrhages found on the inner layer next to blood vessels. There has been a report of blood-filled retinoschises in the macula and elsewhere in battered babies.[12]

Peripheral cystoid degeneration is always found between the anterior edge of the retinoschisis and the ora serrata. The pathogenesis of a retinoschisis seems to be associated closely with cystoid degeneration. The pillars between the cystoid spaces break with progressive degeneration (see Figure 3-60), and a massive coalescence of these spaces is what some authorities believe causes a retinoschisis. It can be very difficult to determine clinically where peripheral cystoid degeneration stops and retinoschisis begins.

For the inexperienced clinician, a retinoschisis can be difficult to differentiate from white-without-pressure in the peripheral retina (see White-Without-Pressure earlier in this chapter). Both conditions obscure underlying choroid detail (retinoschisis

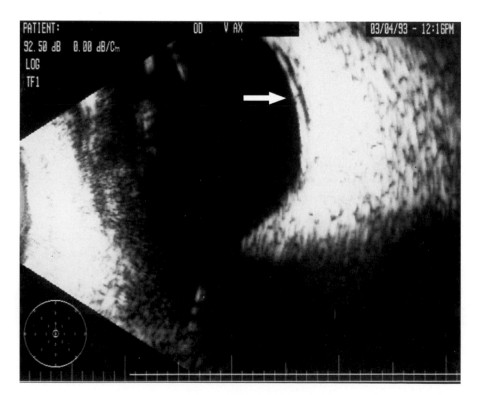

FIGURE 3-63
B-scan of shallow retinoschisis. The inner layer has almost the same curvature as the inner eye wall (*arrow*), which makes the condition difficult to detect during ophthalmoscopy. The fluid layer underneath causes some blurring of underlying choroidal detail.

more so), and both tend to have a whitish appearance (retinoschisis less so). The obscuration of choroidal detail by a retinoschisis is the result of fluid accumulating between the sensory retina and the underlying choroid, and the more fluid that accumulates, the more obscured the choroidal detail becomes. Obscuring of choroidal detail due to fluid accumulation is also found in retinal detachments for the same physiologic reasons. The white-with-out-pressure can slightly haze choroidal detail due to the loss of transparency of the inner retinal layers in this condition. The distinguishing characteristic is the posterior margin, which in a retinoschisis is almost always curved away (convex) from the posterior pole and in white-without-pressure is almost always curved toward (concave) to the posterior pole. The other way to differentiate the two is to perform scleral depression: A retinoschisis is elevated off the roll (a shallow retinoschisis may show the fog bank phenomenon) (see Figure 3-64), and white-without-pressure does not appear elevated on the scleral roll.

Vitreous degeneration is almost always found in association with acquired retinoschisis. It consists of liquefaction of the vitreous gel and PVD, which occurs in 60–85% of cases.[22, 29] The vitreous cortex usually remains attached to the inner layer of the retinoschisis after a PVD. The vitreous gel next to the retinoschisis often displays prominent, taut fibers, some of which are attached to the inner layer of the retinoschisis and appear large and curled. This is one explanation for the clinical finding of snowflakes. The PVD and synchysis of the vitreous are frequent findings associated with retinoschisis, and the prominent fibrous structure of the vitreous gel opposite the retinoschisis cavity may be the source for tractional forces in the formation of retinoschisis.[23, 30] The liquefied vitreous gel becomes a potential source of fluid that enters breaks in the retinoschisis and may be involved in producing a retinal detachment. Breaks in the inner layer of the retinoschisis may be associated with a PVD, and a retinal detachment produced by breaks in the inner and outer layers is almost always associated with a PVD in the region of the inner-layer break.[31] Continued vitreous traction on the inner layer can cause tears, which may greatly enlarge with time and result in the collapse or semicollapse of the retinoschisis. Severe vitreous traction (such as occurs after a PVD) can tear the inner layer into shreds of thin transparent tissue that float in the vitreous cavity.

Most patients with an acquired retinoschisis are asymptomatic until the lesion is in an advanced

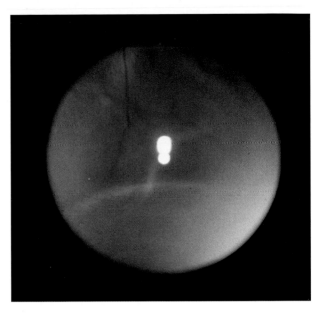

FIGURE 3-64
Shallow retinoschisis on scleral depression displaying a "fog bank" above the roll, which occurs when the split of the retina is on cross-section.

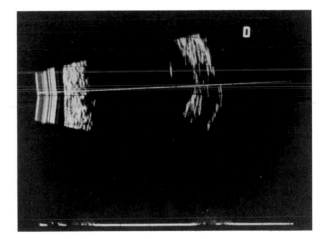

FIGURE 3-65
B-scan ultrasonogram of retinoschisis. Note the small sonic echo sent back by the thin inner layer of the schisis. The white striated area on the left is feedback noise from the eyelid and cornea to the transducer.

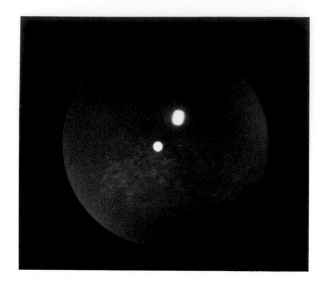

FIGURE 3-66
A very transparent retinoschisis with numerous snowflakes on the inner surface in the superior temporal fundus as seen through the indirect condensing lens.

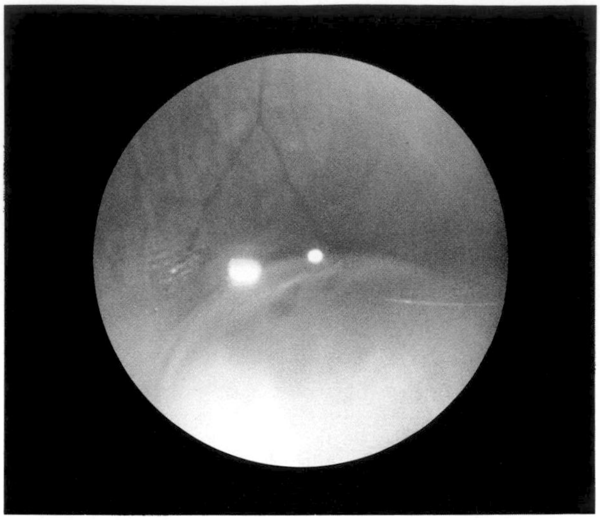

FIGURE 3-67
Inner-layer breaks are seen as clear or grayish defects on the raised retinoschisis during scleral depression. The view is through the indirect condensing lens.

stage. Possible symptoms are flashes and floaters, peripheral field defects, and decreased acuity. The flashes and floaters are the result of vitreous traction. Because the photoreceptors become physically separated from the inner retinal connections at the edge of the retinoschisis, the visual field defects are absolute, with sharp margins, and they progress with advancement of the retinoschisis. This compares to a relative and sloping visual field defect that is found with a retinal detachment. If a retinoschisis and a detachment are found together, then one visual field defect may be superimposed on the other. Often, no visual field defect is detected unless the retinoschisis is posterior to the equator (see Table 3-9).[15, 32]

A retinal detachment can also be differentiated from a retinoschisis by the use of argon laser photocoagulation. Because the energy of the laser beam is mainly absorbed by the pigment epithelium, this tissue and some overlying outer sensory retina suffer protein coagulation. Because the sensory retina no longer closely approximates the pigment epithelium in a retinal detachment, the initial burn spot is not very visible. However, a retinoschisis still has outer sensory retina next to the pigment epithelium, and therefore the laser beam may produce a more observable white spot. This test is not highly

reliable or consistent and therefore is not frequently performed.

More than 25% of the eyes with acquired retinoschisis demonstrate a break in at least one of the layers,[2, 3, 24] and on routine autopsy examinations of eyes with no history of ocular disease, nearly 1% had a retinoschisis with an outer-layer break.[21] There may be multiple breaks, but a single break is most commonly found in either layer. Most breaks are generally thought to be atrophic holes, but some inner-layer breaks are likely to be associated with vitreous traction. Because of the expansion of the inner layer during the formation of a bullous retinoschisis, a more accurate description would be a "stretch break" (Figure 3-67). They are usually found close to the margins of the retinoschisis, especially the posterior margin or in the most bullous region of the retinoschisis.[33] Breaks in the inner layer are seen as clear round or oval areas, and their presence is enhanced during scleral depression. Inner-layer breaks typically do not have rolled margins, and they may slowly enlarge with time due to increases in vitreous traction or physical stretching forces. The outer layer covers the choroid with a faint haze. Outer-layer breaks are typically single and many times larger than inner-layer breaks. They appear red to pinkish, and they may have rolled edges, which is probably due to the more elastic nature of the outer retinal layer (Figure 3-68; see also Figure 3-1). Outer-layer breaks are usually located next to the posterior margin of the lesion and are found in approximately 23% of eyes with retinoschisis.[34] The appearance of a group of these outer layer breaks, which usually is found close to the posterior margin, is sometimes called "frog's eggs."[22]

A traction retinoschisis occurs as the result of marked vitreous traction that pulls the sensory retina into two layers. Its clinical appearance is the same as that of the acquired form, except that large vitreous bands are attached to the inner layer of the retinoschisis. They advance very slowly or remain stationary. Traction retinoschises often occur in eyes that are afflicted with severe uveitis, proliferative diabetic retinopathy, recurrent vitreous hemorrhages, vitreous scarring secondary to trauma, and retrolental fibroplasia.

X-linked retinoschisis (also known as congenital retinoschisis, juvenile retinoschisis, juvenile idiopathic retinoschisis, and juvenile sex-linked retinoschisis) is transmitted as a sex-linked recessive trait and therefore is found exclusively in males,[35, 36] but some questionable exceptions have been reported.[37–39] Almost all eyes affected are hyperopic and show cystoid foveal changes.[27, 35, 36, 40, 41] In rare cases, it has occurred in females as an autosomal recessive disease.[34, 42] The condition is usually first discovered in young adults and children, but it may be present at birth.[15] Patients generally complain of seeing floaters, decreased vision, nystagmus, and strabismus. The strabismus and nystagmus are likely due to the macular changes.[40, 41] In the absence of vitreous hemorrhage, visual acuity may be 20/40 or better, but it often drops below 20/70, and tends to stabilize at 20/200 or worse.[24] The mean visual acuity ranges from about 20/60 to 20/80.[37, 43] In more than half of patients, visual acuity is worse than 20/70. Bilaterality is the rule, but the degree of involvement in the contralateral eye can vary. The vision may get progressively worse with age,[37] but in uncomplicated cases the vision may remain stable.[43–45]

X-linked retinoschisis is usually found in the inferior temporal quadrant, sometimes in two quadrants, and the inner layer is often very bullous.[27] The sensory retina splits in the nerve fiber layer, and the ballooning retinoschisis tends to be very transparent.[46,47] The congenital form does not extend to the ora serrata and is not associated with extensive cystoid degeneration of the retina. Peripheral retinoschises are found in approximately 50–60% of patients.[37, 43, 48, 43–50] Holes are frequently found in

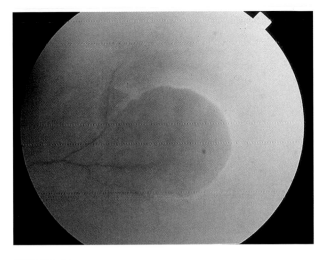

FIGURE 3-68
A large reddish outer-layer break with a surrounding localized retinal detachment can be seen in a retinoschisis. The view is through the indirect condensing lens.

the inner layer but they do not cause a retinal detachment. Holes in the outer layer can cause a retinal detachment, however, and in these cases the prognosis for successful reattachment is good.[27] White or pigmented demarcation lines are seen more frequently in congenital retinoschisis than in the acquired form. Other peripheral findings are vitreous veils (about 30% of cases),[37, 50–53] perivascular sheathing, dendriform patterns,[44] tepetal-like reflex,[40] retinal dragging,[54] subretinal exudates,[55] pigment lines,[42] and tessellated atrophy of the retina.[40, 41, 56, 57] Pigment demarcation lines may be left over from bullous retinoschises that have spontaneously reattached.[58, 59] Vitreous veils are likely the remnants of torn inner-layer membrane.[18, 60] Vascular changes are found in 35% of the eyes.[61]

The most serious complications of X-linked retinoschisis are vitreous hemorrhage and retinal detachment.[40–42, 57, 62, 63] Recurrent vitreous hemorrhages have been reported.[40, 41, 63–67] Vitreous hemorrhage occurs in about 21% of cases.[61] The hemorrhage probably results from vitreous traction on retinal vessels, and retinal vessels that traverse the inner-layer breaks may be at greater risk for hemorrhaging. Another very rare cause for vitreous hemorrhage is neovascularization.[68] The vitreous hemorrhage can set up a vicious cycle, resulting in vitreous scarring and a further increase in vitreous traction. Vitreous hemorrhage is frequent in young patients but is rarely seen in persons over 20 years of age.[24] The incidence of retinal detachment varies from 0 to 20%.[45, 47, 61, 69] Laser photocoagulation has been used to try to collapse these retinoschises, but unfortunately, this has often led to a retinal detachment.[43, 70, 71]

The pathogenesis of congenital retinoschisis appears to be inadequate growth of the vitreous gel: The gel cannot keep up with the circumferential growth of the retina, choroid, and sclera, and so tractional forces are applied to the young retina that cause a split in the nerve fiber layer. More recent studies have suggested that there may be a defect in the Müller's cells responsible for the condition.[72–74] Genetic studies have localized the gene causing the defect to the p22 region of the X chromosome.[75] Most cases of congenital retinoschisis are not discovered until patients reach 5 years of age; this is most likely due to the fact that the upper visual field is usually affected. Visual loss in the upper visual field is generally not appreciated by children nor does it greatly affect their visual performance. Progression of the disease is rapid in the first 5 years of life, after which it advances more slowly and usually becomes stationary by age 20.[24]

Macular involvement is found in all affected people, but the typical foveal changes are seen in only about 68% of the cases.[43, 45, 61] In some cases, the foveal retinoschisis is observable and the patient has 20/20 vision.[61] The macula may be involved and appears as star-shaped areas of edema or cystic degeneration.[37, 41, 62, 76] The tiny cysts that make up the star-shaped pattern are arranged like spokes.[37, 57, 62–64, 76, 77] The foveal findings are considered to be pathognomonic of this condition.[76] Visual acuity is usually mildly to moderately affected. Despite cystic changes in the macula, fluorescein angiography rarely demonstrates macular edema in sex-linked retinoschisis, nor does it demonstrate angiographic anomalies in the senile variety. Macular involvement may be confirmed by showing a reduced b-wave on electroretinogram.[74] Macular involvement is either the direct result of peripheral retinoschisis that is involving or has involved the macula, or it may occur independent of peripheral retinoschisis formation. It has been reported that half the cases demonstrate the foveal involvement only, and in the other half, the foveal changes are accompanied by the peripheral retinoschisis formations.[27] No treatment seems to help this macular condition.[24]

Histopathology

Acquired forms of retinoschisis appear as large cystic cavities in the sensory retina that result from the splitting of the sensory retina at the outer plexiform and inner nuclear layers (Figure 3-69). The inner layer is usually extremely thin and contains patent and hyalinized blood vessels, glial cells, remnants of the inner nuclear and nerve fiber layers, and the internal limiting membrane. Remnants of the glial pillars may be found on the inner surface of the inner layer. The outer layer of the retinoschisis is irregular in thickness and contains remnants of the outer nuclear layer and photoreceptors.[15] The cavity is presumably filled with hyaluronic acid. Vitreous histologic findings are variable. Posterior vitreous detachments are not uncommon.

X-linked retinoschisis also appears as a large cystic cavity that results from the splitting of the sensory retina at the nerve fiber layer. The inner layer contains retinal vessels, nerve fibers, and the internal limiting membrane. The inner layer is very thin and its ability to support blood vessels is diminished; therefore, retinal blood vessels are more often found in the outer layer of a congenital retinoschisis. These retinal vessels may even pass from the inner to the outer layer in the cavity of the retinoschisis.

Clinical Significance

Visual acuity may be reduced if a peripheral retinoschisis invades the macula (a very rare occurrence), if an associated retinal detachment involves the macula, or if there is cystoid macular degeneration associated with a temporal retinoschisis. Even though it is uncommon for a retinoschisis to invade the macula, it occasionally happens (Figure 3-70A). Therefore, it is important to follow a retinoschisis on a yearly schedule and even more frequently if it approaches the temporal arcades. Incidences of a perifoveal retinoschisis associated with peripheral retinoschisis have been reported. In such a case, the patient may have 20/20 foveal vision with a perifoveal scotoma.[16]

Progression of a retinoschisis is very slow and is probably the result of the slow degenerative process of peripheral cystoid degeneration together with the viscous nature of the fluid within the cavity. It seems to grow in a circular and posterior direction and becomes more elevated, but most retinoschises become stationary or progress very slowly.[78] One study of 245 eyes found that only 13.5% had documented growth when observed over time periods ranging from 1 month to 15 years,[32] and others found that the ballooning stage of a retinoschisis has

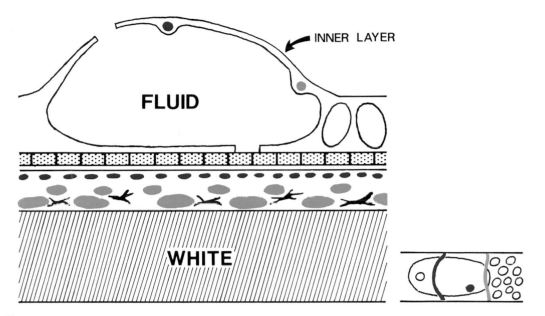

FIGURE 3-69
The intraretinal cavity is filled with a viscous fluid, and there is peripheral cystoid degeneration anterior to the retinoschisis. Note the extreme thinning of the inner and outer layers of the schisis, which can be involved in break formation. An inner-layer hole appears clear because it is in essentially detached retinal and an outer layer hole looks red because it is in attached retina.

a 14% chance of further progression.[24] Sometimes a retinoschisis advances from the periphery to the posterior pole (some actually advancing to the nasal disc margin) and then remain stationary for years. Progression results from either continued vitreous traction or from a secretory mechanism that produces more fluid in the cavity of the retinoschisis. One study found that 85% of senile retinoschises have an associated PVD, but the cortex remains attached to the inner layer of the retinoschisis cavity.[29] Another study found that vitreous liquefaction and PVD are common findings and that prominent fibrous structure in the adjacent gel may be responsible for the peripheral retinal traction and retinoschisis formation.[24] These findings of significant vitreous traction were confirmed in patients undergoing surgery for progressive degenerative retinoschisis.[30] In several cases, once vitreous traction was relieved from the inner layer of a retinoschisis, progression ceased.[18] Therefore, vitreous traction may be the most important factor in progression. Most studies suggest that a retinoschisis is benign in asymptomatic patients.[16, 79]

A break in the inner layer of a retinoschisis does not require treatment because liquefied vitreous is only being allowed into the retinoschisis cavity. The presence of liquefied vitreous in the cavity does not seem to accelerate the progression or increase the size of the retinoschisis. A hole in the outer layer only usually is of little consequence, because it generally produces only a localized retinal detachment around the hole. Two large studies found that retinoschises with outer-layer breaks rarely progressed to retinal detachment.[16, 30] This is most likely due to the limited amount of fluid available to the break or perhaps to the viscosity of the fluid in the cavity. Therefore, treatment is optional for a stationary retinoschisis with only outer-layer breaks. The prevalence of retinal detachment in such cases is only 16%.[22] A hole in both layers can allow a larger amount of fluid from the vitreous cavity to find its way into the subretinal potential space and is therefore more likely to result in a retinal detachment.[16]

There is some debate about the ability of a retinoschisis to produce a detachment, with some experts stating that the presence of breaks in both layers requires immediate treatment because this condition frequently develops into a retinal detachment (especially if a lacuna of fluid vitreous is opposite the inner-layer break). A retinoschisis is responsible for only 3.2% of rhegmatogenous retinal

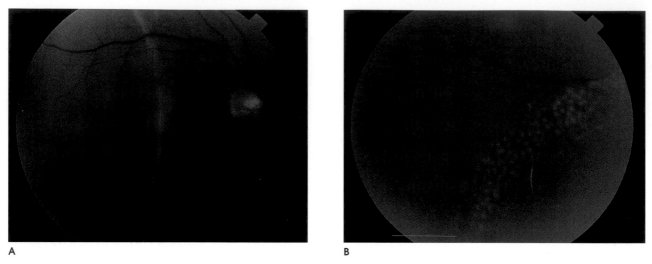

A

B

FIGURE 3-70
A. Large peripheral temporal retinoschisis that has invaded the macula. B. Retinoschisis in fellow eye with fresh argon laser burns placed along the posterior margin in an attempt to halt future progression. (Courtesy of Dr. Arup Das.)

detachments.[80] One report stated that 11% of patients with acquired retinoschises developed a retinal detachment,[22] and another found a 40% chance of developing a retinal detachment in eyes with both inner- and outer-layer breaks.[3]

More recent, long-term observation studies have been less conclusive about the likelihood of a retinal detachment.[7] Hirose et al.[32] followed a large number of patients with senile retinoschisis, and no retinal detachment occurred in any of the eyes with outer-layer breaks or in the 6 eyes with both inner- and outer-layer breaks. They followed another 245 cases of retinoschisis without breaks; of these, nine developed outer-layer breaks, three of which subsequently developed a retinal detachment.

When the retinoschisis cavity collapses over a retinal detachment, the lesion often has the appearance of a typical rhegmatogenous retinal detachment. Sometimes the breaks in a retinoschisis and detachment are difficult to detect; drainage of the subretinal fluid and flattening the retina may make them more visible.[27] Confirmation of a retinoschisis and detachment can be made by the finding of a retinoschisis in the fellow eye; this occurs in 95% of these cases.[81]

A retinoschisis may progress beyond the equator toward the posterior pole and even advance to the macula, although this does not happen often. Another significant finding is the development of cystic macular degeneration, for which there is no treatment. Finally, a vitreous hemorrhage may occur, which could require vitrectomy if recurrent episodes produce extensive chronic vitreous opaci-

fication. A bleeding retinal vessel can be treated with photocoagulation.

Because retinal detachment formation by a retinoschisis is uncommon (and even if a detachment does occur, the progression is very slow), this condition is commonly associated with demarcation lines.[27] Byer[16] followed 14 patients with a localized retinoschisis and detachment, and none progressed to a clinically significant detachment. Therefore, treatment is generally not required even for patients who have outer-layer breaks.[82] Some experts believe that treatment is not necessary unless there is a 25% loss of visual field in at least one quadrant.[4] Treatment may be considered if breaks are large and posterior in location (especially if the breaks are found in both layers), if breaks are found in retinoschisis and there was a retinal detachment caused by a retinoschisis in the fellow eye, the retinoschisis is progressing posteriorly and is threatening the macula, or the retinoschisis is associated with a progressive nonrhegmatogenous retinal detachment.[16, 32, 83, 84] There have been cases of giant (>90 degrees) posterior outer-layer breaks producing a retinal detachment that required surgical repair.[85] However, some now believe that treatment is indicated only if the retinoschisis is associated with a progressive, symptomatic retinal detachment.[16]

A retinoschisis with or without breaks that is progressing in a posterior direction beyond the equator may be treated with photocoagulation and cryotherapy. Photocoagulation is performed by placing at least five rows of laser burns just posterior to the leading margin of the retinoschisis (Figure 3-70B).

Cryotherapy is accomplished by placing cryospots both in healthy retina posterior to the retinoschisis and directly beneath the lesion. This may result in complete flattening of a progressive retinoschisis in about 50% of patients; if the bulla does not flatten, it is likely that vitreous traction is present.[85] Spotty treatment under the bulla may lead to outer-layer holes. Congenital X-linked retinoschisis does not seem to respond to this treatment.

In cases where a retinal detachment is associated with a retinoschisis, photocoagulation, cryoapplication, intraocular gas injection, and a scleral buckle with an encircling band are used in conjunction to treat the condition.[84, 86] Cryotherapy along with scleral buckling is an effective treatment plan for a retinoschisis-retinal detachment, but vision may be reduced due to macular insult from such procedures.[87] Traction retinoschisis is treated in the same manner, and vitreous surgery may also be needed to free vitreous bands. More than 20% of patients with congenital X-linked retinoschisis develop retinal detachment, which seems to occur only after breaks are produced by vitreous traction bands or by an organized vitreous hemorrhage.[24] Treatment is the same as that discussed for a retinal detachment associated with an acquired retinoschisis.

Most retinoschises are stable and usually do not threaten the patient's central visual acuity, and therefore the prognosis is good. The retinoschisis should be drawn on the patient's chart or photographed, if observable with the fundus camera. A stable retinoschisis without holes should be followed yearly, one with an inner-layer stretch break should be followed every 6–12 months, and one with an outer-layer break should be followed every 6 months. Retinoschises with both inner- and outer-layer breaks should be referred to a retinal specialist for possible treatment considerations.

References

1. Wilczek M. Ein fall dernetzaut spaltung mit einer offnung. Z. Augenheiltktd 1935;85:108–116.
2. Straatsma BR, Foos RY. Typical and reticular degenerative retinoschisis. Am J Ophthalmol 1973;75:551–575.
3. Michels RG, Wilkinson CP, et al. Retinal Detachment. Philadelphia: Mosby, 1990.
4. Rutnin U, Schepens CL. Fundus appearance in normal eyes. III. Peripheral degenerations. Am J Ophthalmol 1967;64:1040–1062.
5. Kornsweig AL. Bilateral symmetric cystoid degeneration of the retina. Arch Ophthalmol 1940;23:491–500.
6. Crock GW. A clinical classification of retinoschisis with a preliminary report of three unusual fundus appearances. Trans Ophthalmol Soc NZ 1965;17:18–24.
7. Madjarov B, Hilton GF, et al. A new classification of the retinoschises. Retina 1995;15:282–285.
8. L'Esperance FA, James WA, et al. Diabetic Retinopathy, Clinical Evaluation and Management. St. Louis: Mosby, 1981:214–215.
9. Romayananda N, Golberg MF, et al. Histopathology of sickle cell retinopathy. Trans Am Acad Ophthalmol 1973;77:652–676.
10. Green WR. The Retina. In WH Spencer (ed), Ophthalmic Pathology. An Atlas and Text (3rd ed). Vol. 3. Philadelphia: Saunders, 1985.
11. Schachat AP, Glaser BM. Retinal hamartoma, acquired retinoschisis, and retinal hole. Am J Ophthalmol 1985; 99:604–605.
12. Greenwald MJ, Weiss A, et al. Traumatic retinoschisis in battered babies. Ophthalmology 1986;93:618–625.
13. Wong VG, Bodey GP. Hemorrhagic retinoschisis due to aplastic anemia. Arch Ophthalmol 1968;80:433–435.
14. Brockhurst RJ. Retinoschisis complication of peripheral uveitis. Arch Ophthalmol 1981;99:1998–1999.
15. Yanoff M, Fine BS. Ocular Pathology: A Text and Atlas (2nd ed). Philadelphia: Harper & Row, 1982:510–513.
16. Byer NE. The long-term natural history of senile retinoschisis. Ophthalmology 1986;93:1127–1137.
17. Ballantyne AJ, Michaelson IC. Textbook of the Fundus of the Eye. Baltimore: Williams & Wilkins, 1970:390–396.
18. Byer NE. Clinical study of senile retinoschisis. Arch Ophthalmol 1968;79:36–44.
19. Dul M. Degenerative retinoschisis. Clin Eye Vision Care 1991;3:95–99.
20. Glasgow BJ, Foos RY, et al. Degenerative Diseases of the Peripheral Retina. In TD Duane, EA Jaeger (eds), Clinical Ophthalmology. Vol. 3. Philadelphia: Harper & Row, 1993;26:1–29.
21. Foos RY. Senile retinoschisis: Relationship to cystoid degeneration. Trans Am Acad Ophthalmol 1970;74:33–51.
22. Shea M, Schepens CL, et al. Retinoschisis. I. Senile type: A clinical report of one hundred seven cases. Arch Ophthalmol 1960;63:1–9.
23. Schepens CL. Present-Day Treatment of Retinoschisis: An Evaluation. In A McPherson (ed), New and Controversial Aspects of Retinal Detachment. New York: Harper & Row, 1968:438–442.
24. Schepens CL. Retinal Detachment and Allied Diseases. Philadelphia: Saunders, 1983:557–598.
25. Francois J. Heredity in Ophthalmology. St. Louis: Mosby, 1961:489–494.
26. Hines JL, Jones WL. Peripheral microcystoid retinal degeneration and retinoschisis. J Am Optom Assoc 1982; 7:541–545.
27. Benson WE. Retinal Detachment: Diagnosis and Management (2nd ed). Philadelphia: Lippincott, 1988.
28. DiSclafani M, Wagner A, et al. Pigmentary changes in acquired retinoschisis. Am J Ophthalmol 1988;105: 291–293.
29. Boisdequin D, Croughs P, et al. Vitre et retinoschisis. Bull Soc Belge Ophtalmol 1981;192:75–91.
30. Caspers-Velu LE, Libert J, et al. Vitreous changes in progressive symptomatic retinoschisis. Invest Ophthalmol Vis Sci 1991;32:915.
31. Tolentino FI, Schepens CL, et al. Vitreoretinal Disorders: Diagnosis and Management. Philadelphia: Saunders, 1976:249–266, 360–367.
32. Hirose T, Marcil G, et al. Acquired Retinoschisis: Observation and Treatment. In RC Pruett, CDJ Regan (eds),

Retinal Congress. New York: Appleton-Century-Crofts, 1974:489–504.
33. Pischel DK. Retinal Detachment: A Manual. Am Acad Ophthalmol Otolaryngol 1965:79.
34. Cibis PA. Vitreoretinal Pathology and Surgery in Retinal Detachment. St. Louis: Mosby, 1965:117–119, 124–133.
35. Apple DJ, Rabb MF. Ocular Pathology: Clinical Applications and Self Assessment (3rd ed). St. Louis: Mosby, 1985.
36. Duke-Elder WS. System of Ophthalmology. Congenital Deformities. St. Louis: Mosby, 1958.
37. Forsius H, Krause U, et al. Visual acuity in 183 cases of X-chromosomal retinoschisis. Can J Ophthalmol 1973;8:385–393.
38. Lewis RA, Lee GB, et al. Familial foveal retinoschisis. Arch Ophthalmol 1977;95:1190–1196.
39. Hirose T, Schepens CL, et al. Congenital retinoschisis with night blindness in two girls. Ann Ophthalmol 1980;12:848–856.
40. Bengtsson B, Linder B. Sex-linked hereditary juvenile retinoschisis. Acta Ophthalmologica (Copenh) 1967;45:411–423.
41. Balian JV, Falls HF. Congenital vascular veils in the vitreous: Hereditary retinoschisis. Arch Ophthalmol 1960;63:116–125.
42. Sabates FN. Juvenile retinoschisis. Am J Ophthalmol 1966;62:683–688.
43. Keller U, Brummer S, et al. X-linked juvenile retinoschisis. Graefes Arch Clin Exp Ophthalmol 1990;228:432–437.
44. Ewing CC, Ives EJ. Juvenile hereditary retinoschisis. Eye 1969;89:29–39.
45. Kraushar MF, Schepens CL, et al. Congenital Retinoschisis. In JF Bellows (ed), Contemporary Ophthalmology Honoring Sir Stewart Duke-Elder. Baltimore: Williams & Wilkins, 1972:265–290.
46. Deutman AF. Genetics and retinal detachment. Mod Probl Ophthalmol 1975;15:22–33.
47. Deutman AF. Sex-Linked Juvenile Retinoschisis. In The Hereditary Dystrophies of the Posterior Pole of the Eye. Aspen, CO: Thomas, 1971.
48. Sorsby A, Klein M, et al. Unusual retinal detachment, possibly X-linked. Br J Ophthalmol 1951;35:1-10.
49. Magnus JA. Case of retinal detachment in a child (?cystic ?congenital). Eye 1951;71:728–730.
50. MacRae A. Congenital vascular veils in the vitreous. Eye 1954;74:187–206.
51. Balian JV, Falls HF. Congenital vascular veils in the vitreous. Arch Ophthalmol 1960;63:92–101.
52. Anderson JR. Anterior dialysis of retina: Disinsertion or avulsion at ora serrata. Br J Ophthalmol 1932;16:641, 705.
53. Thompson E. Memorandum regarding family in which neuro-retinal disease of unusual kind occurred only in males. Br J Ophthalmol 1932;16:681–686.
54. Tasman WS, Greven CM, et al. Nasal retinal dragging in X-linked retinoschisis. Graefes Arch Clin Exp Ophthalmol 1991;229:319–322.
55. Greven CM, Moreno RJ, et al. Unusual manifestations of X-linked retinoschisis. Trans Am Ophthalmol Soc 1990;88:211–228.
56. Green JL, Jampol LM. Vascular opacification and leakage in X-linked (juvenile) retinoschisis. Br J Ophthalmol 1979;63:368–373.
57. Hung JY, Hilton GF. Neovascular glaucoma in a patient with X-linked juvenile retinoschisis. Ann Ophthalmol 1980;12:1054–1055.
58. George NDL, Yates JRW, et al. Infantile presentation of X-linked retinoschisis. Br J Ophthalmol 1995;79:653–657.
59. Kawano K, Tanaka K, et al. Congenital hereditary retinoschisis: Evolution at initial stage. Graefes Arch Clin Exp Ophthalmol 1981;217:315–323.
60. Basmadjian G, Labelle P, et al. The natural evolution of juvenile retinoschisis. Can J Ophthalmol 1973;8:33–37.
61. George NDL, Yates JRW, et al. Clinical features in affected males with X-linked retinoschisis. Arch Ophthalmol 1996;114:274–280.
62. Burns RP, Lovrien EW, et al. Juvenile sex-linked retinoschisis. Clinical and genetic studies. Trans Am Acad Ophthalmol Otolaryngol 1971;75:1011–1021.
63. Odland M. Congenital retinoschisis. Acta Ophthalmol (Khb) 1981;59:649–658.
64. Schulman J, Peyman GA, et al. Indications for vitrectomy in congenital retinoschisis. Br J Ophthalmol 1985;69:482–486.
65. Carr RE, Siegel IM. The vitreo-tapeto-retinal degenerations. Arch Ophthalmol 1970;84:436–445.
66. Alexander RL, Shea M. Clinical sciences. Wagner's disease. Arch Ophthalmol 1965;74:310–318.
67. Conway BP, Welch RB. X-chromosome-linked juvenile retinoschisis with hemorrhagic retinal cyst. Am J Ophthalmol 1977;83:853–855.
68. Pearson R, Jagger J. Sex-linked retinoschisis with optic disc and peripheral retinal neovascularization. Br J Ophthalmol 1989;73:311–313.
69. Schepens CL. Congenital retinoschisis. Klin Oczna 1988;90:127–132.
70. Brockhurst R. Photocoagulation in congenital retinoschisis. Arch Ophthalmol 1970;84:158–165.
71. Turut P, Francois P, et al. Analysis of the results in the treatment of peripheral retinoschisis in sex-linked congenital retinoschisis. Graefes Arch Clin Exp Ophthalmol 1989;227:328–331.
72. Manschot WA. Pathology of juvenile retinoschisis. Arch Ophthalmol 1972;88:131–137.
73. Condon GP, Brownstein S, et al. Congenital hereditary (juvenile X-linked) retinoschisis: Histopathologic and ultrastructural findings in three eyes. Arch Ophthalmol 1986;104:576–583.
74. Peachey NS, Fishman GA, et al. Psychological and electroretinographic findings in X-linked juvenile retinoschisis. Arch Ophthalmol 1987;105:513–516.
75. Sieving PA, Bingham EL, et al. Linkage relationship of X-linked juvenile retinoschisis with Xp22.3 probes. Am J Hum Genet 1990;47:616–621.
76. Harris GS, Yeung JW-S. Maculopathy of sex-linked juvenile retinoschisis. Can J Ophthalmol 1976;11:1–10.
77. Harris GS. Retinoschisis. Pathogenesis and treatment. Can J Ophthalmol 1968;3:312–317.
78. Lean JS. Diagnosis and Treatment of Peripheral Retinal Lesions. In WR Freeman (ed), Practical Atlas of Retinal Disease and Therapy. New York: Raven, 1993;12:211–220.
79. Byer NE. The natural history of retinoschisis. Arch Ophthalmol 1972;88:207–209.
80. Hagler WS, Woldoff HS. Retinal detachment in relation to senile retinoschisis. Trans Am Acad of Ophthalmol Otolaryngol 1973;72:99–113.
81. Schachat A, Beauchamp G, et al. Retinal Detachment: Preferred Practice Pattern. Chicago: American Academy of Ophthalmology, 1990.
82. Sneed SR, Blodi DF, et al. Pars plana vitrectomy in the management of retinal detachments associated with degenerative retinoschisis. Ophthalmology 1990;97:470–474.
83. Messmer EP. Prevention of retinal detachment and treatment of retinoschisis. Fortschr Ophth 1990;87:S62–69.

84. Sulonen JM, Wells CG, et al. Degenerative retinoschisis with giant outer layer breaks and retinal detachment. Am J Ophthalmol 1985;99:114–121.
85. Okun E, Cibis PA. The role of photocoagulation in the management of retinoschisis. Arch Ophthalmol 1964;72:309–314.
86. Amber JS, Meyers SM, et al. The management of retinal detachment complicating degenerative retinoschisis. Am J Ophthalmol 1989;107:171–176.
87. Forest A, Girard P, et al. Surgical treatment of retinoschisis. J Fr Ophtalmol 1979;2:109–114.

Lattice Degeneration

Clinical Description

Lattice degeneration of the retina, also known as equatorial, circumferential, and palisade retinal degeneration, is a vitreoretinal degeneration that was found in 5%, 6%, 8%, 9.5% and 10.7% of autopsied eyes.[1-6] Clinical studies showed a prevalence of 6%, 7.1%, and 8%.[7-10] Thus, lattice degeneration is not an uncommon finding in the general population. It occurs more frequently in younger than older persons and usually becomes evident in the second decade of life.[7, 8, 11] The disease seems to reach a maximum prevalence prior to 10 years of age.[8] This indicates that the disease develops fairly early in life; lattice degeneration was demonstrated histologically in a 17-month-old infant.[7] There does not seem to be an increasing incidence of lattice degeneration with age over 10 years.[11, 12] The sexes are equally affected, and there seems to be no racial preference among Caucasian, Asians, and Africans.[6, 8, 13-16] Some have suggested that myopia has a greater association with lattice degeneration,[6, 8, 11, 17] but others believe that refractive errors are not an important factor.[4, 7, 8, 18, 19] Karlin and Curtin[20] found an increasing prevalence of lattice degeneration with increasing axial length in myopic eyes, reaching a prevalence of 11% in eyes over 26.5 mm and 16% at the longest axial length of 36.6 mm in a clinical study of 1,437 eyes. Pierro et al.[21] also found an increasing frequency (13.2%) of lattice lesions in 513 eyes with longer axial lengths. The higher incidence of lattice degeneration in eyes with very long axes is likely due to the dynamic condition of the vitreous on the peripheral retina. Some propose that myopia may predispose to increased frequency of lattice lesions, but its occurrence in patients with low myopia is nearly the same as in those with high myopia.[22]

It is unclear whether heredity is a factor in lattice degeneration. Several reports cite heredity as a possible explanation of the existence of some cases of lattice,[23-29] but the hereditary pattern in some of these families is unclear.[12] In general, the transmission pattern appears to be autosomal dominant, either regular or irregular. Falls[30] believes that lattice degeneration is transmitted as a recessive trait with pseudodominance. In one report, a pedigree demonstrated a probable autosomal dominant mode of transmission,[31] and in another, two generations of three families had lattice degeneration and no significant refractive errors.[18]

Lattice degeneration tends to be both fairly symmetric and bilateral, affecting both eyes 33.0–48.1% of the time.[3, 8, 11] The number of lesions per eye can vary from 1 to 19 or more,[6, 8] and the average number per eye is 2.4, 2.3, or 2.0.[5, 6, 8] Lattice lesions usually grow adjacent to each other either on the same equatorial line or lined up in rows parallel to the ora serrata (Figure 3-71). Their size usually varies from 0.5 to 1.75 (range 0.25–0.66 clinical and 0.10–3.33

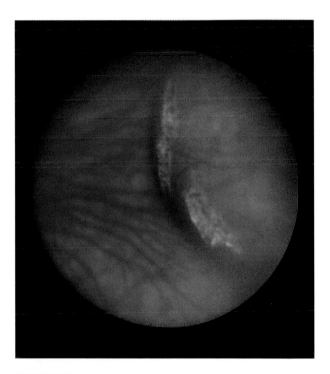

FIGURE 3-71
Two adjacent areas of typical lattice degeneration at different distances to the superior ora serrata as seen through the indirect condensing lens. Note the whitish lesions with very irregular surfaces, both displaying atrophic holes. (Courtesy of William Townsend.)

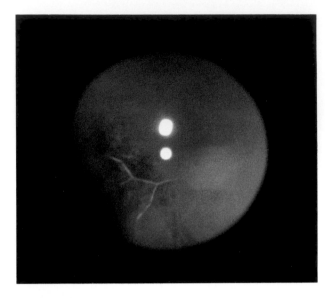

FIGURE 3-72
Typical lattice degeneration in a pigmented broad band, with white sclerotic vessels just posterior to the inferior ora serrata seen through the indirect condensing lens. Also note tiny off-white areas of retinal degeneration within the lesion.

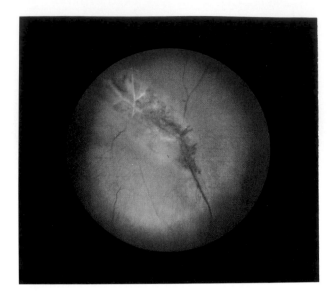

FIGURE 3-73
Perivascular lattice degeneration with pigmentation and white sclerotic vessels in a radial growth pattern in the midperiphery of the superior fundus.

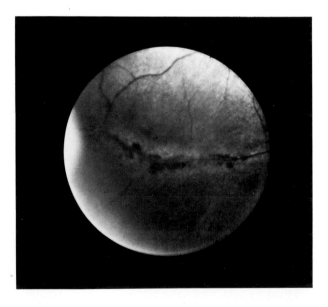

FIGURE 3-74
Perivascular lattice degeneration near the equator with an orientation almost parallel to the ora serrata.

0.10–3.33 autopsy) disc diameters in width and 1–4 (range 0.5–12.0 clinical and 0.12–12.00 autopsy) disc diameters in length; however, the length can extend to an entire quadrant.[6, 8] Sometimes the lattice lesions are so thin that they appear to be a thin line in the retina. Rarely, lattice degeneration can coalesce to extend circumferentially around the retina. The temporal half of the fundus is affected most frequently, and the highest concentration of lattice lesions are clustered around the vertical meridians (11–1 o'clock and 5–7 o'clock), which contained 66% of 286 lesions in an autopsy study and 78.6% of 393 lesions in a clinical study.[6, 8] The retinal area next to the temporal horizontal meridian is next most commonly affected; least affected is the nasal horizontal meridian.[32] It is not clear whether the superior or inferior temporal quadrant is most frequently involved.[8, 11]

Lattice degeneration is usually seen as a small, elongated patch of inner retinal thinning (often very thin) with its long axis generally parallel to the ora serrata (Figure 3-72). Lesions located at or posterior to the equator usually have a radial or oblique directional pattern (Figure 3-73; see also Figure 3-1). Lattice lesions located in the equatorial region of the retina tend to be wider than those near the ora serrata. Lattice degeneration can develop on either side of a large retinal vessel (most often seen in the equatorial region); this is known as perivascular lattice degeneration (Figure 3-74; see also Figures 3-72, 3-73). Lesions close to the ora serrata tend to be narrow and linear (see Figure 3-71) and those at the equator are wider and more oval or even round. Lattice degeneration is seen as a well-demarcated area

Table 3-10. Lattice Degeneration vs. Prominent Vitreous Base vs. Retinal Pigment Clump

Lattice degeneration	Prominent vitreous base	Retinal pigment clump
Flat	Flat	Flat
Usually hyperpigmented	Hyperpigmented	Hyperpigmented
Usually oblong; length ranges from 1 diopter to an entire quadrant; the long axis is parallel to the ora serrata	Usually seen circumferentially but may be present in isolated areas	Small and irregularly shaped but usually somewhat circular
Located posterior to ora serrata, with fairly normal-looking retina between the lesion and the ora, but sometimes found at the equator, where they tend to have a radial orientation	Located posterior and adjacent to the ora serrata	Usually found between the ora serrata and the equator
White sclerotic vessels are often present	White vessels not frequently seen	White vessels not frequently seen
Whitish flecks may be seen within the lesion	Not seen	Not seen
Thin retina	No thinning	No thinning
Retinal degeneration present	Normal peripheral retina	Retinal degeneration present
Vitreous traction present	Vitreous traction present	Vitreous traction present
May have multiple lesions	May have multiple lesions but usually fairly contiguous	May have multiple lesions
Vitreous lacunae present over lesion	Vitreous lacunae not present over lesion	Vitreous lacunae not present over lesion
Chorioretinal atrophy may be associated with the lesions	Chorioretinal atrophy may be associated with the lesions	Chorioretinal atrophy may be associated with the lesions
Atrophic holes within and tears along the margins of the lesion	Atrophic holes within the base are infrequently seen and tears along the margin may be found	Retinal tears are associated with these lesions
Retinal detachments are commonly associated	Not generally associated with retinal detachments	May cause a retinal detachment

of retinal degeneration that has a dull, rough appearance. The lesion is composed of tiny jagged areas of degenerating retinal tissue across a base that is uneven in thickness, a "moth-eaten" appearance.

There is always fairly normal-appearing retina between lattice degeneration and the ora serrata; this is a key difference from a prominent vitreous base. On occasion, only the posterior margin of a pigmented area in the far periphery may be seen during ophthalmoscopy, which may give rise to the presumptive diagnosis of lattice degeneration. The pigmented area should be placed under scleral depression to make the anterior part of the lesion visible. If the pigmented area is adjacent to the ora serrata, the diagnosis would most likely be a prominent vitreous base, but if retina is found anterior to the lesion, the most likely diagnosis is lattice degeneration (if it has the other characteristics). A fairly large pigment clump also can have the appearance of an atypical round lattice lesion (Table 3-10).

White lines may display a criss-crossing pattern, the appearance that is responsible for the term lattice degeneration. White lines need not be present, however, to make the diagnosis. The involved vessels are surrounded by glial proliferation or hyaline deposits.[4] There may be a single straight white vessel within the lesion, but usually there is more than one and they often branch (see Figures 3-72 and 3-73). Sometimes, a white sclerotic vessel travels down the center of a lattice lesion, giving off small branches, resulting in a "fishbone" appearance (Figure 3-75). Lattice degeneration with white lines is more commonly found in the inferior half of the retina.[9] The earliest changes demonstrated are localized narrowing of the vessels in the area of the lattice lesion; many of these lesions remain in an arrested state.[9] Some of these vessels may progress to showing parallel white sheathing, however, and some may even advance to typical white lines. The white lines are most often sheathed or occluded blood vessels, most frequently venules that are continuous with normal-appearing vessels outside of the lesion.[33] White lines are not commonly seen in young patients, being found in 3.3% of the 10- to 19-year-old age group, but they do increase in frequency with advancing age, reaching a maximum prevalence of 42.9% after age 50 years.[8] Another report found white lines in 11.9–42.9% of patients with lattice degeneration.[12] When lattice lesions have been followed for years, new white lines can develop. This has been documented in 14% of 204 patients in one study.[9]

Abnormal pigmentation is the most common finding in lattice degeneration, occurring in 81.7%

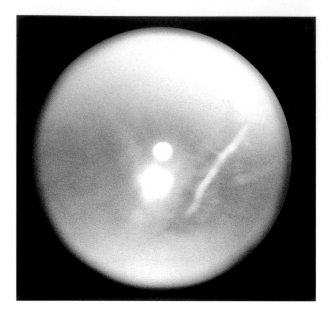

FIGURE 3-75
Perivascular lattice degeneration with large sclerotic vessel down the center of the lesion and small sclerotic vessel branches perpendicular, giving the lesion a "fishbone" appearance.

and 92% of lesions.[6,8] The increase in pigmentation is found in the retina and choroid and seems to increase with age. The hyperpigmentation is the result of pigment epithelial hyperplasia and migration into the overlying sensory retina. The second most common feature is tiny white or yellow flecks (in 80% of lesions) located between the retinal surface and the vitreous cortex.[9] In the early stages of lattice degeneration these flecks are located over the entire surface, but later they seem to concentrate at the borders of the lesions.[12] They give the retinal surface of the lesion a granular appearance. Sometimes these white flecks are arranged in a line, producing a pseudo–white line appearance.

White-with- or -without-pressure sometimes shows up along the borders of the lesion (especially the posterior border), which indicates vitreous traction (see Figure 3-54). Another condition that sometimes occurs concomitantly is chorioretinal atrophy. On occasion, tiny, snowflake-like opacities may be adjacent to the lattice lesion. If the retinal areas adjacent to lattice lesions are viewed with magnification with a three-mirror fundus lens or a 90-diopter or 60-diopter precorneal lens, small areas of snow-flakelike degeneration can sometimes be seen a short distance away. These areas are usually not visible with binocular indirect ophthalmoscopy. It may be surmised that they are the precursor to typical lattice degeneration.

The vitreous over areas of lattice degeneration shows liquefaction of the vitreous gel that forms a lacuna (Figure 3-76). This vitreous degeneration is not uniformly distributed throughout the vitreous body, and it has been reported that the incidence of PVD is the same in eyes with and without lattice degeneration.[34] The lacuna is lined by a condensed membrane of vitreous that is attached at the edge of the lattice lesion. The condensed vitreous membranes are very transparent and therefore only occasionally seen during ophthalmoscopy (Figure 3-77). Glial cells proliferate along the vitreal surface and form tight vitreoretinal adhesions.[35, 36] Posterior vitreous detachment is not uncommon, and it generally does not involve the area of lattice degeneration due to the strong vitreoretinal adhesions. An early lattice lesion may have a small isolated lacuna over it, but an advanced lesion tends to have a large lacuna with communication to other lacunae within the vitreous body. This can make available a large quantity of liquefied vitreous to enter a retinal break and possibly cause a retinal detachment, but it is more likely that a retinal detachment will occur following a posterior vitreous detachment when more fluid is available and more vitreous traction is present.

Lattice degeneration is a slowly progressive disease that results in gradual retinal thinning and loss of transparency. With time, punched-out areas, retinal cysts and breaks, and occasionally, a small retinal hemorrhage may appear within the lesion.

Fluorescein angiography displays delayed leakage of dye from the choroidal vessels in the area of the lattice lesion and avascularity both within and proximal to the lesion. The retinal vessels proximal to the lesion exhibited dye leakage in 61%, delayed filling in 54%, arteriovenous shunts in 33%, and microaneurysm in 16% of eyes.[37] These findings have led some to believe that degeneration of the retinal vessels is responsible for most of the pathogenesis of this condition and that choroidal changes may also have some part in the disease process. Others have found that there was filling of the retinal vessels in the lattice lesion but no leakage of dye outside the vessels[2] and that the arterioles and venules peripheral to the lattice lesion would perfuse, which suggests that there is perfusion to the retina with the lattice lesion.[38] One suggestion is that only the vessels limited to the lesion itself may be part of the disease process. Due to defects in the pigment epithelium, areas of hyperfluorescent window defects are seen in the lesion during the angiogram.

The pathogenesis of lattice degeneration is still unclear. Localized retinal ischemia may produce retinal and vitreal degeneration,[6, 15, 37, 39, 40] but some have

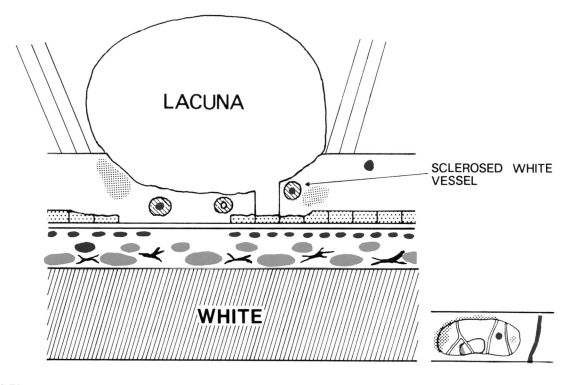

FIGURE 3-76
Lattice degeneration with sclerosed white vessels (center vessel is totally occluded), pigment migration into the sensory retina, a red atrophic hole, chorioretinal atrophy, a vitreous lacuna, and vitreous traction on the edges of the lesion. Note that the retina has degenerated to about one-third its normal thickness.

doubts about the ischemic theory.[12, 38, 41] The condition may be primarily the result of vitreous degeneration causing localized areas of vitreoretinal traction with secondary loss of inner retinal tissue. Other theories propose genetic predisposition and developmental factors.[4] There may be abnormalities in the internal limiting membrane, and it may be that the disease process locus is in the Müller cells.[5, 6, 12, 36, 42]

There seems to be no correlation of the severity of appearance of the lesion and the increasing age of the patient, as seen in one study of autopsied eyes,[5] but another study found statistically significant changes in the degree of vitreoretinal attachments, pigment abnormalities, white lines, retinal holes and tears, and posterior vitreous detachment in autopsied eyes with increasing age.[6] In the latter study, however, there was no age-related correlation of the size, location, or orientation of the lesions. From a clinical standpoint, it is not possible to draw any conclusions about a particular lesion in regard to its age based on the ophthal-

moscopic appearance.[8] There is frequently a large disproportion between the severity of the lesion and the age of the patient; younger patients may show advanced changes in the lattice lesions and older patients may show only mild clinical changes. This disproportion may be the result of the lattice lesions being in a clinically arrested state for the entire life of the patient; many patients show no noticeable change of their lesions for years.[9] If clinical changes do occur, they progress very slowly, except in the presence of a tractional tear.[12] New lesions sometimes occur, and they have been documented in 5% of patients with pre-existing lattice degeneration. Most of these new lesions (95%) occur before age 19 years.[9]

Histopathology

Based on autopsied eyes,[5, 43] the early changes consist of a localized area of vitreous liquefaction over a localized area of degeneration of the innermost

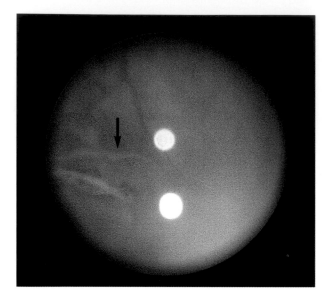

FIGURE 3-77
Small peripheral pigmented lattice degeneration lesion with a visible lacuna above it (*arrow*). The wall of the lacuna is composed of compressed vitreous fibrils.

retinal layers. Further progression causes increased vitreoretinal adhesions at the margins of the lesion and an increased thinning of the retina down to the middle layers (outer nuclear and sensory cells) of the retina. Next, the pigment epithelium undergoes atrophy and proliferative changes. Last, the entire retinal area tends to be become a fibrous gliosed plate that is invaded by pigment cells and has irregularly dispersed clumps of pigment.

Lattice degeneration shows variable retinal thinning, with the greatest amount generally in the center (see Figure 3-76). The retinal surface is irregular and has amorphous gray-white particles.[18] There is loss of the inner retinal layers down to the outer nuclear and outer limiting membranes, which are often replaced in part by glial elements. Often, a conspicuous loss of photoreceptors occurs within the lesion.[44] Advanced degeneration can affect the entire sensory retina, the pigment epithelium, and the basal lamina (Bruch's membrane). Pigment granules are often seen in macrophages throughout the lesion.

Retinal vessel walls are thickened and display hyaline degeneration. Some vessels may be completely obliterated and replaced by dense cords of connective tissue. Obliterated vessels are generally found in the center of the lattice lesion. Retinal degeneration often occurs around a hyalinized vessel, leaving a sclerotic vessel exposed on the surface of the lesion.

The vitreous within the margins of the lattice degeneration shows a loss of vitreoretinal attachments and the presence of liquefied vitreous gel. The edges of the lesion demonstrate an exaggerated adhesion to the vitreous. Often, a thin translucent membrane appears between the lattice lesion and the vitreous; it is believed to be the result of vitreous condensation and glial cell proliferation.

Clinical Significance

Lattice degeneration is the most important clinical entity of the peripheral retina, especially as it relates to retinal detachment. Lattice degeneration frequently leads to the formation of retinal breaks due to progressive retinal thinning, exaggerated vitreoretinal adhesions at the margins of the lesion, and the liquefied vitreous that is produced above the lesion. Breaks may either be solitary or multiple, small or large. Retinal breaks occur in about 25% of affected eyes.[2] Most retinal breaks in lattice degeneration occur in the superior half of the fundus, which accords with reports that most breaks (95%, 73%, and 82%) are found in the upper half of the retina.[33, 45, 46] The complications of atrophic holes and traction tears are statistically rare, considering the high prevalence of lattice degeneration in the population.[12]

Atrophic holes may form in a lesion due to the loss of all the sensory retinal tissue, occurring in 18.2–28.7% of cases.[9, 18] Due to this simple loss of tissue in the production of holes in lattice degeneration, atrophic holes are asymptomatic, and they occur earlier in life than do traction tears. Retinal holes may either occur inside the lattice lesion or in adjacent retinal tissue. Atrophic holes in lattice are generally small, typically around one-fourth disc diameter, rarely reaching one disc diameter. Many of these holes are as small as one-fifth disc diameter and may be difficult to identify.[12] Most atrophic holes in lattice are solitary, but occasionally they are multiple. Foos[47] studied 5,600 autopsied eyes and found that 2.4% of them had atrophic holes and that 75% of these holes were found in lattice lesions; therefore, 3% of cases (1.8% of the eyes) had lattice degeneration with holes. A clinical study found retinal holes in 16.3–18.2% of eyes with lattice degeneration.[12, 48] Another study found retinal holes in 13.3% of patients 10–19 years old with lattice degeneration, and the prevalence slowly increased with time. It has been reported that 65% of the patients who develop new retinal holes are younger than 35 years of age.[9] Statistically, most atrophic holes are found in the inferior half of the retina in a ratio greater than 2:1 inferior to superior.[9] The preferred quadrant is the inferior temporal retina.[9, 23, 49]

Atrophic holes are red and usually round or oval (Figure 3-78; see also Figure 3-1). Many of these holes have a small surrounding retinal detachment that appears white to dirty white. The localized detachments are almost always found within the borders of the lattice lesion, but occasionally, the localized retinal detachment spreads less than a disc diameter from the lattice lesion, where it may produce a small pigmented demarcation line.[12] Rarely, the localized detachment extends farther than one disc diameter from the lattice lesion and becomes a subclinical retinal detachment, but this occurs in only 1.5% of lattice cases followed over a period of years.[9] The subclinical detachments tend to remain stable, which is most likely due to the limited source of fluid in the lacuna over the lattice lesion. However, if the small overlying lacuna becomes interconnected with a larger, nearby vitreous lacuna, a significant retinal detachment may develop. Eisner[50] does not believe that this free communication with the vitreous body is sufficient to produce a clinically significant detachment. Whatever the cause of localized retinal detachments associated with atrophic holes in lattice degeneration, the fluid entering the subretinal space almost always remains stable and confined to the margins or spreads a minute distance from the margin of the lesion; this is one of the prominent clinical behavioral features of lattice degeneration.[12]

Even though atrophic holes are much more common than tractional tears in lattice degeneration, they are far less able to cause a retinal detachment. The frequency of retinal detachment caused by atrophic holes in lattice degeneration is fairly low (2.8%, 13.9%).[49, 51] In these two studies, 50% of the patients were under 30 years of age, more than 75% had myopia greater than 3.00 diopters, inferior detachments were most common (often showing signs of slow progression), and successful surgical repair was excellent. Others have reported that 30–45% of retinal detachments caused by lattice degeneration are the result of atrophic holes.[9, 52] Of these types of detachments, 70% occur in myopic eyes and 70% occur in patients younger than 40 years of age.[49, 52] Detachments caused by atrophic holes usually progress slowly and therefore are commonly associated with demarcation lines.[49, 52] In a long-term clinical study by Byer,[9] none of 137 atrophic holes in eyes with lattice degeneration led to a clinically significant detachment. Byer has calculated the risk of a retinal detachment secondary to

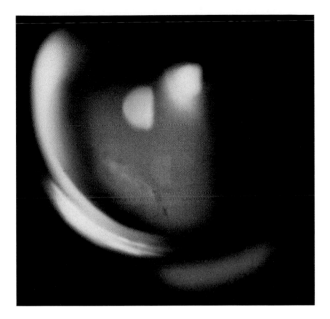

FIGURE 3-78
Lattice degeneration with white sclerotic vessels and hyperpigmentation in the inferior temporal fundus as seen through the 90-diopter condensing lens. Note the large flap tear at one lateral edge and the three atrophic holes at the opposite lateral edge. The lesion has produced a retinal detachment (note the obscuration of underlying choroidal detail). Yellow tinge is due to the yellow color of the condensing lens.

atrophic holes at 1 in 365 patients who have such lesions. Byer[12] also found that the incidence of retinal detachments due to lattice degeneration with holes actually decreases with age.

One study found retinal tears in 2.4% in 125 autopsied eyes with lattice degeneration,[6] and another study found 1.5% in a clinical study of 289 patients with lattice lesions followed for 3–10 years.[9] Other studies found retinal tears in 1.0% of eyes with lattice degeneration.[12, 48] Tears are most frequently located at the posterior and lateral edges of the lesion (Figures 3-78, 3-79, and 3-80), although they occasionally occur at the anterior edge of the lesion. Tears tend to be linear along the margin of the lesion but may appear as a horseshoe tear. The risk of a retinal tear is greater if the lattice lesion is juxtabasal or extrabasal in relation to the vitreous base.[4, 48] Retinal tears do not occur across the lesion due to the strength of the involved fibrotic area. Because lattice degeneration causes a degeneration of the sensory retina, the resultant fibrosis of the lesion produces an area of retina that is stronger than the surrounding normal retina. Sometimes an operculated tear develops inside a lattice lesion and a vitreous strand might be seen attached to the operculum. Rarely, a giant retinal tear may develop

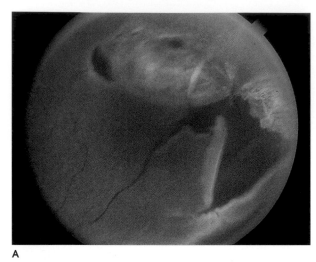

A

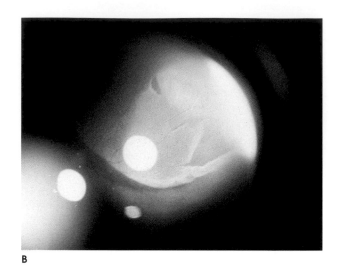

B

FIGURE 3-79
A. Two adjacent peripheral lattice lesions are seen on a retinal detachment in the superior temporal region of the fundus. The lattice lesion on the left has a small tear at the lateral edge and an atrophic hole at the middle of the anterior margin. The lattice lesion to the right has a large tear along the posterior margin. Note that the lattice lesions have areas of hyperpigmentation and white sclerotic vessels. B. The same lattice lesion as seen through the QuadrAspheric lens shows almost all the retinal detachment and its relation to the optic disc.

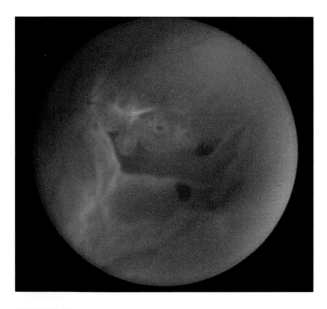

FIGURE 3-80
A lattice lesion is located on a retinal detachment in the superior fundus. There is a large linear retinal tear along the posterior margin with retinal hemorrhages caused by a torn blood vessel on either side of the gap and an atrophic hole in the center of the lesion. Note that the lattice has areas of hyperpigmentation and a white sclerotic vessel.

along the posterior margin of extensive lattice degeneration.

When a retinal tear is associated with lattice degeneration, it is common to find a PVD that ends

at the posterior margin of the lesion.[53] The tear is probably the result of sudden tractional forces produced by the PVD at the margins of the lattice lesions and, because the tractional forces are sudden, most but not all of these tears are symptomatic. The tears can either be small or very large. Tiny areas of lattice degeneration most frequently lead to a retinal tear because vitreous tractional forces applied to a small retinal area are much more destructive than those spread over a larger area. Lattice lesions that are found within the vitreous base (intrabasal) are protected from the risk of developing a traction tear.[33, 54] The existence of a retinal break is not usually sufficient in itself to cause a retinal detachment in these cases because there must be vitreous traction and liquefied vitreous or aqueous available to detach the retina.

In a series of 100 eyes having a symptomatic retinal detachment, Dumas and Schepens[33] found that 30 eyes had lattice degeneration and 33 flap tears were associated with the lattice lesions. This study also found that 54.5% of the lattice lesions with flap tears were found in the superior temporal region, which accords with the finding that most breaks occur in the superior temporal quadrant of eyes with retinal detachment. They also found that 88% of these flap tears were in the superior half of the retina, which is most likely explained by the tractional forces applied by the vitreous being dragged downward by gravity. Of the 40 horseshoe tears found in the 30 eyes with lattice, 82.5% were adjacent to the lattice; so not all tractional tears in eyes with lattice are directly associated with lattice degeneration. In another study of fellow eyes with lattice, 15 eyes developed new retinal breaks over the study period, and only 67% of these breaks were associated with the lattice lesions, leaving 33% of the tractional breaks occurring in previously normal-looking retina.[55] A cited report by Foos[12] of 6,800 autopsied eyes, 139 eyes had tractional tears, 18% of these eyes had lattice degeneration, and only 28% of the eyes had the tears adjacent to the lattice lesions. Lattice with tractional tears or a mixture of breaks was responsible for retinal detachments in 16–27% of all primary detachments.[49, 51] Two reports found that 55–70% of retinal detachments in eyes with lattice degeneration were caused by tears at the posterior edge of the lattice lesions (see Figures 3-79 and 3-80).[9, 52] In these types of retinal detachments, 90% were found in patients older than 50, and only 43% occurred in myopic eyes.[52] Retinal detachments caused by lattice with tears progress more rapidly than those produced by atrophic holes; therefore, they are not usually associated with demarcation lines.[56]

Lattice degeneration and retinal detachment have a significant association: 20–41% of patients undergoing surgery for a rhegmatogenous retinal detachment have lattice degeneration.[4, 6, 51, 57–59] This does not mean that all patients with lattice degeneration are likely to develop a retinal detachment; in fact, this occurs in only 0.3–0.5% of patients or 1 in 200–300 patients with the disease.[8, 9] In a study by Hyams et al.[60] of 278 eyes with either lattice or snail-track degeneration, only 1.4% developed a retinal detachment over a 1- to 6-year period; Folk et al.[61] found an incidence of 5.1% in 112 eyes with lattice lesions followed without treatment for 7 years. The prevalence of lattice degeneration in the fellow eye of patients with a retinal detachment has been reported as 9.2–35%.[3, 46, 62–64] One study reported the incidence of retinal detachment in fellow eyes with lattice was 16%, which accounts for approximately 4% of fellow eye detachments in general.[12, 55] According to a study by Foos and Simons,[34] the higher prevalence of retinal detachments in eyes with lattice degeneration is not related to PVD, even though it is well accepted that retinal tears with lattice are associated with PVD.

No clinical studies have shown that patients with myopia and lattice degeneration are more likely to develop a retinal detachment than myopes with no lattice lesions. Extensive lattice degeneration is no more likely to produce a retinal detachment than are solitary lattice lesions. Lattice degeneration with and without breaks is less commonly associated with aphakic retinal detachments than phakic detachments.[12]

Management of lattice degeneration without breaks consists of recording the location and pertinent characteristics of the lesion and following the patient on a yearly basis. The treatment of lattice degeneration without breaks is definitely unjustified, and so-called prophylactic surgery gave a very doubtful protection from the development of a retinal detachment.[12, 65] Prophylactic treatment of lattice lesions should not be given unless the fellow eye has had a retinal detachment; the eye with the lattice degeneration has symptomatic tears; there is a strong family history of retinal detachment; or the eye with lattice is highly myopic, aphakic, or soon to become aphakic.[12, 66] There has been no cumulative evidence that the prophylactic treatment of lattice lesions in the fellow eye of a patient who has had a retinal detachment is of much value in preventing a retinal detachment. An argument for the treatment of lattice in these fellow eyes can be made, but there may be only a small therapeutic advantage gained by performing treatment procedures.[12] One of the main arguments for the limited value of treatment in lattice degeneration is the fact that new breaks often occur away from the areas of pre-existing lattice lesions. Schepens[67] reported that in 55% of the eyes with subclinical detachments, some of the breaks occurred in unpredictable sites. In a study of 388 fellow eyes, Folk et al.[65] found that 29.2% of the new retinal breaks after prophylactic treatment occurred away from visible areas of lattice degeneration. Many other authors have made this discovery and suggest a conservative attitude toward prophylactic treatment.[33, 53, 68, 69]

Patients with symptoms of floaters and photopsia must be examined at 6-month intervals. It is important to perform the examination with binocular indirect ophthalmoscopy and scleral depression. Patients with asymptomatic small retinal holes need not be treated unless there are coexisting circumstances that enhance the possibility of a retinal detachment, such as aphakia, high myopia, or vitreous scarring. No prophylactic treatment is without some potential complications, and there are statistical grounds for concluding that the very treatment modalities used may even bring about the natural complications (retinal detachment) that they are supposed to prevent.[12, 46] The risk of retinal detachment following cryopexy treatment of eyes

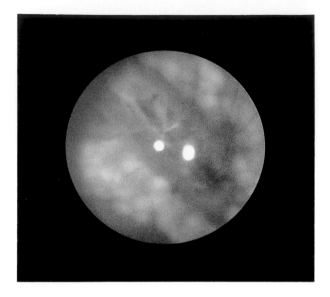

FIGURE 3-81
Fresh argon laser photocoagulation spots are bright white areas around the perivascular lattice degeneration shown in Figure 3-73. The view is through the indirect condensing lens.

The treatment of lattice degeneration with significant breaks and without a retinal detachment is photocoagulation (Figure 3-81) and cryopexy. Because the lesion is within an area of very thin retina, the tensile strength of the chorioretinal adhesion produced by the treatment is low, and a flap tear following a PVD may occur at the margin of the lesion even after treatment. The retinopexy should completely surround the lattice lesion anteriorly, so that even if a flap tear occurs, a retinal detachment is not likely to develop.[66] In a study by Benson et al.,[74] prophylactic treatment with cryopexy sometimes leads to new flap tears that may extend beyond the area of treatment, and so it is advisable to treat the margins of the lattice adequately and to include the area adjacent to the ora serrata. The development of a retinal detachment usually requires the additional procedure of scleral buckling with or without an encircling band. Retinal detachment from an atrophic hole in lattice degeneration has a surgical success rate of 98–100%.[52, 49]

with lattice is reported to be 3.3%[67] and 1.8%.[70] Okun and Cibis[71] treated 66 eyes with holes in the lattice lesions and 6% later detached. Tasman and Jaeger[72] treated a similar group of 176 eyes and 2.8% subsequently detached. Folk et al.[61] treated 164 fellow eyes of patients with unilateral phakic lattice retinal detachments and found a 1.8% rate of retinal detachment in those eyes over a 7-year period.

Prophylactic treatment of lattice does seem to be effective in preventing retinal detachments in eyes with less than 1.25 diopters of myopia, but it is far less effective in reducing the same risk in the 1.25- to 6.00-diopter myopes; therefore, it is difficult to recommend a specific treatment for this group. Prophylactic treatment did not reduce the risk of retinal detachment in eyes with more than 6.00 diopters of myopia and more than 6 clock hours of lattice; therefore, it may be prudent to follow these eyes and consider treatment only if breaks occur.[67]

The existence of flap tears with lattice degeneration may create a higher risk of producing a retinal detachment; thus, some authors suggest prophylactic treatment.[46] However, it has also been found that flap tears associated with lattice may have a higher risk of posttreatment problems.[73] Because these reported rates are not very different from the natural incidence of retinal detachments with lattice degeneration, there seems to be little justification for treatment in many cases.[12]

References

1. Boniuk M, Butler FC. An Autopsy Study of Lattice Degeneration, Retinal Breaks and Retinal Pits. In A McPherson (ed), New and Controversial Aspects of Retinal Detachment. New York: Harper & Row, 1968: 59–75.
2. Straatsma BR, Zeegen PD, et al. Lattice degeneration of the retina. Trans Am Acad Ophthalmol Otolaryngol 1974; 78:87–113.
3. Everett WG. Bilateral retinal detachment and degeneration. Trans Am Ophthalmol Soc 1966;64:543–585.
4. Straatsma BR, Allen RA. Lattice degeneration of the retina. Trans Am Acad Ophthalmol Otolaryngol 1962;66:600–613.
5. Daicker B. Anatomie und pathologie der menschlichen retino-ziliaren fundusperipherie. Basel: Karger, 1972:247–253.
6. Straatsma BR, Zeegen PD, et al. Lattice degeneration of the retina. Trans Am Acad Ophthalmol Otolaryngol 1974; 77:619–649.
7. Halpern JI. Routine screening of the retinal periphery. Am J Ophthalmol 1966;62:99–102
8. Byer NE. Clinical study of lattice degeneration of the retina. Trans Am Acad Ophthalmol Otolaryngol 1965;69:1064–1081.
9. Byer NE. Changes in and prognosis of lattice degeneration of the retina. Trans Am Acad Ophthalmol Otolaryngol 1974;78:114–125.
10. Bohringer HR. Statistisches zu Haufigheit und Risiko der Netzhautablosung. Ophthalmologica 1956;131:331–334.
11. Karlin DB, Curtin BJ. Peripheral chorioretinal lesions and axial length of the myopic eye. Am J Ophthalmol 1976; 81:625–635.
12. Byer NE. Lattice degeneration of the retina. Surv Ophthalmol 1979;23:213–247.
13. Kojima K. Equatorial degeneration. Ganka Ophthalmol (Tokyo) 1967;9:24–35.
14. Kojima K. Equatorial degeneration (I). Nippon Ganka Kiyo, Folia Ophthalmolgica Japonica 1968;19:647–656.

15. Sato K. Shunt formation in lattice degeneration and retinal detachment. Mod Probl Ophthalmol 1972;10:133–134.

16. Av-Shalom A, Berson D, et al. The vitreo-retinopathy associated with retinal detachment among Africans. Am J Ophthalmol 1967;64:387–391.

17. Morse PH. Lattice degeneration of the retina and retinal detachment. Am J Ophthalmol 1974;78:930–934.

18. Tolentino FI, Schepens CL, et al. Vitreoretinal Disorders: Diagnosis and Management. Philadelphia: Saunders, 1976;16:340–349.

19. Celorio JM, Pruett RC. Prevalence of lattice degeneration and its relation to axial length in severe myopia. Am J Ophthalmol 1991;111:20–23.

20. Karlin DB, Curtin BJ. Axial Length Measurements and Peripheral Fundus Changes in the Myopic Eye. In RC Pruett, CDJ Regan (eds), Retina Congress. New York: Appleton-Century-Crofts, 1972:629–641.

21. Pierro FI, Camesasca MM, et al. Peripheral retinal changes and axial myopia. Retina 12:12–17.

22. Schepens CL. Retinal Detachment and Allied Diseases. Philadelphia: Saunders, 1983;8:167–169.

23. Aaberg TM, Stevens TR. Snail-track degeneration of the retina. Am J Ophthalmol 1972;73:370–376.

24. van Balen ATM, Falger ELF. Hereditary hyaloideoretinal degeneration and palatoschisis. Arch Ophthalmol 1970;83:152–162.

25. Cibis PA. Vitreoretinal Pathology and Surgery in Retinal Detachment. St. Louis: Mosby, 1965:111–133.

26. Delaney WV, Podedworny W, et al. Inherited retinal detachment. Arch Ophthalmol 1963;69:44–50.

27. Gonin II. Familiare netzhautablosung. Deutsch Gesundh 1966;21:1662–1665.

28. Haut MM, Limon S. et al. Degenerescence retinienne peripherique familiale et decollement de la retine. Bull Soc Ophthalmol Fr 1973;73:27–37.

29. Lewkonia I, Davies MS, et al. Lattice degeneration in a family. Br J Ophthalmol 1973;57:566–571.

30. Falls HF. The Genetics of Lattice Degeneration. In SJ Kimura, WM Caygill (eds), Retinal Diseases: Symposium on Differential Diagnostic Problems of Posterior Uveitis. Philadelphia: Lea & Febiger, 1966:162–163.

31. Gartner J. Erbbedingte aquatoriale degenerationen nict-myoper. Solitarformen und oraparallele bander. Klin Monatsbl Augenheilkd 1960;136:523–539.

32. Glasgow BJ, Foos RY, et al. Degenerative Diseases of the Peripheral Retina. In TD Duane, EA Jaeger (eds), Clinical Ophthalmology. Vol. 3. Philadelphia: Harper & Row, 1993;26:1–29.

33. Dumas J, Schepens CL. Chorioretinal lesions predisposing to retinal breaks. Am J Ophthalmol 1966;61:620–630.

34. Foos RY, Simons KB. Vitreous in lattice degeneration of the retina. Ophthalmology 1984;91:452–457.

35. Robinson MR, Streeten BW. The surface morphology of retinal breaks and lattice retinal degeneration: A scanning electron microscopic study. Ophthalmology 1986;93:237–246.

36. Streeten BW, Bert M. The retinal surface in lattice degeneration of the retina. Am J Ophthalmol 1972:1201–1209.

37. Sato K, Tsunakawa N, et al. Fluorescein angiography of retinal detachment and lattice degeneration. Part II. Acta Soc Ophthalmol Jap (Tokyo) 1973;89:293–295.

38. Tolentino FI, Lapus JV, et al. Fluorescein angiography of degenerative lesions of the peripheral fundus and rhegmatogenous retinal detachment. Int Ophthalmol Clin 1976;16:13–29.

39. Amalric P. L'angiographie fluoresceineque dans le decollement juvenile. Ann Ocul 1968;201:1178–1196.

40. Heinzen H. Die prophyladtische behandlung der metzhautablosung. Stuttgart, Germany: Ferinand Ende Verlag, 1960:38–45.

41. Wessing A. New aspects of angiographic studies in retinal detachment. Mod Probl Ophthalmol 1974;12:202–206.

42. Ricci A. Classification des degenerescences vitreo-retiniemmes et chorio-retiniennes en relation avec le decollement de retine. Mod Probl Ophthalmol 1969;8:183–205.

43. Draicker B. Discussion of Pau H. Histologie von zum einrisz disponierenden degenerativen bzw. sklerotischen arealen der netzhaut. Die Prophylaxe der idiopathischen netzhautabhebung. Munchen: Bergmann, 1971:45–46.

44. Yanoff M, Fine BS. Ocular Pathology: A Text and Atlas (2nd ed). Philadelphia: Harper & Row, 1982;11:567–569.

45. Colyear BH, Pischel DK. Preventive treatment of retinal detachment by means of light coagulation. Trans Pac Coast Oto-Ophthalmol Soc 1960;41:193–215.

46. Davis MD. Natural history of retinal breaks without detachment. Arch Ophthalmol 1974;92:183–194.

47. Foos RY. Retinal holes. Am J Ophthalmol 1978;86:354–358.

48. Sigelman J. Vitreous base classification of retinal tears: Clinical application. Surv Ophthalmol 1980;25:59–70.

49. Tillery WV, Lucier AC. Round atrophic holes in lattice degeneration—an important cause of aphakic retinal detachment. Trans Am Acad Ophthalmol Otolaryngol 1976;81:509–518.

50. Eisner G. Autoptische spaltlamperuntersuchung des glaskorpers. IV. Der glasskorper an aequatorialen degenerationen. Graefe's Arch Klin Exp Ophthalmol 1973;187:1–4.

51. Morse PH, Sheie HG. Prophylactic cryoretinopexy of retinal breaks. Arch Ophthalmol 1974;92:204–207.

52. Benson WE, Morse PH. The prognosis of retinal detachment due to lattice degeneration. Ann Ophthalmol 1978;10:1097–1200.

53. Tasman WS. Posterior vitreous detachment and peripheral retinal breaks. Trans Am Acad Ophthalmol Otolaryngol 1968;72:217–224.

54. Dumas J. Equatorial chorioretinal lesions predisposing to retinal breaks. Can J Ophthalmol 1966;1:128–133.

55. Davis MD, Segal PP, et al. The Natural Course Followed by the Fellow Eye in Patients with Rhegmatogenous Retinal Detachment. In RC Pruett, DJ Regan (eds), Retina Congress. New York: Appleton-Century-Crofts, 1974:643–659.

56. Benson WE. Retinal Detachment. Diagnosis and Management (2nd ed). Philadephia: Lippincott, 1988:33–52.

57. Michaelson IC. Retinal detachment: clinical evidence of the role of the choroid. Acta XVII Concilium Ophthalmolgicum 1954:392–403.

58. Michels RG, Wilkinson CP, et al. Retinal Detachment. Philadelphia: Mosby, 1990.

59. Ashrafzadeh MT, Schepens CL, et al. Aphakic and phakic retinal detachment. Arch Ophthalmol 1973;89:476–483.

60. Hyams SW, Meir E, et al. Chorioretinal lesions predisposing to retinal detachment. Am J Ophthalmol 1974;78:429–437.

61. Folk JC, Arrindell EL, et al. The fellow eye of patients with phakic lattice retinal detachment. Ophthalmology 1989;96:72–79.

62. Everett WG. The fellow-eye syndrome in retinal detachment. Am J Ophthalmol 1968;56:739–748.

63. Merin S, Feiler V, et al. The fate of the fellow eye in retinal detachment. Am J Ophthalmol 1971;71:477–481.

64. Meyer-Schwickerath G. Light coagulation (translated by SM Drance). St. Louis: Mosby, 1960:56–65.
65. Folk JC, Bennett SR, et al. Prophylactic treatment to the fellow eye of patients with phakic lattice retinal detachment: Analysis of failures and risks of treatment. Retina 1990;10:165–169.
66. Lean JS. Diagnosis and Treatment of Peripheral Retinal Lesions. In WR Freeman (ed), Practical Atlas of Retinal Disease and Therapy. New York: Raven, 1993;12: 211–220.
67. Schepens CL. Part XIV. In Symposium: Preventive treatment of idiopathic and secondary retinal detachment. Acta XVIII Concilium Ophthalmologicum, Belgica, Vol. 1, 1958:1019–1027.
68. Malbran E. Preventive treatment of retinal detachment. Mod Probl Ophthalmol 1966;4:183–192.
69. Spira C. Prevention of Retinal Detachment: Indications and Limitations. In A McPherson (ed), New and Controversial Aspects of Retinal Detachment. New York: Harper & Row, 1968.
70. Boniuk I, Okun E, et al. Xenon photocoagulation versus cryotherapy in the prevention of retinal detachment. Mod Probl Ophthalmol 1974;12:81–92.
71. Okun E, Cibis PA. Photocoagulation in "Limited" Retinal Detachment and Breaks Without Detachment. In A McPherson (ed), New and Controversial Aspects of Retinal Detachment. New York: Harper & Row, 1968:164–172.
72. Tasman W, Jaeger KR. A Retrospective Study of Xenon Photocoagulation and Cryotherapy in the Treatment of Retinal Breaks. In RC Pruett, CD Regan (eds), Retinal Congress. New York: Appleton-Century-Crofts, 1972:557–564.
73. Robertson DM, Norton EWD. Long-term follow-up of treated retinal breaks. Am J Ophthalmol 1973;75:395–404.
74. Benson WE, Morse PH, et al. Late complications following cryotherapy of lattice degeneration. Am J Ophthalmol 1977;84:514–516.

Snail-Track Degeneration

Clinical Description

Snail-track degeneration, also known as *Schneckenspuren*, appears as a glistening white area in the retina that derives its distinctive name from the mucus track left behind by a mollusk. The appearance is sometimes likened to white-without-pressure or frostlike changes on the retina, and other names, such as Milky Way–like and galaxy-like degeneration, probably represent snail-track degeneration. The shape of these lesions can vary from an elongated oval or spindle (Figure 3-82; see also Figure 3-1) to a band that encompasses an entire quadrant. Snail-track degeneration's distinctive white to silver-white glistening appearance and whitish frosting appearance is composed of white dots. During scleral depression, the snail-track lesions appear even whiter, and the full extent of retinal involvement is better appreciated. They are usually found between the equator and the ora serrata; 80% occur two disc diameters anterior to the equator.[1] The lesions seem to be most frequent in the temporal half of the fundus.

The vitreous reveals evidence of fibrillar degeneration and pockets of liquefaction of the vitreous gel (lacunae). Vitreoretinal adhesions over the lesions (particularly at the margins) have been described,[1] but others have found no obvious vitreoretinal adhesions.[2] Some families have snail-track degeneration and significant frequency of myopia.[1]

Many authorities believe that snail-track degeneration is an early form of lattice degeneration that precedes the development of white vessels and pigmentary degeneration. The shape and location of these lesions are similar to those of lattice degeneration, but snail-track degeneration has not been known to turn into a typical latticelike lesion and therefore may be a distinct variant.[3] Also, snail-track degeneration is not found nearly as frequently as lattice degeneration. Bec et al.[4] found that the ultrastructure of snail-track degeneration is distinct from lattice and should not be considered a variant of lattice degeneration.

Histopathology

Snail-track degeneration is characterized by very small, glistening, yellow-white flecks that were first thought to represent cholesterin deposits.[5] Later studies discovered that these particles were microglial cells containing lipoid or lipoprotein material, and the surrounding retina was always primarily or secondarily atrophic.[6]

Clinical Significance

As with lattice degeneration, snail-track degeneration can result in retinal breaks, such as holes,

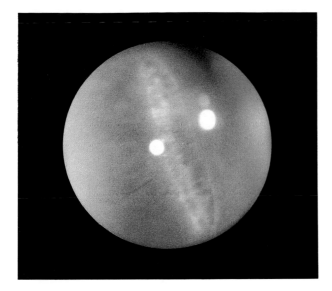

FIGURE 3-82
Snail-track degeneration in the superior temporal fundus just posterior to the ora serrata.

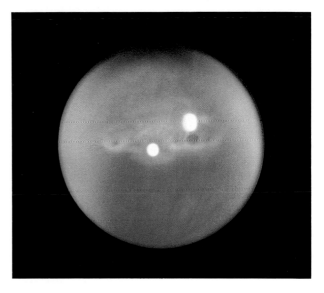

FIGURE 3-83
Fellow eye of that in Figure 3-82 shows a patch of snail-track degeneration of the inferior temporal fundus with two red holes at each end of the lesion with scleral depression. View is through the indirect condensing lens.

but the holes tend to be larger and are more likely to cause a retinal detachment (Figure 3-83). Flap tears are not likely to be associated with this condition.[2] Snail-track degeneration without atrophic holes is generally not treated, unless there is a personal or family history of retinal detachment, high myopia, aphakia, physical sports with sudden head movements, or some vitreoretinal degeneration that predisposes the patient to retinal break formation. When large retinal holes are found with this condition, prophylactic retinopexy may be considered; some retinal specialists preventively treat snail-tracking with holes.[2] Treatment of breaks and retinal detachment is the same as for lattice degeneration.

The prognosis for most patients with snail-track degeneration is good because only a very small percentage of patients develop a retinal detachment. Patients with this condition without retinal breaks should be followed on a routine yearly basis. They should be educated about the symptoms of a retinal tear or detachment and told to return immediately if these symptoms occur. If these patients have pho-topsia, they should have follow-up visits every 2–3 months with binocular indirect ophthalmoscopy. They should return immediately if the symptoms increase in severity, if they notice a curtain invading their vision, or if they experience a loss of vision.

References

1. Aaberg TM, Stevens TR. Snail-track degeneration of the retina. Am J Ophthalmol 1972;73:370–376.
2. Lean JS. Diagnosis and Treatment of Peripheral Retinal Lesions. In WR Freeman (ed), Practical Atlas of Retinal Disease and Therapy. New York: Raven, 1993;12:211–220.
3. Shukla M, Ahuja OP. A possible relationship between lattice and snail track degenerations of the retina. Am J Ophthalmol 1981;92:482–485.
4. Bec P, Malecaze F, et al. Lattice degeneration of the peripheral retina: Ultrastructural study. Ophthalmologica 1985;191:107–113
5. Gonin J. Le decollement de la retine pathogenie-traitement. Lausanne, Switzerland: Librarie Payot, 1934.
6. Daicker B. Zur kenntnis von substrat und bedeutung der sogennanten schneckenspuren der retina. Ophthalmologica 1972;165:360–365.

Peripheral Retinal Excavation

Clinical Description

Peripheral retinal excavations, also known as retinal pits, erosion, and rarefaction, are small, round to oval depressions in the retina (Figure 3-84).[1, 2] They are a developmental variation of the peripheral retina, like enclosed ora bays and meridional folds. Developmental variations of the peripheral retina

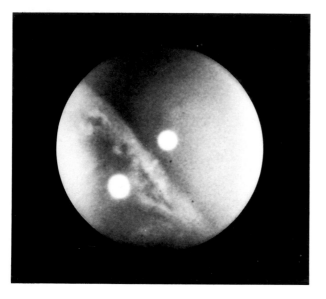

FIGURE 3-84
Areas of vitreous base excavations with evidence of vitreous traction at the nasal ora serrata seen through the indirect condensing lens with scleral depression.

are found in approximately 20% of all eyes and share common features, such as presence at birth, tendency to occur symmetrically in both eyes, persistence throughout life, and association with other developmental anomalies.[3] They are most easily seen with scleral depression during indirect ophthalmoscopy. There is little white-with-pressure on scleral depression, and small white flecks or tags may be visible on their surface. The excavation appears transparent even though there is erosion of the inner half of the retina.

The retinal vessels look normal in color and size, but their course is altered when they dip down into an excavated area. The lesions generally occur within a region that is about four disc diameters posterior to the ora serrata and frequently in the superior nasal quadrant. Peripheral excavations tend to be found in a straight line directly posterior to an enclosed ora bay, a meridional fold, or meridional complex (see Enclosed Ora Bay and Meridional Folds and Complexes). They occur in 10% of the population, are bilateral in 43% of cases, and therefore are present in 8% of all eyes. Two or more excavations were found in one-half of the eyes.[4]

Histopathology

Peripheral retinal excavations show a loss of the inner retinal layers, but the outer sensory layers, the pigment epithelium, and the underlying choroid are intact (Figure 3-85).

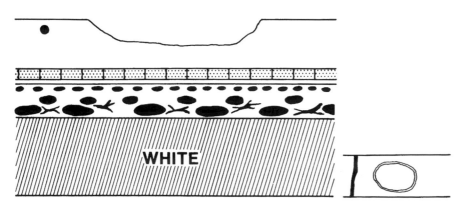

WHITE

FIGURE 3-85
Peripheral retinal excavation shows degeneration of the inner layers of the retina.

Clinical Significance

The peripheral excavation may be mistaken for a retinal hole; however, a full-thickness retinal hole is red and not transparent as is the case with most excavations. This condition may predispose an eye to full-thickness retinal breaks after a posterior vitreous detachment.[5] Because retinal breaks do occur frequently in areas posterior to meridional folds,[6] it is possible that an excavation could progress to the formation of a full-thickness hole. Therefore, if a rhegmatogenous retinal detachment is found, a thorough examination during ophthalmoscopy is suggested to determine whether there is an associated retinal break with a developmental anomaly, such as a retinal excavation. No treatment is usually necessary for a peripheral retinal excavation.

References

1. Meyer E, Kurz GH. Retinal pits. Arch Ophthalmol 1963;70;640–646.
2. Spencer LM, Foos RY. Paravascular vitreoretinal attachments. Arch Ophthalmol 1970;84:557–564.
3. Spencer LM, Foos RY, et al. Meridional folds and meridional complexes of the peripheral retina. Trans Am Ophthalmol Otolaryngol 1969;73:204.
4. Glasgow BJ, Foos RY, et al. Degenerative Diseases of the Peripheral Retina. In TD Duane, EA Jaeger (eds), Clinical Ophthalmology. Vol. 3. Philadelphia: Harper & Row, 1993;26:1–29.
5. Goldbaum MH. Retinal Examination and Surgery. In GA Peyman, DR Sanders, et al. (eds), Principles and Practice of Ophthalmology. Vol. 2. Philadelphia: Saunders, 1980;15:1023.
6. Dumas J, Schepens CL. Chorioretinal lesions predisposing to retinal breaks. Am J Ophthalmol 1966;61:620–630.

Snowflake Vitreoretinal Degeneration

Clinical Description

Snowflake vitreoretinal degeneration appears as tiny yellow-white spots in the far peripheral retina (Figures 3-86 and 3-87). The spots are often brilliant and almost seem crystalline as light reflects off them, especially during scleral depression. Their appearance seems to be identical to that of the snowflakes found in retinoschisis. The superficial layers of the retina are involved, and retinal transparency is lost. The anterior margin of the degeneration can extend to the ora serrata, and the posterior margin tends to disappear gently into the retina, usually just anterior to the equator. The posterior margin is poorly demarcated and irregular in shape. If there is involvement posterior to the equator, it is not unusual to see the snowflakes distributed radially along retinal vessels. The distribution of the degeneration can be circumferential, sectorial, or in oval to elongated patches with their long axes parallel to the ora serrata. The last configuration is very similar in appearance to snail-track degeneration. This condition should be differentiated from peripheral cystoid degeneration (Table 3-11).

Snowflake degeneration is located most frequently in the superior temporal quadrant (95%) and least frequently in the inferior nasal quadrant (68%).[1] Yet other reports suggest that there may be a predilection for the inferior retina or for even distribution throughout the entire circumference of the retina.[2] Some cases demonstrate sheathing of the major peripheral retinal vessels in the area of degeneration but not the criss-crossing pattern seen in typical lattice degeneration of the retina. Sheathing of the retinal vessels on or near the optic disc can occur. Other retinal findings include attenuated arterioles, occlusion of small vessels, white-without-pressure, lattice degeneration, and annular macular pigmentary defects. Pigment clumps of irregular or round shapes (sometimes bone spicule in shape) are commonly seen and seem to develop late in the progression of the disease, as do the sheathed vessels.[2] The pigment clumping can occur slightly posterior or within the degeneration.[1, 3] Neovascular retinal tufts adjacent to areas of snowflake degeneration have been described in a few patients.[4]

Vitreous changes consist of fibrillar degeneration and liquefaction of the gel. Fine vitreous strands float in the liquefied vitreous above the degenerated areas of the retina, but recognizable vitreous degenerative changes may not be present in this condition.[2] Visual field studies have shown peripheral defects more pronounced in the inferior field, showing irregular annular scotomas.[5, 6] Electroretinographic studies can be abnormal, a more typical finding in the late stages of the disease. The electroretinogram may show abnormalities in both the a-wave and b-wave, the electro-oculogram may show decreased light-to-dark ratios, and dark adaptation may show elevated rod thresholds. One author has suggested that the similarities of these electroretinographic findings to those of retinitis pigmentosa may indicate that snowflake degeneration is a variant of retinitis pigmentosa.[5, 6] Myopia is a common finding.[1] Heredity also plays a role in snowflake degeneration; transmission appears to be autosomal dominant.[1, 2, 4, 6]

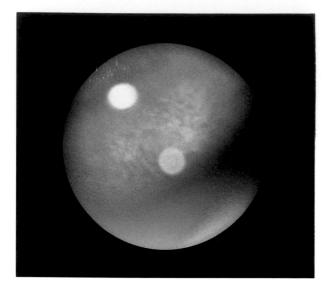

FIGURE 3-86
Snowflake vitreoretinal degeneration in the inferior far peripheral retina seen through the indirect condensing lens.

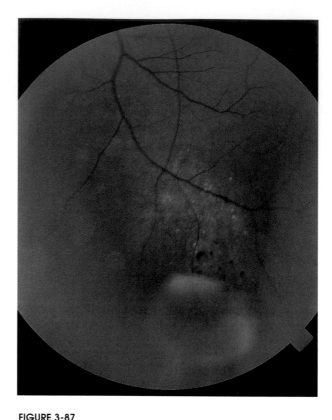

FIGURE 3-87
Snowflake vitreoretinal degeneration around retinal vessel with pigment clumping.

Histopathology

Snowflake degeneration is composed of granular deposits that are up to 100–200 μ in size and are found in areas of localized retinal thickening.[2]

Clinical Significance

Snowflake vitreoretinal degeneration can lead to the formation of retinal breaks, such as holes and tears. Retinal detachment may follow the development of these breaks; in one family, 17% of the eyes that were affected with this condition had a retinal detachment.[1] The prognosis for successful reattachment surgery is generally poor; therefore, prophylaxis with laser therapy or cryopexy of retinal breaks in snowflake degeneration is recommended.

Table 3-11. Snowflake Retinal Degeneration vs. Peripheral Cystoid Degeneration

Snowflake Retinal Degeneration	Peripheral Cystoid Degeneration
Flat	Flat
White specks and sometimes associated pigment spots	White with dark circular spots within the involved area
Retinal breaks may be present	Retinal atrophic partial or full thickness holes may be present
Usually located slightly away from the ora serrata to the equator	Located directly adjacent to the ora serrata

References

1. Hirose T, Lee KY, et al. Snowflake degeneration in hereditary vitreoretinal degeneration. Am J Ophthalmol 1974;77:143–153.
2. Robertson DM, Link TP, et al. Snowflake degeneration of the retina. Ophthalmology 1982;89:1513–1517.
3. Schepens CL. Retinal Detachment and Allied Diseases. Philadelphia: Saunders, 1983:614–615.
4. Pollack A, Uchenik D, et al. Prophylactic laser photocoagulation in hereditary snowflake vitreoretinal degeneration. Arch Ophthalmol 1983;101:1536–1539.
5. Hirose T, Wolf E, et al. Retinal functions in snowflake degeneration. Ann Ophthalmol 1980;12:1135–1146.
6. Chen CJ, Everett TK, et al. Snowflake degeneration: An independent entity or a variant of retinitis pigmentosa? Southern Med J 1986;79:1216–1223.

Hereditary Hyaloideoretinopathies: Wagner's Disease and Stickler's Hereditary Vitreoretinal Degeneration

Clinical Description

Hereditary hyaloideoretinopathies are potentially blinding inherited disorders manifested by abnormal-appearing vitreous gel and associated retinal changes. These syndromes include Wagner's disease,[1, 2] Stickler's syndrome,[3, 4] Goldmann-Favre syndrome,[5] and erosive vitreoretinopathy.[6]

Wagner's Disease

Wagner's disease was first describe by Wagner in 1938 in a Swiss family with myopia, cataracts, vitreous liquefaction, retinal vessel changes, and RPE changes.[1] This family had been followed for years by other ophthalmologists, during which time only one member had had a rhegmatogenous retinal detachment.[2, 7, 8] Wagner's hereditary vitreoretinal degeneration, also called hyaloideoretinalis hereditaria and Wagner's disease, is a rare ocular condition characterized by marked vitreoretinal changes. Wagner's disease is considered an abnormality in the secondary vitreous.[1, 9–11] It is an autosomal dominant trait with 100% penetrance, therefore, 50% of offspring will have the disease.[1, 12] As with erosive vitreoretinopa-

thy, Wagner's disease has no known systemic manifestations and can be distinguished from Stickler's disease by the absence of such findings as cleft palate or lip, joint pains, and radiologic abnormalities.

Wagner's disease demonstrates fibrous condensation of the vitreous, consisting of whitish bands and membranes that cross a vitreous cavity (Figure 3-88), together with extensive liquefaction of the central and posterior portions of the vitreous body, making it appear optically dark.[13–15] The resultant large vitreous lacuna appears as an optically empty space that may contain free-floating vitreous fibers. A thin layer of cortical gel along the retinal surface may have vitreous strands attached to it. The cortex may be replaced by a transparent membrane that remains translucent and may float above the retina in the vitreous.[13, 16, 17] This membrane can develop holes, but because there are no blood vessels in the membrane, it can be easily differentiated from a retinal detachment with holes. The vitreous membranes can exert considerable traction on the peripheral retina, and so it is not unusual to find white-without-pressure, meridional folds, and retinal breaks. Posterior vitreous detachment generally does not develop in Wagner's disease.[16] Maumenee has described anthro-ophthalmopathies in which

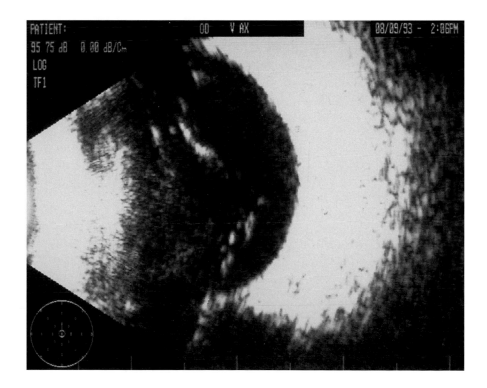

FIGURE 3-88
B-scan ultrasonogram of vitreous bands in a patient with Wagner's disease.

vitreous liquefaction, collagen condensation, and vitreous syneresis is associated with dysplastic connective tissue disease that primarily involves the joints. It may well be that Wagner's disease is included in these type II collagen diseases described by Maumenee.[17] Wagner's syndrome is an allelic disorder linked to chromosome 5q13–14.[18]

Early fundus changes consist of prominent choroidal tessellation that is seen as elongated patches of chorioretinal atrophy (see Chorioretinal Atrophy earlier in this chapter).[1, 10, 13, 14, 19] Small clumps of pigment scattered throughout the peripheral retina are often found along retinal vessels, especially veins, which can give the appearance of retinitis pigmentosa.[1, 13, 14, 20] In one study, retinal pigmentation was present in 61% of cases.[21] With time, these vessels become sheathed and obliterated.[1, 13, 17, 19, 20] Lattice degeneration and peripheral cystoid degeneration are frequently found and may be a predisposing factor for retinal breaks. Therefore, even mild ocular trauma may result in a retinal break in patients with Wagner's disease.

Other ocular findings associated with Wagner's disease are a subnormal electroretinogram, night blindness, retinoschisis, optic atrophy, contraction of the visual fields, glaucoma, myopia, and cataracts.[12, 13, 19, 20, 22] Early punctate lens opacities are seen in patients younger than 22 years of age, and cataract surgery is not uncommon after the age of 40 years.[10, 13, 14, 17, 19] Electroretinograms are often moderately depressed,[13, 19] and dark adaptation may be abnormal.[1, 11] The frequency of myopia is high (84% of cases).[13] No extraocular components have been identified in Wagner's disease[2]; however, there have been reports of patients with this type of vitreoretinopathy demonstrating flat faces, cleft palate, arthritis, and hypermobility of joints. The term *Stickler's syndrome* is usually used to describe these patients.[3]

Wagner's disease is a slowly progressive, relentlessly degenerative condition. Changes occur bilaterally, but they may be more advanced in one eye than the other. In the early stages, the patient is often asymptomatic, and a routine fundus examination may first uncover the disease. Signs of the disease have been found in patients under 10 years of age.[1] Usually, it is discovered only when the patient seeks attention for decreased vision secondary to a cataract or retinal detachment.

ciates in 1965.[3] This syndrome has an incidence of about 1 in 10,000.[23] It is an autosomal dominant trait with 100% penetrance[24] or incomplete penetrance[25, 26] and variable expressivity and is caused by a mutation in the COL2A1 gene on chromosome 12q14.3.[24, 27–31] Because collagen type II is the most common protein of collagen and is found in the vitreous gel, it may be that mutations in type II procollagen is found at COL2A1.[17, 32] Stickler's syndrome is the most common of the hereditary vitreoretinopathies, and orofacial, skeletal, and auditory abnormalities are found in almost every patient with the syndrome. These patients are identified by marfanoid skeletal habitus and orofacial and ocular manifestations. A subgroup with short stature, Weill-Marchesani habitus, thoracic kyphoscoliosis, and genu valgum has been identified. Systemic findings include progressive sensorineural hearing loss, cleft palate, mandibular hypoplasia, hypotonia, and relative muscle hypoplasia.[17, 26, 31] In cases involving cleft palate, there may be chronic otitis leading to conductive hearing loss.[24] The skeletal findings accepted as characteristic of Stickler's syndrome are radiologic evidence of flat epiphyses, broad metaphyses, and especially spondyloepiphyseal dysplasia; these conditions can lead to hypomotility or hypermotility.[3, 17, 24, 31, 33, 34] The joint problems can lead to arthritis developing in individuals in their 40s.[20]

Ocular abnormalities include vitreous changes (vitreous liquefaction, fibrillar collagen condensation) and retinal findings (perivascular latticelike degeneration in the peripheral retina, giant tears, and retinal detachment). The lattice lesions are commonly seen along blood vessels and have a radial orientation in the fundus. Stickler's syndrome patients have difficulty with night vision, visual field defects, and abnormal electroretinographic, electro-oculogram, and visual evoked response findings.[18, 31] There is an incidence of myopia over 10 diopters in 72% of these patients,[34] and the degree of myopia is higher than is typically found in Wagner's disease. It is most likely that high myopia and the perivascular lattice degeneration are responsible for the high incidence of retinal detachment in these patients. Other ocular findings include glaucoma; cataracts; amblyopia; and strabismus, membrane, or iris root anomalies in the anterior chamber.[12, 25, 31, 34]

Stickler's Disease

Stickler's disease is a hereditary vitreoretinal degeneration that was first described by Stickler and asso-

Erosive Vitreoretinopathy

In 1994, Brown et al.[6] described a new entity labeled erosive vitreoretinopathy. It has a greater incidence of rhegmatogenous retinal detachment and a poorer visual prognosis than Wagner's disease. Erosive vitreoretinopathy has no known systemic manifestations and can be distinguished from Stickler syndrome by the absence of such findings as cleft palate or lip, joint pains, or radiologic abnormalities. The genetic defect that produces the disease is found on chromosome 5q13–14, as with Wagner's disease, and it appears that the different clinical features in these two diseases arise from different mutations in a single gene or from mutations in two different but tightly linked genes.[18]

Goldmann-Favre Vitreoretinal Dystrophy

Goldmann-Favre disease is an autosomal recessive vitreoretinopathy. This disease was first described by Goldmann in 1957.[35] The ocular findings include chorioretinal atrophy, peripheral retinoschisis, vitreous degeneration with veils, and epiretinal membranes.[36] Other findings are microcystic macular changes (macular schisis), cataracts, night blindness, nonrecordable electroretinogram early in the disease, and visual field defects similar to retinitis pigmentosa.[5, 9, 17, 37, 38] Francois et al.[39] described the condition as a vitreous syneresis with fibrillar degeneration with strand formation and punctate deposits. The retinal changes show bone spicule hyperpigmentation characteristic of retinitis pigmentosa along with attenuated blood vessels.[5, 38] Fluorescein angiography shows the presence of cystoid macular edema and vascular occlusive disease demonstrating leakage in areas of peripheral retinoschisis.[5] The cystoid macular edema is believed to occur as a result of vitreous degeneration causing posterior vitreous traction of the macula.[40] Organized vitreous attaches to the areas of peripheral retinoschisis.[5, 11, 38]

Histopathology

In Wagner's disease, there is a preretinal membrane of unknown origin that is thickest at the equator.[41] This membrane is sometimes coated with a unicellular layer also of unknown origin that occasionally has a fine network of capillaries. Vitreous strands can be found extending from the membrane into the vitreous cavity. The vitreous body has extensive liquefaction in the central and posterior regions. There are localized areas of chorioretinal atrophy and pigment proliferation. Peripheral retinal blood vessels are decreased in

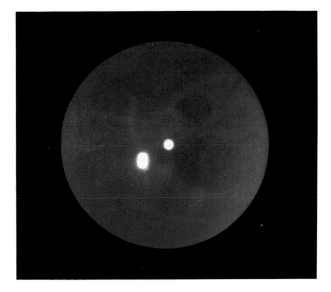

FIGURE 3-89
Wagner's vitreoretinal degeneration shows two large retinal tears on one side and lattice degeneration on the opposite side. View is of the superior fundus through the indirect condensing lens.

number and have thick walls. The choroid is atrophic-looking and heavily pigmented. In Goldmann-Favre disease, the outer nuclear layer is attenuated and photoreceptors are absent, which indicates that it is primarily a retinal dystrophy.[38]

Clinical Significance

The two most clinically significant aspects of Wagner's disease are cataracts and retinal breaks with detachment (Figure 3-89); in Stickler's syndrome they are breaks and detachment. Cataracts are found in more than 50–75% of Wagner's cases that develop after adolescence.[13, 19, 21] They are often posterior subcapsular lens opacities, but nuclear sclerosis and mature cataracts also occur. After the age of 40, nearly all patients have cataracts. These are frequently mature and obscure the fundus.

Retinal breaks with or without detachment occur in 75% of the eyes with Wagner's disease, usually located in the superotemporal quadrant.[42] The incidence of rhegmatogenous detachment has been found to be uncommon in Wagner's disease by some[18] and not uncommon by others.[42] If the traction from the vitreous membrane is on a small localized area of the retina, an operculated tear or a horseshoe tear may result. If the membrane adheres circumferentially to the peripheral retina, traction may lead to the formation of a giant tear. The prognosis for retinal repair is poor because of marked vitreous degeneration with traction, extensive vitreous liquefaction, multiple breaks, large breaks, and cataracts that may obscure the fundus. In Stickler's syndrome and erosive vitreoretinopathy, the incidence of retinal detachment is approximately 50%.[18, 43]

Treatment of small retinal breaks without retinal detachment or extensive vitreous traction is by cryopexy or photocoagulation. In the presence of a retinal detachment or extensive vitreous traction, scleral buckling with an encircling band and cryotherapy are the procedures of choice. The vitreous membranes sometimes prevent settling of the retinal detachment and therefore may require a pars plana vitrectomy.[13, 15] One study found the surgical success rate for reattachment to be 68%.[13]

Differential diagnosis includes Goldmann-Favre's vitreoretinal degeneration and congenital retinoschisis. Other entities include Turner's, Marfan's, and Ehlers-Danlos syndromes.

References

1. Wagner H. Ein bisher unbekanntes erbleiden des auges (digeneratio hyaloideoretinalis hereditaria), biobachtet im Kanton Zurich. Klin Monatsbl Augenheilkd 1938;100: 840–857.
2. Maumenee IH, Stoll HU, et al. The Wagner syndrome versus hereditary arthroophthalmopathy. Trans Am Ophthalmol Soc 1982;81:349–365.
3. Stickler GB, Belau PG, et al. Hereditary progressive arthroophthalmopathy. Mayo Clin Prog 1965;40:443–455.
4. Weingeist TA, Hermsen V, et al. Ocular and Systemic Manifestations of Stickler's Syndrome: A Preliminary Report. In E Cotlier, IH Maumenee, ER Berman (eds), Genetic Eye Diseases: Retinitis Pigmentosa and Other Inherited Eye Disorders. New York: Liss, 1982:539–560.
5. Fishman GA, Jampol LM, et al. Diagnostic feature of the Favre-Goldmann syndrome. Br J Ophthalmol 1976;60: 345–353.
6. Brown DM, Kimura AE, et al. Erosive vitreoretinopathy: A new clinical entity. Ophthalmology 1994;101:694–704.
7. Bohringer HR, Dieterle P, et al. Aur klinik und pathologie der degeneratio hyaloideo-retinalis hereditaria (Wagner). Ophthalmologica 1960;139:330–338.
8. Ricci A. Clinique et transmission genetique des differentes formes de degenerescences vitreo-retiniennes. Ophthalmologica 1960;139:338–343.
9. Apple DJ, Rabb MF. Ocular Pathology. Clinical Applications and Self-Assessment (3rd ed). St Louis: Mosby 1985.
10. Van Nouhuys CE. Chorioretinal dysplasia in young subjects with Wagner's vitreoretinal degeneration. Int Ophthalmol 1981;3:67–77.
11. Sebag J. The Vitreous Structure, Function, and Pathobiology. New York: Springer-Verlag, 1989.
12. Spencer WH (ed). Ophthalmic Pathology. An Atlas and Textbook (3rd ed). Philadelphia: Saunders, 1983.
13. Hirose T, Lee KY, et al. Wagner's hereditary vitreoretinal degeneration and retinal detachment. Arch Ophthalmol 1973;89:176–185.
14. Carr RE, Siegel IM. The vitreo-tapeto-retinal degenerations. Arch Ophthalmol 1970;84:436–445.
15. Brown GC, Tasman WS. Vitrectomy in Wagner's vitreoretinal degeneration. Am J Ophthalmol 1978;86:485–488.
16. Tolentino FI, Schepens CL, et al. Vitreoretinal Disorders: Diagnosis and Management. Philadelphia: Saunders, 1976;13:242–249.
17. Maumenee IH. Vitreoretinal degeneration as a sign of generalized connective tissue diseases. Am J Ophthalmol 1979;88:432–449.
18. Brown DM, Graemiger RA, et al. Genetic linkage of Wagner disease and erosive vitreoretinopathy to chromosome 5q13–14. Arch Ophthalmol 1995;113:671–675.
19. Manning LM. Wagner's hereditary vitreoretinal degeneration. Aust J Ophthalmol 1980;8:29–33.
20. Alexander RL, Shea M. Clinical sciences. Wagner's disease. Arch Ophthalmol 1965;74:310–318.
21. Tasman W. The Vitreous. In TD Duane, EA Jaeger (eds), Clinical Ophthalmology. Vol. 3. Philadelphia: Harper & Row, 1980;38:10–11.
22. Anderson JR. Anterior dialysis of retina. Disinsertion or avulsion at ora serrata. Br J Ophthalmol 1932;16:641, 705.
23. Pyeritz RE. Heritable and Developmental Disorders of Connective Tissue and Bone. In DJ McCarty (ed), Arthritis and Allied Conditions: A Textbook of Rheumatology. Philadelphia: Lea & Febiger, 1989:1323–1359.
24. Hall JG, Herrod H. The Stickler syndrome presenting as a dominantly inherited cleft palate and blindness. J Med Genet 1975;12:397–400.
25. Nielsen CE. Stickler's syndrome. Acta Ophthalmol (Kbh) 1981;59:286–295.
26. Morse PH. Vitreoretinal Disease (2nd ed). Chicago: Year Book, 1989.
27. Francomano CA, Liberfarb RM, et al. The Stickler syndrome. Genomics 1987;1:293–296.
28. Ahmad NN, Ala-Kokko L, et al. Stop codon in the procollagen II gene (COL2A1) in a family with the Stickler syndrome (arthroophthalmopathy). Proc Natl Acad Sci U S A 1991;88:6624–6627.
29. Brown DM, Nichols BE, et al. Procollagen II gene mutation in stickler syndrome. Arch Ophthalmol 1992;110: 1589–1593.
30. Ashmad NN, Dimascio J, et al. Stickler syndrome. A mutation in the nonhelical 3' end of type II procollagen gene. Arch Ophthalmol 1995;113:1454–1457.
31. Blair NP, Albert DM, et al. Hereditary progressive arthroophthalmopathy of Stickler. Am J Ophthalmol 1979;88: 876–888.
32. Kuhn K. The Classical Collagens: Types I, II and III. In R Mayne, RE Burgeson (eds), Structure and Function of Collagen Types. New York: Academic, 1987:1–42.
33. Optiz JM, France T, et al. The Strickler syndrome. N Engl J Med 1972;286:546–546.
34. Herrmann J, France TD, et al. The Stickler syndrome (hereditary arthro-ophthalmopathy). Birth Defects 1975; 11:76–103.
35 Goldmann H. Biomicroscopie du corps vitre et du fond de l'oeil. Bull Mem Soc Fr Ophthalmol 1957;70:265–272.
36. Frave M. A propos de deux cas de degenerescence hyaloideo-retinienne. Ophthalmologica 1958;135:604–609.

37. Carr RE, Heckenlively JR. In TD Duane, EA Jaeger (eds), Clinical Ophthalmology. Vol. 3. Philadelphia: Harper & Row, 1986;24:11.
38. Peyman GA, Fishman GA, et al. Histopathology of Goldmann-Favre syndrome obtained by full-thickness eye-wall biopsy. Ann Ophthalmol 1977;9:479–484.
39. Francois J, de Rouck A, et al. Degenerescence hyaloideo-tapeto-retinienne de Goldmann-Favre. Ophthalmologica 1974;168:81–96.
40. Sebag J. Vitreous Pathology. In TD Duane, EA Jaeger (eds), Clinical Ophthalmology. Vol. 3. Philadelphia: Harper & Row, 1992;39:3–4.

41. Kraushar MF. Hereditary, Developmental and Congenital Disorders Affecting the Retina, Choroid and Vitreous. In PH Morse (ed), Vitreoretinal Disease: A Manual for Diagnosis and Treatment. Chicago: Year Book, 1979; 11:349.
42. Schepens CL. Retinal Detachment and Allied Diseases. Philadelphia: Saunders, 1983; 27:599–608.
43. Spencer WH. Vitreous. In WH Spencer (ed), Ophthalmic Pathology: An Atlas and Text. Vol. 2. Philadelphia: Saunders, 1985:548–588.

Chorioretinal Scar

Clinical Description

Chorioretinal scars are the result of an inflammatory process in the choroid and retina, usually associated with trauma or infection. They are white fibrotic areas in the fundus, often with pigmented margins from reactive pigment proliferation and migration (Figure 3-90; see also Figure 3-13).[1] These scars can be found in any region of the fundus and are frequently close to retinal blood vessels. The vitreous is often firmly attached to the scar as a result of the inflammatory reaction. Fairly dense vitreous bands often travel from the surface of the scar into the vitreous (Figure 3-91). The resultant scarring can result in contraction with pulling of retinal vessels into the scar (Figure 3-92) or dragging the disc or macula toward it. Intraocular foreign bodies are commonly associated with scarring (Figure 3-92 and 3-93).

Males are more likely to have chorioretinal scars because they have a higher incidence of ocular trauma.[2] Males and females are probably equally likely to have postinfective chorioretinal scars. Older patients have a higher incidence of these scars because they have had more time to be exposed to trauma.

Histopathology

There is destruction of the retinal and choroidal tissue, with fibrotic tissue replacing it. The margins of the scar may demonstrate reactive pigment epithelial hyperplasia, and pigment migration can be found in the scar and adjacent retina (Figure 3-94). Usually, only the choriocapillaris and the inner layers of the choroidal vessels are involved in the destructive process, except in a toxoplasmosis scar, where the choroid is totally destroyed, leaving a view of the white underlying sclera.

Clinical Significance

Because scarring is the healing phase of some inflammatory event, the scar is generally stable and quiescent. Rarely, a retinal tear or detachment is associated with a chorioretinal scar after a posterior vitreous detachment. The vitreous attachment to the chorioretinal scar may be extremely firm, much more adherent than the vitreous attachment to the normal retinal surface. In a PVD, the vitreous remains adherent to the scar but detaches itself from

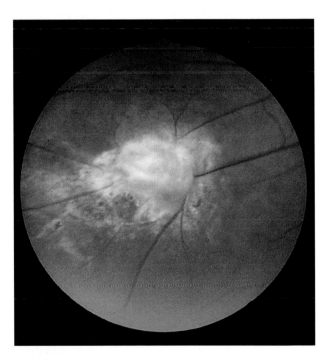

FIGURE 3-90
Chorioretinal scar from a perforating foreign body in the mid-periphery of the fundus. Note the gliotic scar and the reactive pigment proliferation and migration. Contraction of the gliotic mass has pulled the retinal vessels toward the scar.

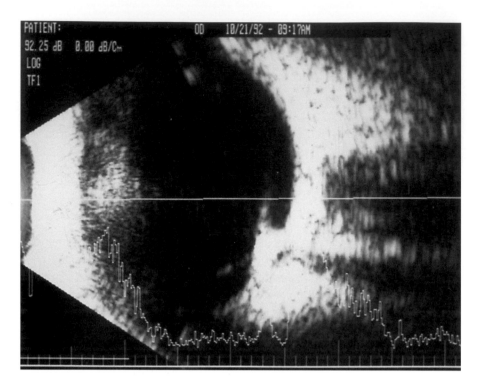
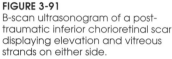

FIGURE 3-91
B-scan ultrasonogram of a post-traumatic inferior chorioretinal scar displaying elevation and vitreous strands on either side.

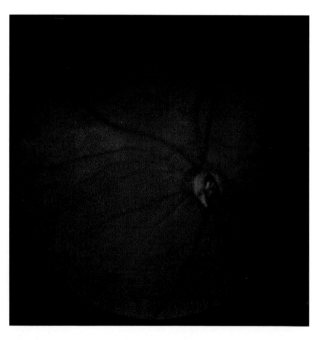

FIGURE 3-92
Perforating metallic foreign body produced a retinal scar which contracted and pulled the retinal vessels towards it.

the retina around the scar. This firm attachment with traction may lead to the formation of a retinal tear at the edge of the scar that can be either round or horseshoe-shaped. Occasionally, the break can be in the form of an operculum that contains the entire scar, and sometimes the scar can be seen on the flap of a horseshoe tear.

If the scar is secondary to an infection, such as *Toxoplasmosis gondii*,[3] histoplasmosis capsulatum,[4, 5] or cytomegalovirus retinitis secondary to AIDS,[6] there may be future inflammatory scarring episodes. In the case of toxoplasmosis, the sites of reactivation occur either at the edge or at a short distance away from the original scar. Vision may be reduced by the associated vitritis or cystoid macular edema caused by the retinal inflammation[7] or secondary to a retinal detachment.[8] Histoplasmosis can reactivate in any part of the fundus (9–16% of patients develop new histoplasmic spots),[9–11] and sometimes it can occur in the macular area. Reactivation in the macular area may result in a subretinal neovascular membrane that can bleed and subsequently scar, thus resulting in a loss of central vision. Cytomegalovirus retinitis is found in 15–40% of patients with AIDS,[12–15] and up to 22% of these patients treated with ganciclovir develop a retinal detachment.[16] Chorioretinal scars are asymptomatic (except if they occur in the macula) and may become symptomatic if there is reactivation.

Early detection of scars due to systemic infection can allow for an early diagnosis of certain conditions. The patient should be educated about possible future complications. Patients with a chorioretinal scar should have routine eye examinations with pupillary dilation. The prognosis is good for most of these scars because they are stable and quiescent; therefore, a failure to detect is usually of no consequence. If the scar is the result of some under-

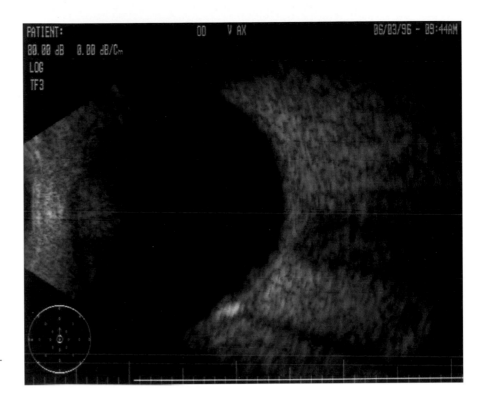

FIGURE 3-93
B-scan ultrasonogram of a foreign body embedded in the inferior posterior eye wall from a mortar explosion in World War II.

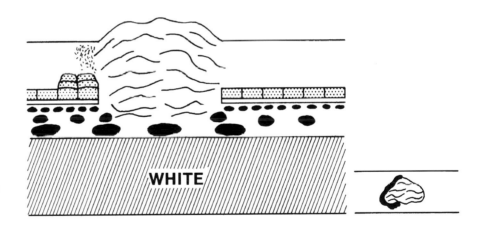

FIGURE 3-94
Chorioretinal scar shows hyperplasia of the pigment epithelium, pigment migration, and scar tissue from the retina to the middle of the choroid.

lying chronic systemic infection, however, failure to detect could delay the diagnosis, which might result in untoward ocular complications, such as loss of vision from macular edema or scarring.

References

1. Foos RY. Anatomy and pathologic aspects of the vitreous body. Trans Am Acad Ophthalmol Otolaryngol 1973;77: 171–183.
2. Schepens CL. Retinal Detachment and Allied Diseases. Philadelphia: Saunders, 1983.
3. Doft BH, Gass JDM. Punctate outer retinal toxoplasmosis. Arch Ophthalmol 1986;103:1332–1336.
4. Smith RE, Gamley JP, et al. Presumed ocular histoplasmosis: Patterns of peripheral and peripapillary scarring in persons with nonmacular disease. Arch Ophthalmol 1972;87:251–257.
5. Becker M, Tessler HH. In TD Duane, EA Jaeger (eds), Clinical Ophthalmology. Vol. 4. Philadelphia: Harper & Row, 1991;48:1–10.
6. Freeman WR. Infectious Retinitis. In TD Duane, EA Jaeger (eds), Clinical Ophthalmology. Vol. 4. Philadelphia: Harper & Row, 1992;45:1–29.
7. Schlaegel TF Jr, Webber JC. The macula in ocular toxoplasmosis. Arch Ophthalmol 1984;102:697–698.
8. Braunstein RA, Gass JDM. Branch artery obstruction caused by acute toxoplasmosis. Arch Ophthalmol 1980; 98:512–513.

9. Schlaegel TF. The natural history of histo spots in the disc and macular area. Int Ophthalmol Clin 1972;15:19–28.

10. Lewis LM, Van Newkirk MR, et al. Follow-up study of presumed ocular histoplasmosis syndrome. Ophthalmology 1980;87:393–399.

11. Watzke RC, Klaussen R. The long term course of multifocal choroiditis (presumed ocular histoplasmosis). Am J Ophthalmol 1981;91:750–760.

12. Henderly DE, Freeman WR, et al. Cytomegalovirus retinitis and response to therapy with ganciclovir. Ophthalmology 1987;94:425–434.

13. Freeman WR, Lerner CW, et al. A prospective study of the ophthalmologic findings in the acquired immune deficiency syndrome. Am J Ophthalmol 1984;97:133–142.

14. Holland GN, Pepose JS, et al. Acquired immune deficiency syndrome: Ocular manifestations. Ophthalmology 1983;90:859–873.

15. Palestine AG, Rodriguez MM, et al. Ophthalmic involvement in acquired immune deficiency syndrome. Ophthalmology 1984,91:1092–1099.

16. Freeman WR, Henderly DE, et al. Prevalence, pathophysiology, and treatment of rhegmatogenous retinal detachment in treated cytomegalovirus retinitis. Am J Ophthalmol 1987;103:527–536.

Pars Planitis (Intermediate Uveitis)

Clinical Description

Pars planitis, also known as intermediate uveitis (IU), cyclitis, chronic cyclitis, basal uveitis and peripheral uveitis, is a chronic inflammatory disease of the peripheral retina and pars plana ciliaris. The incidence of pars planitis in two eye clinic populations was reported to be 7.6% and 8%,[1, 2] although the incidence in the general population would be expected to be much smaller. Of patients referred for uveitis, 4.3–15.4% have pars planitis.[1–6] The disease seems to occur more commonly in Caucasians than in African-Americans.[2, 4, 6] There have been reports of familial occurrence of pars planitis.[6–10]

There appears to be no gender predilection,[11] but one report found a 2:1 preponderance for males.[12] It has been found that 66–80% of patients have bilateral involvement.[2, 8, 9, 13–15] It begins at an early age and can be either asymptomatic or minimally symptomatic, with such complaints as asthenopia, floaters, occasional mild ocular injection, and blurred vision. Pars planitis usually affects children and young adults and seldom occurs before age 5 years or after 30 years of age; most cases develop in the 20s.[2, 11] Children do not often complain of a slow progressive loss of vision, especially if it involves the upper visual field, and usually the disease is not discovered until extensive damage has already occurred. Approximately 16% of children with uveitis have pars planitis.[6] Nearly half of all patients have serious loss of vision at the time of diagnosis.[13] Most investigators have found that the incidence of pars planitis is higher in Caucasians than in African-Americans,[6, 13] and the disease has been found in Hispanics.[4, 6]

Patients with pars planitis have either no or minimal inflammation, seldom form posterior synechia; pupillary block or seclusion do not occur, and there are usually inflammatory cells in the vitreous.[2, 16]

Symptoms are generally that of blurred vision and floaters, and there are seldom complaints of pain, redness, or photophobia.[16] Often patients with the disease are totally asymptomatic, and the condition is discovered on a routine eye examination.[13, 15] In the anterior chamber, aqueous flare is usually low grade and cells rarely greater than 2+,with more cells found posterior to the lens than in the aqueous.[17] There are no keratic precipitates (KP), but there may be a fine dusting of cellular debris and fibrin on the endothelium of the cornea. If KP are numerous, the diagnosis of IU should be reconsidered.[16] Band keratopathy may develop in patients who acquired the disease in childhood or the early teens.[2, 6]

Early fundus changes consist of a few yellowish gray aggregates of exudates on the peripheral retina, ora serrata, pars plana, or vitreous (Figure 3-95). When a spherical clump of inflammatory material is seen in the vitreous separate from the exudative inferior membrane, they are called "snowball" opacities.[18, 19] Sometimes, snowball opacities can be seen floating in the vitreous and may cause the patient to see a dark floater (Figure 3-96). These exudates are most frequently found in the inferior region of the fundus, presumably due to gravitational forces. Inflammation results in the presence of white cells in the anterior vitreous (Figure 3-97); the diagnosis of pars planitis should not be made in the absence of cells in the vitreous.[11, 18] The vitritis can result in a definite haze shown by the direct ophthalmoscope, which may vary from 1+ to 4+.[17] The chronic inflammation can result in the presence of inflammatory cells in the vitreous along with the aggregation of collagen fibrils into linear structures called elongated cylindroids. These cylinders are composed of condensations of vitreous collagen fibrils that are coated with inflammatory cells and inserted into the vitreous base.[20] There is often a peripheral vasculitis, usually affecting the

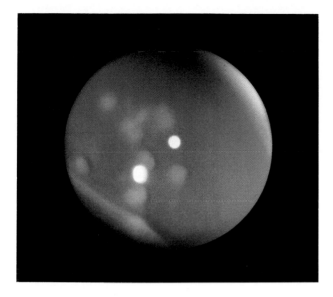

FIGURE 3-95
A group of exudates on the inferior retina just posterior to the ora serrata in a patient with pars planitis. View is through the indirect condensing lens during scleral depression.

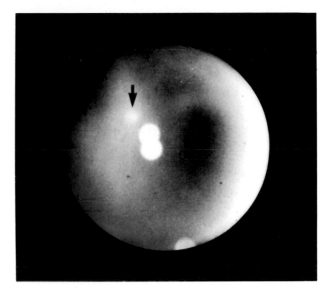

FIGURE 3-96
A white snowball can be seen floating in the vitreous of a patient with pars planitis (*arrow*). View is through an indirect condensing lens.

veins (periphlebitis), that is seen as attenuated and sheathed retinal vessels.[16]

Progression of the disease can lead to a continued obliteration of the vessels toward the posterior pole together with the development of optic atrophy and severe loss of vision. Fluorescein angiography demonstrates diffuse arterial, venous, and capillary leakage and venular wall staining, which suggest a diffuse vasculitis rather than a primary uveal inflammation.[21] Dye studies and vitreous fluorophotometry show little evidence that the disease primarily involves the inferior fundus.[22]

Further progression leads to a coalescence of these exudates into a plaque "snowbank" that covers the area just anterior and posterior to the ora serrata and hides all underlying detail and this is the hallmark of pars planitis (Figure 3-98). Sometimes scleral depression is necessary to discover the exudates and snowbank.[18, 19] When the inflammation is active, the snowbank has a soft and slightly raised appearance, but in quiescent stages it looks thin and membranous.[15, 18] In the early stages of the disease process, the exudates in the inferior fundus are discontinuous clumps composed of cells, fibrin, and cellular debris.[13] With time, these clumps coalesce in an organized smooth white membrane. In patients with asymmetric involvement, the less involved eye often displays a broken band, compared to a continuous band in the more affected eye.[16] In

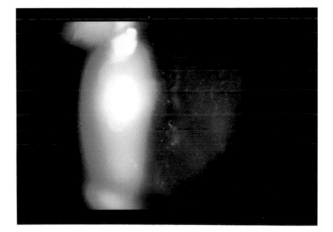

FIGURE 3-97
Slit-lamp view of anterior vitreous shows numerous white blood cells and a few vitreous strands in a patient with pars planitis.

advanced stages, there can be neovascularization of this membrane.[23] The membrane may in fact may play a role in the pathogenesis of the disease.[24] The snowbanking could be formed by glial elements of the peripheral retina.[10] The presence of pars plana exudates or membrane is frequently but not always associated with the more severe form of vitritis and cystoid macular edema (CME).[25] The membrane may form in the inferior fundus secondary to grav-

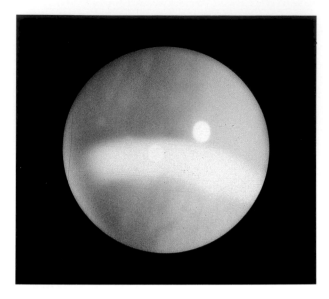

FIGURE 3-98
A bright white snowbank on the inferior ora serrata in a patient with pars planitis. View is through the indirect condensing lens during scleral depression.

itational forces settling inflammatory cells and debris from the inflamed vitreous and blood vessels in the inferior region, or it may be because more vitreous cells are found in the inferior vitreous.[26]

The etiology of pars planitis is unknown, but an autoimmune mechanism is suggested. One experimental study proposed that patients might be allergic to their own retinas;[27-31] another suggested an immune reaction to vitreous cells.[32] Present histologic studies show that the inflammation mainly involves the vitreous and suggest that the pathogenesis begins in the vitreous.[10, 33] There have been some cases of idiopathic age-related vitritis that resemble pars planitis.[34-36] Some believe that foreign proteins deposited in the vitreous may lead to pars planitis.[37, 38] Even the endothelium of vessels in the peripheral retina may play a role in this disease.[10] Some reports describe a relationship between pars planitis and multiple sclerosis,[4, 11, 33, 39-42] but the exact mechanism for the pathogenic relationship is unknown. Pars planitis is linked to an autoimmune etiology, which is supported by the finding of patients with the disease having a positive HLA-DR2 (found in patients with multiple sclerosis). The hyposensitivity of these patients to skin tests suggests a decrease in cell-mediated immunity that is also seen in lepromatous leprosy and sarcoid[43]; in one report, patients with suspected clinical pars planitis had a 9.7% incidence of sarcoidosis.[44]

Pars planitis is associated with systemic diseases. One study found that 26 of 83 patients (31.3%) had a systemic disease: 13 patients had presumed sarcoidosis, six had multiple sclerosis, two had isolated optic neuritis, two had inflammatory bowel disease, four had isolated thyroid abnormalities, and two had histories suggestive of Epstein-Barr virus infection.[33] There are case reports of such an appearance in a patient with inflammatory bowel disease[45] and one with Whipple's disease.[46] Patients with pars planitis should have a workup to rule out tuberculosis, occult sarcoidosis, collagen vascular disease, and Lyme disease.[47, 48] Patients with syphilis, reticulum cell, and sarcoma may have a clinical appearance resembling pars planitis.[41, 44] Chronic iridocyclitis and intermediate uveitis secondary to sarcoidosis can closely resemble pars planitis.[49] There have been reports of familial occurrence of pars planitis.[27] Unfortunately, no specific laboratory test can diagnose the condition. The differential diagnosis includes nematode over ciliary body, multiple sclerosis, and other conditions involving characteristic low-grade chronic inflammation. Unilateral cases should be carefully evaluated for the possibility of toxoplasmosis and toxocariasis.[50]

Useful laboratory tests are chest x-ray, serum lysozyme, angiotensin-converting enzyme, fluorescein treponemal absorption test, immunofluorescent antibody, and enzyme-linked immunosorbent assay.

Histopathology

Pars planitis is a chronic granulomatous inflammation of the anterior retina and the pars plana ciliaris (Figure 3-99). Peripheral periphlebitis is composed of mural cells and lymphocytic cuffing (mostly T-helper cells) around the venules.[24] The retinal arterioles are not involved. The snowbank is composed of glial elements, type IV collagen, and laminin.[19] There is cellular proliferation from the retina and hyperplasia of the nonpigmented epithelium.[51] There is usually collapse of the vitreous (PVD). Multinucleated giant cells and epithelioid cells have been found in vitreous snowballs.[52] The choroid seems to be free of the disease process and does not show epithelioid cells and multinucleated giant cells.[10, 52] Extensive fibroglial proliferation and fibrous astrocytelike cells are found in the region of the vitreous base.[24, 53] If fibrovascular tissue is in the snowbank, it is composed of well-differentiated capillaries, which probably originate from the peripheral retina.[53] The CME shows histologic findings that are consistent with typical clinical edema of the fovea.[24]

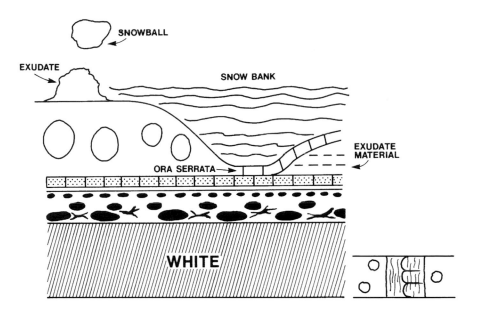

FIGURE 3-99
Pars planitis shows an exudate on the retina, a snowball in the vitreous, a snowbank covering the ora serrata, and exudative detachment of the nonpigmented epithelium of the pars plana and cystoid degeneration of the peripheral retina. Lower drawing shows an exudate on the pars plana.

Clinical Significance

Pars planitis is in most cases a diagnosis by exclusion. It is a chronic smoldering disease with remissions and exacerbations, which may last for 20–30 years but usually seems to burn out after about 10 years. Most patients undergo remission in the mid- to late 30s.[16] A study by Smith and colleagues[2] of 100 patients with IU found that the clinical course can be divided into three categories: (1) a benign self-limited course of slow improvement without episodes of exacerbations (10%), (2) a prolonged smoldering course without exacerbations (59%), and (3) a prolonged course with episodes of exacerbations (31%). Increased cellular reaction in the anterior chamber and vitreous was the common indication of exacerbation. Spontaneous remission in pars planitis is rare (4% of cases).[2] The severity of the disease is not associated with the longevity of the illness. Unilateral cases may present with the milder form of the disease than do bilateral cases.[16] Areas of the peripheral fundus may demonstrate active inflammatory deposits while others appear quiescent.

Ocular complications include yellowish, gelatinous exudates on the trabeculum of the filtration angle in 20% of cases.[54] Exudates can also occur on the anterior surface of the iris, and peripheral anterior synechiae are sometimes noted. In severe cases, a cyclitic membrane may develop behind the iris. Cataracts (usually posterior subcapsular) occur frequently and are the result of chronic inflammation and corticosteroid treatment (42%).[2, 55] PVD is quite

common, and preretinal membranes may be found.[30] Rarely, there can be neovascularization of the optic disc and in the subretinal space.[15, 23, 39, 56, 57] Sometimes neovascular glaucoma may occur.[58] There also can be neovascularization of the peripheral retina.[59] Sometimes a vitreous hemorrhage, retinal tears and detachment, and dragging of the disc occurs, but these are fairly rare events (< 5% of cases).[2, 13, 23, 60] Disc edema also can be seen in cases of pars planitis. Late sequelae are band keratopathy, glaucoma, and retinoschisis.[2, 61]

Vitreous degeneration with subsequent shrinkage can produce tractional forces that may result in macular edema, retinal folds, and retinal breaks.[33] Retinal breaks produced by this vitreous traction can be operculated, linear, horseshoe shaped, or retinal dialysis. Proliferation of the membrane at the vitreous base in a posterior direction may result in a sealing off of breaks, thus preventing a retinal detachment.[51]

Rhegmatogenous retinal detachments may occur[62] and are noted in about 50% of cases of retinal detachment in pars planitis.[63] Exudative retinal detachments and choroidal effusions can also occur in these eyes, and it is not unusual to discover a rhegmatogenous detachment superimposed on an exudative retinal detachment. A tractional detachment may form without retinal breaks being present. The retinal detachments tend to be slowly progressive, and therefore multiple pigmented demarcation lines are often seen (see the section on Demarcation Lines). Due to the advanced degree of vitreous traction, marked fixed retinal folds may

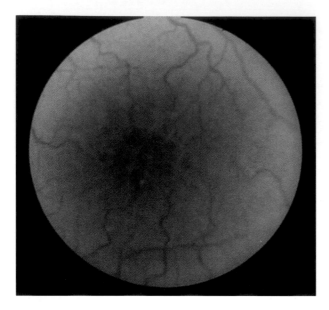

FIGURE 3-100
Cystoid macular edema can be seen as a petaloid area made of cyst-like lesions in the macular area. Note the absence of the foveal reflex.

occur in the detached retina, and can extend from the ora serrata to the posterior pole.

CME (Figures 3-100 and 3-101) is a complication of pars planitis and is most likely the leading cause of reduced vision.[64] CME is found in 28% of cases, and with increased duration of the disease, there is increased frequency of CME.[2] It appears that in pars planitis, partial PVD that results in increased vitreoretinal traction in the macular area produces a higher incidence of macular edema and decreased vision.[65, 66] CME, together with cataract formation, can cause early reduction in vision before a retinal detachment occurs. If there is a reduction in the patient's vision and a cataract does not seem to be completely responsible, the patient should have a fluorescein angiogram to rule out CME. CME shows a characteristic petaloid appearance during the late stages of the angiogram (Figure 3-102). The presence of pars plana exudates is often associated with a more severe vitreous disease and therefore increases the incidence of CME.[25]

Many patients with pars planitis do not require any form of treatment because the disease is often self-limiting. Hogan[67] reported that 80% of cases have a benign course and do not need treatment. Ciliary spasm is an infrequent finding, and therefore cycloplegic medications are seldom necessary. Suggested drug treatments for pars planitis include corticosteroids, antimetabolites, and immunosuppressive agents, but corticosteroid remains the mainstay. Treatment can consist of both oral and subtenon injection of corticosteroids. Improvement with corticosteroids is agonizingly slow. Steroids may be used to eliminate cells in the vitreous, but the cells tend to return after withdrawal of the medication. In the case of visual complaints caused by large or numerous vitreous floaters, a trial of steroids may be attempted to determine if the

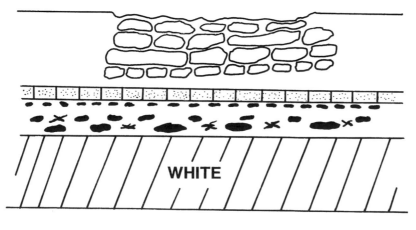

WHITE

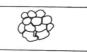

FIGURE 3-101
Diagram of cystoid macular edema demonstrating many fluid filled compartments that are found throughout the sensory retina. Note that normal macular morphology is distorted.

patient's vision can be improved.[16] One should not try to totally eliminate a snowbank but attempt to decrease retinal exudates that may cause a cyclitic membrane or retinal detachment and try to prevent CME. The treatment best suited for CME is a posterior subtenon injection of repository steroids. The subtenon injection is preferred due to its lower systemic toxicity compared to oral administration. The use of corticosteroids may hasten the formation of cataracts; thus, careful monitoring of the patient is critical. Ultrasonography may be used to facilitate more accurate placement of the injection opposite the macular region.[68] The injection is best placed superior to the macula to favor gravitational forces in the spreading of the depo-steroid.

Retrobulbar and subconjunctival injections are less effective due to the further distance from the macula.[16] If the subtenon injection is ineffective or if a steroid-induced glaucoma occurs, a trial of oral prednisone may be initiated. Intravenous pulse therapy of methylprednisolone has met with success in one case of severe pars planitis.[69] If no improvement occurs after 4–5 months of corticosteroid treatment, treatment should be halted because permanent macular damage has probably occurred.[16]

The ultimate goal of corticosteroid treatment should be to prevent further loss of vision. A reasonable goal is 20/30 to 20/40.[70–72] The 5-year projected visual prognosis is excellent for 80% of patients without treatment. Most of the remaining 20% do well on alternate-day oral prednisone or periocular steroid injections.[14] The best approach is to stabilize the condition with steroid treatment until the disease runs its natural course. Carbonic anhydrase inhibitors have been of some use in the treatment of CME, and some improvement of CME has been reported in three of six cases of uveitis with CME using these drugs.[73]

Abstinence from smoking may have a beneficial effect because of the vasoconstrictive effects of nicotine. Cryotherapy and diathermy have had limited success in selected cases. Cryotherapy has been used for peripheral retinal ablation in cases that are refractory to steroid treatment.[71, 74–76] This treatment reduces the vascular component of the disease by destroying tissue that is producing an ischemic neovascular response; it also results in less retinal exudation. Patients treated with cryotherapy have displayed an improvement of three lines of Snellen acuity.[75] Cryotherapy of the vitreous base reduced inflammation by 57–67%,[77–79] but fewer than 50% of patients have a complete or permanent recovery from the inflammation.[80] Generally, cryotherapy has a tem-

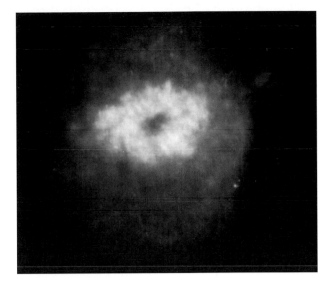

FIGURE 3-102
Fluorescein angiography of a patient with cystoid macular edema. Note the characteristic flower pattern, which is produced with time due to accumulation of the dye in the cystoid spaces.

porizing effect, and the snowbank usually returns 3–6 months after treatment.[71] Cryotherapy may be considered before attempting invasive vitrectomy or immunosuppressive therapy, both of which have a higher risk of complications. More recently, cryoablation has been advocated for the treatment of neovascularization of the vitreous base, and it is believed that the treatment reduces the ischemic tissue response and therefore causes the regression of the neovascularization.[78, 81] Cryotherapy of the vitreous base is thought to reduce intraocular inflammation by destroying the tissue that contains the inflammatory stimulus.[26, 74, 82] Peripheral scatter photocoagulation has been used to treat the same condition and was found to be just as effective as cryotherapy. Photocoagulation has the additional benefit of not seeming to induce rhegmatogenous retinal detachments; on the contrary, it produces a barrier to the development of a subsequent detachment.[83]

In some patients, treatment with immunosuppressive drugs has met with favorable results,[84] with such agents as chlorambucil,[85] azathioprine,[86] cyclophosphamide,[66] and methotrexate.[87, 88] There is not clear evidence that these agents are effective when corticosteroids have failed, but they may be used in patients who are unable to take periocular or systemic steroids.[16] Cyclosporine has been reported to improve CME in patients unresponsive to steroid treatment.[89, 90] Caution is needed when using this drug, for 75% of the patients taking for an extended period of time develop nephrotoxicity[91]; therefore, it should be administered only in severe cases.

Sometimes, a vitrectomy is required for patients with pars planitis,[92] especially if there is extensive vitreous hemorrhaging that has not resolved in 6 months. Its beneficial effect may result from mechanically removing inflammatory mediators, which results in stabilizing the inflammation and improving visual acuity,[93–98] but there may be an additional advantage of allowing better penetration and distribution of corticosteroids.[99, 100] This procedure is of benefit in some cases of chronic CME and has had some success in improving and stabilizing visual functioning.[32, 93, 96, 98, 101, 102] Some patients with a total PVD have had a better response to therapy for CME than did patients with a partial PVD[16]; relief of vitreous traction on the macula or removal of vitreous with toxic antigens from the macular area is believed responsible for this effect. In patients with vitreous opacification and neovascularization, a combined cryotherapy and vitrectomy has been used.[99, 102] One problem with cryotherapy and pars plana vitrectomy is that it may precipitate a rhegmatogenous detachment.[103]

Retinal breaks without detachment can be treated with cryoapplication and photocoagulation. In one study, retinal detachment occurred in 12% (12 of 102 eyes), seven of which were rhegmatogenous and five were tractional. After cryotherapy, retinal detachment occurred in 21% (nine of 43 eyes), but this happened in only 5% (three of 59 eyes) of eyes not receiving cryotherapy. Five of seven eyes that had both a pars plana vitrectomy and cryotherapy suffered a retinal detachment. This suggests that such therapies may have greater inherent risks than the disease itself. The recent use of indirect laser scatter for peripheral retinal ablation may be just as effective as cryotherapy without such a high risk of retinal detachment.[103] If substantial vitreous traction is present, scleral buckling with an encircling band may be necessary. Patients should be referred to a primary care physician for a complete medical evaluation to rule out systemic disease.

The prognosis for pars planitis is guarded because it is a chronic disease condition and most patients suffer some reduction in vision, although some report that the prognosis for vision is good.[40] The condition usually goes into remission in patients in their mid to late 30s. The patient should be told about the severity of the condition and educated about the symptoms of a retinal tear or detachment. Patients with this condition should have follow-up examinations every 6 months with indirect ophthalmoscopy including scleral depression, and if they notice a significant vision loss or experience the symptoms of a retinal tear or detachment, they should return immediately.

References

1. Schlaegel TF Jr. Differential diagnosis of uveitis. Ophthalmol Digest (audiotape) 1973.
2. Smith RE, Godfrey WA, et al. Chronic cyclitis. I. Course and visual prognosis. Trans Am Acad Ophthalmol Otolaryngol 1973;77:760–768.
3. Van Metre TE Jr. The role of the allergist in diagnosis and management of patients with uveitis. JAMA 1966;195:167–172.
4. Godfrey W. Chronic iridocyclitis. In W Tasman, EA Jaeger (eds), Clinical Ophthalmology. Vol. 4. Philadelphia: Harper & Row, 1987;42:7.
5. Henderly DE, Genstler AJ, et al. Changing patterns of uveitis. Am J Ophthalmol 1987;103:131–136.
6. Hogan MJ, Kimura SJ, et al. Peripheral retinitis and chronic cyclitis in children. Trans Ophthalmol Soc UK 1965;85:39–45.
7. Culbertson WW, Conrad GL, et al. Familial pars planitis. Retina 1983;3:179–181.
8. Augsburger JJ, Annesley WH Jr, et al. Familial pars planitis. Ann Ophthalmol 1981;13:553–557.
9. Doft BH. Pars planitis in identical twins. Retina 1983;3:32–33.
10. Wetzeg RP, Chan CC, et al. Clinical and immunopathological studies of pars planitis in a family. Br J Ophthalmol 1988;72:5–10.
11. Schlaegel TF Jr. Ocular Toxoplasmosis and Pars Planitis. New York: Grune & Stratton, 1978:263–360.
12. Martenet AC. Chronic cyclitis. Arch Ophthalmol (Paris) 1973;33:533–540.
13. Brockhurst RJ, Schepens CL, et al. Uveitis. II. Peripheral uveitis. Pathogenesis, etiology, complications and differential diagnosis. Am J Ophthalmol 1960;49:1257–1266.
14. Hogan MJ. Discussion. Gills JP Jr, Buckley CE. Oral cyclophosphamide in the treatment of uveitis. Trans Am Acad Ophthalmol Otolaryngol 1070;74:505–508.
15. Kimura SJ, Hogan MJ. Chronic cyclitis. Arch Ophthalmol 1964;71:193–201.
16. Lam S, Tessler HH. Intermediate Uveitis. In W Tasman, EA Jaeger (eds), Clinical Ophthalmology. Vol. 4. Philadelphia: Harper & Row, 1991;43:1–15.
17. Tessler HH. Classification and Symptoms and Signs of Uveitis. In W Tasman, EA Jaeger (eds), Clinical Ophthalmology. Vol. 4. Philadelphia: Harper & Row, 1987;32:1–10.
18. Welch RB, Maumenee AE, et al. Peripheral posterior segment inflammation, vitreous opacities and edema of the posterior pole: Pars planitis. Arch Ophthalmol 1960;64:540–549.
19. Schepens CL. L'inflammation de la region de l'ora serrata et ses sequelae. Bull Soc Ophthalmol Fr 1950;63:113–125.
20. Roizenblatt J, Grant S, et al. Vitreous cylinders. Arch Ophthalmol 1980;98:734–739.
21. Pruett RC, Brockhurst RJ, et al. Fluorescein angiography of peripheral uveitis. Am J Ophthalmol 1974;77:448–453.
22. Mahlberg PA, Cunha-Vaz JG, et al. Vitreous fluoropho-

tometry in pars planitis. Am J Ophthalmol 1983;95: 189–196.

23. Felder KS, Brockhurst RJ. Neovascular fundus abnormalities in peripheral uveitis. Arch Ophthalmol 1982;100: 750–754.

24. Pederson JE, Kenyon KR, et al. Pathology of pars planitis. Am J Ophthalmol 1978;86:762–764.

25. Henderly DE, Haymond RS, et al. The significance of the pars plana exudate in pars planitis. Am J Ophthalmol 1987;103:669–671.

26. Gartner J. The fine structures of the vitreous base of the human eye and pathogenesis of pars planitis. Am J Ophthalmol 1971;71:1317–1327.

27. von Sallmann L, Meyers RE, et al. Retinal and uveal inflammation in monkeys following inoculation with homologous retinal antigen. Arch Ophthalmol 1969;81: 374–382.

28. Rahi AH, Addison DJ. Autoimmunity and the outer retina. Trans Ophthalmol Soc UK 1983;103:428–437.

29. Nussenblatt RB, Gery I, et al. Cellular immune responsiveness of uveitis patients to retinal S-antigen. Am J Ophthalmol 1980;89:173–179.

30. Abrahams IW, Gregerson DS. Longitudinal study of serum antibody responses to bovine retinal S-antigen in endogenous granulomatous uveitis. Br J Ophthalmol 1983;67:681–684.

31. Gregerson DS, Abrahams IW, et al. Serum antibody levels of uveitis patients to bovine retinal antigens. Invest Ophthalmol Vis Sci 1981;21:669–680.

32. Eisner J. The fine structure of the vitreous base of the human eye and pathogenesis of pars planitis. Am J Ophthalmol 1971;71:1317–1327.

33. Boskovich SA, Lowder CY, et al. Systemic diseases associated with intermediate uveitis. Cleve Clin J Med 1993;60:460–465.

34. Brinton GS, Osher RH, et al. Idiopathic vitritis. Retina 1983;3:95–98.

35. Gass JDM. Vitiliginous chorioretinitis. Arch Ophthalmol 1981;99:1778–1787.

36. Gass JDM. Idiopathic Diffuse Nonnecrotizing Retinitis and Vitritis Without Vitreous Base Exudation and Organization (Idiopathic Vitritis). In Stereo Atlas of Macular Diseases: Diagnosis and Management (3rd ed). Vol. 2. St. Louis: Mosby, 1988:526–527.

37. Hultsch E. Peripheral uveitis in the owl monkey. Experimental model. Mod Probl Ophthalmol 1977;18: 247–251.

38. Zimmerman LE, Solverstein AM. Experimental ocular hypersensitivity: Histopathologic changes observed in rabbits receiving a single injection of antigen into the vitreous. Am J Ophthalmol 1959;48:447–465.

39. Chester CH, Black RK, et al. Inflammation in the region of the vitreous base: pars planitis. Trans Ophthalmol Soc UK 1976;96:151–157.

40. Giles CL. Peripheral uveitis with multiple sclerosis. Am J Ophthalmol 1970;70:17–19.

41. Malinowski S, Pulido JS, et al. Long-term visual outcome and complications associated with pars planitis. Ophthalmology 1993;100:818–824.

42. Berger BC, Leopold IH, et al. The incidence of uveitis in multiple sclerosis. Am J Ophthalmol 1966;62:540–545.

43. Papageorgiou PS, Glade RR. Impaired cell-mediated immunity and antibody titers. N Engl J Med 1971; 285:580–581.

44. Zierhut M, Foster CS. Multiple sclerosis, sarcoidosis and other diseases in patients with pars planitis. Dev Ophthalmol 1992;23:41–47.

45. Zaidman GW, Cules RS. Peripheral uveitis and ulcerative colitis. Ann Ophthalmol 1981;13:73–76.

46. Glickman RN, Sleisenger MH. Malabsorption. In JB Wyngaarden, LH Smith (eds), Cecil Textbook of Medicine (17th ed). Philadelphia: Saunders, 1985:719–740.

47. Fujikawa LS. Advances in immunology and uveitis. Ophthalmology 1989;96:1115–1120.

48. Winward KE, Smith JL, et al. Ocular Lyme borreliosis. Am J Ophthalmol 1989;108:651–657.

49. Tessler HH. What is Intermediate Uveitis? In TJ Ernest (ed), The Year Book of Ophthalmology. Chicago: Year Book, 1985:155–157.

50. Hogan MJ, Kimura SJ, et al. Visceral larva migrans and peripheral retinitis. JAMA 1965;194:1345–1347.

51. Yanoff M, Fine BS. Ocular Pathology: A Text and Atlas (2nd ed). Philadelphia: Harper & Row, 1982:73.

52. Green WR, Kincaid MC, et al. Pars planitis. Trans Ophthalmol Soc UK 1981;101:361–367.

53. Kenyon KR, Pederson JE, et al. Fibroglial proliferation in pars planitis. Trans Ophthalmol Soc UK 1975;95:391–397.

54. Brockhurst RJ, Schepens CL, et al. Uveitis. I. Gonioscopy. Am J Ophthalmol 1956;42:545–554.

55. Smith RE, Godfrey WA, et al. Complications of chronic cyclitis. Am J Ophthalmol 1976;82:277–282.

56. Shorb SR, Irvine AR, et al. Optic disk neovascularization associated with chronic uveitis. Am J Ophthalmol 1976; 82:175–178.

57. Arkfeld DF, Brockhurst RJ. Peripapillary subretinal neovascularization in peripheral uveitis. Retina 1985;5:157–160.

58. Campo RV, Reiss GR, et al. Glaucoma associated with retinal disorders and retinal surgery. In TD Duane, EA Jaeger (eds), Clinical Ophthalmology. Vol. 3. Philadelphia: Harper & Row, 1990;54E:18.

59. Brown GC, Brown RH, et al. Peripheral proliferative retinopathies. Int Ophthalmol 1987;11:41–50.

60. Phillips WB, Bergren RL, et al. Pars planitis presenting with vitreous hemorrhage. Ophthalmic Surg 1993; 24:630–631.

61. Brockhurst RJ. Retinoschisis complication of peripheral uveitis. Arch Ophthalmol 1981;99:1998–1999.

62. Brockhurst RJ, Schepens CL, et al. Uveitis. IV. Peripheral uveitis: The complications of retinal detachment. Arch Ophthalmol 1968;80:747–753.

63. Schepens CL. Retinal Detachment and Allied Diseases. Philadelphia: Saunders, 1983:673–683.

64. Henderly DE, Genstler AJ, et al. Pars planitis. Trans Ophthalmol Soc UK 1986;105:227–232.

65. Hikichi T, Tempe CL. Role of the vitreous in the prognosis of peripheral uveitis. Am J Ophthalmol 1993;116:401–405.

66. Hirokawa H, Takahashi M, et al. Vitreous changes in peripheral uveitis. Arch Ophthalmol 1985;103:1704–1707.

67. Gills JP, Buckley CE. Oral cyclophosphamide in the treatment of uveitis. Trans Acad Am Ophthalmol Otolaryngol 1970;74:505–508.

68. Freeman WR, Green RL, et al. Echographic localization of corticosteroids after periocular injection. Am J Ophthalmol 1987;103:281–288.

69. Wakefield D, McCluskey P, et al. Intravenous pulse methylprednisolone therapy in severe inflammatory eye disease. Arch Ophthalmol 1986;104:847–851.

70. Kaplan HJ. Intermediate uveitis (pars planitis): A four-step approach to treatment. In KM Saari, ed. Uveitis Update. Amsterdam: Excerpta Medica, 1984:169–172.

71. Nussenblatt RB, Palestine AG. Uveitis: Fundamentals and Clinical Practice. Chicago: Year Book, 1989:185–197.
72. Smith RE, Nozik RA. Uveitis. A Clinical Approach to Diagnosis and Management (2nd ed). Baltimore: Williams & Wilkins, 1989:166–170.
73. Cox SN, Hay E, et al. Treatment of chronic macular edema with acetazolamide. Arch Ophthalmol 1988;106:1190–1195.
74. Aaberg TM, Cesarz TJ, et al. Treatment of peripheral uveoretinitis by cryotherapy. Am J Ophthalmol 1973;75:685–688.
75. Aaberg TM. Editorial. The enigma of pars planitis. Am J Ophthalmol 1987;103:828–830.
76. Kalsika G, Kaluzny J, et al. Use of transconjunctival cryoapplication in chronic pars planitis with involvement of peripheral retina and choroid. Klin Oczna 1993;95:44–46.
77. Okinami S, Sunakawa M, et al. Treatment of pars planitis with cryotherapy. Ophthalmologica 1991;202:180–186.
78. Devenyi RG, Mieler WF, et al. Cryopexy of the vitreous base in the management of peripheral uveitis. Am J Ophthalmol 1988;105:136–138.
79. Verma L, Kumar A, et al. Cryopexy in pars planitis. Can J Ophthalmol 1991;26:313–315.
80. Bonnet M, Moron MF. Diathermy and cryotherapy of the pars plana in the treatment of pars planitis: Long-term evaluation. J Fr Ophtalmol 1985;8:37–41.
81. Mieler WF, Aaberg TM. Further observations of cryotherapy of the vitreous base in the management of peripheral uveitis. Dev Ophthalmol 1992;23:190–195.
82. Josephberg RG, Kanter ED, et al. A fluorescein angiographic study of patients with pars planitis and peripheral exudation (snowbanking) before and after cryopexy. Ophthalmology 1994;101:1262–1266.
83. Park SE, Mieler WF, et al. Peripheral scatter photocoagulation for neovascularization associated with pars planitis. Arch Ophthalmol 1995;113:1277–1280.
84. Nozik RA, Godfrey WA, et al. Immunosuppressive treatment of uveitis. Mod Probl Ophthalmol 1974;16:305–293.
85. Kanski JJ. Care of children with anterior uveitis. Trans Ophthalmol Soc UK 1981;101:387–390.
86. Charamis I, Skouras I. Treatment with azathioprine of peripheral chronic cyclitis with cystoid edema of the macula. Klin Monatsbl Augenheilkd 1977;170:362–365.
87. Lazar M, Weiner MJ, et al. Treatment of uveitis with methotrexate. Am J Ophthalmol 1969;67:383–387.
88. Wong VG, Hersh EM. Methotrexate in the therapy of cyclitis. Trans Am Acad Ophthalmol Otolaryngol 1965;69:279–293.
89. Nussenblatt RB, Palestine AG, et al. Cyclosporine therapy for uveitis. Long-term follow-up. J Ocul Pharmacol 1985;1:369–382.
90. Nussenblatt RB, Palestine AG, et al. Cyclosporin A therapy in the treatment of intraocular inflammatory disease resistant to systemic corticosteroids and cytotoxic agents. Am J Ophthalmol 1983;96:275–282.
91. Nussenblatt RB, Palestine AG, et al. Cyclosporine. Immunology, pharmacology and therapeutic uses. Surv Ophthalmol 1986;31:159–169.
92. Smiddy WE, Isernhagen RD, et al. Vitrectomy for nondiabetic vitreous hemorrhage. Retinal and choroidal vascular disorders. Retina 1988;8:88–95.
93. Diamond JG, Kaplan HJ. Lensectomy and vitrectomy for complicated cataract secondary to uveitis. Arch Ophthalmol 1978;96:1798–1804.
94. Kaplan HJ, Diamond JG, et al. Vitrectomy in experimental uveitis. Arch Ophthalmol 1979;97:331–335.
95. Algvere P, Alanko H, et al. Pars plana vitrectomy in the management of intraocular inflammation. Acta Ophthalmol 1981;59:727–736.
96. Diamond JG, Kaplan HJ. Uveitis: Effect of vitrectomy combined with lensectomy. Ophthalmology 1979;86:1320–1327.
97. Dangel ME, Stark WJ, et al. Surgical management of cataract associated with chronic uveitis. Ophthalmic Surg 1983;14:145–149.
98. Nolthenius PAT, Deutman AF. Surgical management of the complications of chronic uveitis. Ophthalmologica 1983;186:11–16.
99. Mieler WF, Aaberg TM. Vitrectomy surgery in the management of peripheral uveitis. Dev Ophthalmol 1992;23:239–250.
100. Dugel PU, Rao NA, et al. Pars plana vitrectomy for intraocular inflammation-related cystoid macular edema unresponsive to corticosteroids. Ophthalmology 1992;99:1535–1541.
101. Limon S, Bloch-Michael E, et al. 100 Vitrectomies in Uveitis. In KM Saari (ed), Uveitis Update, Proceedings of First International Symposium on Uveitis. Amsterdam: Excerpta Medica, 1984:521–524.
102. Mieler WF, Will BR, et al. Vitrectomy in the management of peripheral uveitis. Ophthalmology 1988;95: 859–864.
103. Mieler WF, Malinowski SM. Current evaluation and therapy of pars planitis. Vitreoretinal Surg Techn 1994; 6:3–4.

Chapter 4

Vitreous Degeneration Related to Peripheral Retinal Breaks and Retinal Detachment

Synchysis and Syneresis

The vitreous body slowly degrades with age, undergoing liquefaction (synchysis) and shrinkage (syneresis); this can be readily seen after 45–50 years of age.[1–10] In one large study of autopsied eyes, half the vitreous body was liquefied in 25% of people 40–49 years of age; synchysis increased to 62% in those 80–89 years of age.[5] An ultrasound study also found progressive liquefaction with age.[11] Other researchers found that liquefaction occurs much earlier in life than can be seen clinically, that evidence of liquid vitreous can be seen at 4 years of age, and that 10–12.5% liquefaction occurs in adult eyes 14–18 years of age.[8, 12] This same study of 610 autopsied eyes found a steady increase in liquefaction of the vitreous gel after the age of 40 and, by ages 80–90, more than half the vitreous body was liquefied.

In synchysis, degeneration starts in the central region of the vitreous body, with cortical layers the last to be affected. The liquefaction usually starts in the central posterior vitreous, where vitreous fibrils are first seen clinically.[13–15] The posterior vitreous tends to form large pockets of liquid vitreous.[16] The areas of liquefaction, called lacunae, can be small and with time coalesce into large pockets that occupy most of the vitreous cavity. Liquefied vitreous can travel between lacunae, thus making available large quantities of fluid to enter retinal breaks. The cavity of the lacuna contains liquefied vitreous gel that may be the result of the breakdown of hyaluronic acid (HA). This cavity appears empty because its optical density is less than that of the surrounding gel. The fluid within the lacuna resembles aqueous humor and may contain delicate remnants of vitreous fibrils. It is thought that a dissolution of the HA-collagen complex leads to liquefaction and allows for the fibrils to aggregate into bundles.[14, 17] The walls of the lacuna are the result of vitreous condensation, which forms a membrane-like structure that is occasionally seen clinically. High myopia is known to result in earlier onset of liquefaction of the vitreous.[18–20]

Syneresis describes the physical contraction of the vitreous body over time due to aging or to episodes of vitritis. The time-related aging aspect of syneresis may be associated with vitreous changes secondary to the passage of light energy through the vitreous body, which could alter the HA or collagen structure and result in the dissociation of collagen and depolarization and precipitation of HA molecules that leads to liquefaction.[6, 9, 21] The aging of the collagen leads to cross-linking, as manifested by decreased solubility and an increase in collagen "stiffness."[22] Syneresis also results in condensation of the vitreous fibers, which become much more visible. The fibers can become so compacted that they resemble bundles of yarn. Consolidation of vitreous fibers is most prominent in the anterior vitreous behind the lens or over the vitreous base. Further degeneration may lead to the formation of vitreous membranes that criss-cross the vitreous body, but usually they are found above the vitreous base. These membranes may float freely in the vitreous or attach to the retina or pars plana (see Vitreous Bands and Membranes later in this chapter).

Clinical Significance

The degree of synchysis is important in determining how much movement the vitreous makes during eye movements, for with a more liquid vitreous comes a greater rotational motion. Such movements are much like what is seen in a washing machine, with the water lagging behind the rotator blade on a partial rotation and then spinning back in the other direction on opposite rotation of the blades. The movement of the vitreous allows for pulling of the vitreous cortex on the underlying retinal surface, and the more the vitreous moves, the greater the force trying to separate the cortex from the retina. The degree of liquefaction found over a retinal break is important in the development of a retinal detachment, although vitreous traction is probably the most important factor in the formation of a detachment. A small amount of fluid may result in a limited retinal detachment at the margins of the break (see Figures 5-6, 5-17, and 6-24). A continued supply of small amounts of fluid, and more important, continued vitreous traction may lead to slow progression of the retinal detachment with multiple demarcation lines (see Figure 6-28). This may explain why a retinal detachment can be so slow in forming even after a retinal dialysis. A large reservoir of fluid along with strong vitreous traction can lead to a clinically significant retinal detachment that progresses rapidly.

The existence of vitreoretinal degeneration results in a far greater degree of vitreous liquefaction than that produced in normal eyes. Therefore, patients with such diseases as Wagner's vitreoretinal degeneration, lattice degeneration, and myopia are much more likely to experience a retinal detachment.

Syneresis is usually a very slow process that leads to tractional forces on the underlying retina and, along with synchysis, sufficient tractional forces can be generated to separate the vitreous cortex from the retinal surface. Therefore, both synchysis and syneresis can lead to a posterior vitreous detachment and possible rhegmatogenous retinal detachment.

References

1. Busacca A. La structure biomicroscopique du corps vitre normal. Annales d'Oculiste 1958;91:487–491.
2. Goldmann H. Senescenz des Glaskorpers. Ophthalmologica 1962;143:253–279.
3. Michaels RG, Wilkinson CP, et al. Retinal Detachment. St. Louis: Mosby, 1990.
4. Lindner B. Acute posterior vitreous detachment and its retinal complications: A clinical biomicroscopic study. Acta Ophthalmol Scand Supp 1966;87:9.
5. O'Malley P. The Pattern of Vitreous Syneresis: A Study of 800 Autopsy Eyes. In AR Irvine, P O'Malley (eds), Advances in Vitreous Surgery. Springfield, IL: Thomas, 1976;17–33.
6. Flood MT, Balazs EA. Hyaluronic acid content in the developing and aging human liquid and gel vitreous. Invest Ophthalmol Vis Sci 1977;16(suppl):67.
7. Foos RY, Wheeler NC. Vitreoretinal juncture: Synchysis senilis and posterior vitreous detachment. Ophthalmology 1982;89:1502–1512.
8. Balazs EA, Denlinger JL. Aging Changes in the Vitreous. In R Sekuller, D Kline, K Dismukes (eds), Aging and Human Visual Function. New York: Alan R Liss, 1982;45–57.
9. Larsson L, Osterlin S. Posterior vitreous detachment: A combined and psychochemical study. Graefes Arch Clin Exp Ophthalmol 1985;223:92–95.
10. Sebag J. Aging of the vitreous. Eye 1987;1:254–262.
11. Oksala A. Ultrasonic findings in the vitreous body at various ages. Graefes Arch Clin Exp Ophthalmol 1978;207:275–280.
12. Balazs EA, Flood MT. Age-related changes in the physical and chemical structure of human vitreous. In Proceedings of the Third International Congress for Eye Research, Osaka, Japan, 1978.
13. Sebag J, Balazs EA. Human vitreous fibres and vitreoretinal disease. Trans Ophthalmol Soc UK 1985;104:123–128.
14. Sebag J, Balazs EA. Morphology and ultrastructure of human vitreous fibers. Invest Ophthalmol Vis Sci 1989;30:1867–1871.
15. Sebag J. Age-related changes in human vitreous structure. Graefes Arch Clin Exp Ophthalmol 1987;225:89–93.
16. Kishis S, Shimizu K. Posterior precortical vitreous pocket. Arch Ophthalmol 1990;108:979–982.
17. Armand G, Chakrabarti B. Conformational differences between hyaluronates of gel and liquid human vitreous: fractionation and circular dichroism studies. Curr Eye Res 1987;6:445–450.
18. Akiba J. Prevalence of posterior vitreous detachment in high myopia. Ophthalmology 1993;100:1384–1388.
19. Rieger H. Über die bedeutung der aderhautveranderungen fur die entstehung der glaskorperabhebung. Graefes Arch Ophthalmol 1937;136:118–165.
20. Singh A, Paul SD, et al. A clinical study of vitreous body (in emmetropia and refractive errors). Orient Arch Ophthal 1970;8:11–17.
21. Uneo N, Sebag J, et al. Effects of visible–light irradiation on vitreous structure in the presence of a photosensitizer. Exp Eye Res 1987;44:863–870.
22. Schnider SL, Kohn RR. Effects of age and diabetes mellitus on the solubility of collagen from human skin, tracheal cartilage, and dura mater. Exp Gerontol 1982;17:185–194.

Posterior Vitreous Detachment

A posterior vitreous detachment (PVD) occurs when the vitreous cortex separates from the posterior retina and optic disc. If it extends to the ora serrata, it is known as a complete PVD (Figure 4-1); if it involves only the posterior region, it is known as an incomplete or partial PVD. Another report states that in adult eyes of all ages, occurrence is 2% for incomplete PVD and 12% for complete PVD. The frequency after age 65 increases to 3% for incomplete and 31% for complete PVD.[1] One study of autopsied eyes found that a PVD in people younger than 30 years was rare, but the prevalence increased to 10% in people 30–59 years of age, 27% in people 60–69 years of age, and 63% of people more than 70 years.[2] Clinical studies found that a PVD occurred in 58% of patients over 50 years of age[3] and in 65% of patients aged 65–85.[4] Aphakic eyes have a higher incidence of PVD; in aphakic eyes at autopsy, incomplete PVD was seen in 6–24.5% and complete PVD in 66–77%[4, 5] and a clinical study of aphakic eyes found an 80% incidence.[6] The greatest risk of PVD is soon after cataract surgery.[7] An ultrasonography study found that 75% of patients over age 80 had a PVD.[8] Generally, patients present with bilateral involvement. One study found 90% bilaterality with very symmetric findings in each eye,[4] but on the initial presentation, bilateral involvement was found in only 14% of cases.[7] But if presentation is unilateral, it is typical for the other eye to develop a PVD within a few years. Byer[7] found in one study that the fellow eye developed a PVD within 3 months in 27% of cases, 52% in 1 year, 80% in 2 years, and 100% in 7 years.

High myopia is associated with an increased incidence of PVD; this was first reported by Rieger[9] in 1937. Myopes have a higher incidence of PVD, likely because of the increase in axial length, which adds stress to the vitreoretinal interface; there also may be myopic degenerative changes in the structure of the vitreous.[10] In myopes over 3.00 diopters, PVD has been found to occur about 10 years earlier than in the emmetropes or hyperopes, and it has been found in patients in their twenties.[7, 11–14] Morita et al.[15] reported the youngest patients with high myopia who had a PVD were 21–29 years of age. In 196 patients with myopia over 8.25 diopters, they also reported an incidence of 12.5% in patients aged 20–29, 24.1% in patients aged 30–39, 54.4% in patients aged 40–49, 69.4% in patients aged 50–59, 71.2% in patients aged 60–69, and 92.9% in patients aged 70–79. In this last study, the control

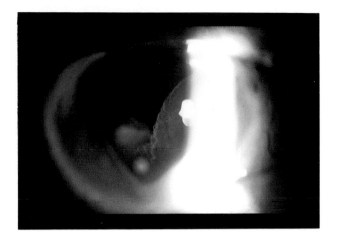

FIGURE 4-1
Posterior vitreous detachment with total collapse into the anterior vitreous cavity, seen during biomicroscopy. Note the sharp delineation of the posterior vitreous face against the optically dark liquefied vitreous.

group of patients who had less than 3.00 diopters of myopia, emmetropia, and hyperopia had a PVD incidence of 1.5% in patients aged 40–49, 21.3% in patients aged 50–59, 39.7% in patients aged 60–69, and 61.1% in patients aged 70–79. In 1970, a report by Singh et al.[16] found that myopia over 6.00 diopters was associated with PVD formation occurring in the fourth decade and increased with age. A study by Akiba[11] found that a PVD occurred earlier in myopic eyes over 10.25 diopters than in myopic eyes from 6.00 to 10.00 diopters. This association was particularly strong for patients aged 50–69.[7] In a study of 513 myopic eyes with axial lengths of 24 mm to more than 33 mm, myopes had a 47.7% incidence of PVD.[17] Another study also found an increase in PVD with increase in axial length, reporting an incidence of 33.3% in eyes 26.0–26.9 mm, 51.0% in eyes 30.0–30.9 mm, and 78.9% in eyes 32.0–32.9 mm.[15] A study of cataract extraction (presumably intracapsular) in eyes over 6 diopter in myopia found that all but one of 103 eyes had a postsurgical PVD.[18] The incidence of liquefaction and lacuna formation increases with the degree of myopia,[8, 14, 16, 19–22] and highly myopic eyes have large lacunar degeneration at the posterior pole prior to the development of a PVD.[19–21] Morita et al.[15] found in highly myopic patients that large lacunae were seen over the temporal vascular arcades in 18.8% of all eyes, in 18.1% of patients aged 20–29, and 22.2% of patients aged 30–39. These findings did not hold in patients aged 20–39 with myopia less

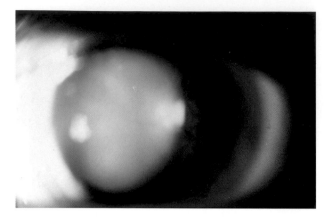

FIGURE 4-2
The light gray diaphanous posterior vitreous face with many folds can be seen behind the lens during biomicroscopy.

than 3.00 diopters. It is evident that the early vitreous degeneration in high myopes is instrumental in PVD formation.

Studies have found that PVD occurs more frequently in females than males, which may be due to postmenopausal hormonal changes on the vitreous as well as on other body organs and tissues and that HA (stabilizer of vitreous gel) is in lower concentrations in females. The synthesis of HA is known to be influenced by gonadal hormones, and a PVD may in part be the consequence of hormonal withdrawal.[1, 11, 12, 23–31] Other studies,[14, 32] including a study by Byer,[7] found insufficient evidence for any gender predilection.

The occurrence of equatorial degeneration of the retina does not seem to affect the time of onset of PVD.[11] Trauma can also induce a PVD. In a study of asymptomatic amateur boxers, 20% were found to have a PVD.[33] Two patients developed an acute PVD after air-puff noncontact tonometry.[34] Other traumatic causes for premature PVD can be eye surgery and postoperative yttrium–aluminum–garnet laser capsulotomy.

A PVD can be seen with an ophthalmoscope as a very thin and transparent membrane or with a biomicroscope as a more dense, transparent membrane in the central portion of the vitreous cavity. The posterior vitreous face is the curtain that separates the vitreous proper from the optically opaque posterior vitreous space. The reason the vitreous is visible is that it contains particulate material that scatters light, but the retrovitreous space is very low in particulate matter (consisting of liquefied vitreous and aqueous) and therefore appears optically dark as light passes through

without significant scattering. During biomicroscopy, the posterior vitreous face (cortex) is seen as a thin grayish-white membrane with numerous folds (a "pleated appearance") that moves freely on eye movements (Figure 4-2). The posterior vitreous face can be photographed with a photographic biomicroscope, but because the vitreous face is so transparent and is a fair distance behind the lens, it is difficult to illuminate the posterior cortex sufficiently due to the light flash entering at an angle that does not allow enough reflected light to expose the film adequately in most cases. Photographing prominent vitreous floaters (including the prepapillary annulus) with the fundus camera is generally not very difficult. Photographing the posterior vitreous face close to the retinal surface is possible but also difficult due to the transparent vitreous being close to the colorful retinal and choroidal background. Photographs of partial PVDs and other vitreous opacities have been documented.[35–39] Highly sensitive monochromic charged coupled cameras (CCD) can image the posterior vitreous and as well as the vitreous in dynamic motion.[40, 41] The posterior vitreous face can also be shown with ultrasonography as a very thin, just discernible membrane in the vitreous cavity (Figures 4-3 and 4-4). Sometimes the posterior vitreous face is close to the retinal surface and other times is far anterior.

Often the prepapillary ring can be seen in the center of the posterior face, which is pathognomonic of a PVD. Because the vitreous has broken free from the posterior inner wall of the globe, it can move easily on eye movements. Therefore, when the vitreous in one eye is seen to move much more rapidly than in the fellow eye, that eye should be suspected of having a PVD. The ascension-descension phenomenon can be used to detect the posterior cortical face because a clear membrane in the vitreous moves at a different speed than the posterior retinal surface.[3] When the vitreous fibrils are stretched across the vitreous cavity, they are thin and fairly transparent; after a PVD, however, they become thicker (like a rubber band after tension is released) and more transparent.[42] Therefore, more obvious vitreous strands in one eye should alert the clinician to the possibility of a PVD. A PVD allows for vitreous strands to twine around each other during eye movements, which also causes them to become more visible and aids in the diagnosis of a PVD (Figure 4-5). Collapsing vitreous may cause collection of vitreous strands and parts of vitreous cortex in the inferior vitreous

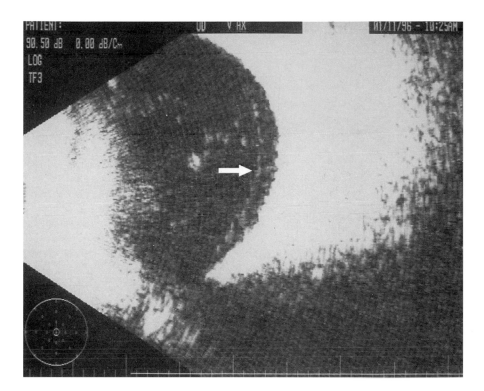

FIGURE 4-3
B-scan of typical PVD showing the posterior vitreous cortex close to the retinal surface (*arrow*) and floaters seen more anterior in the vitreous gel.

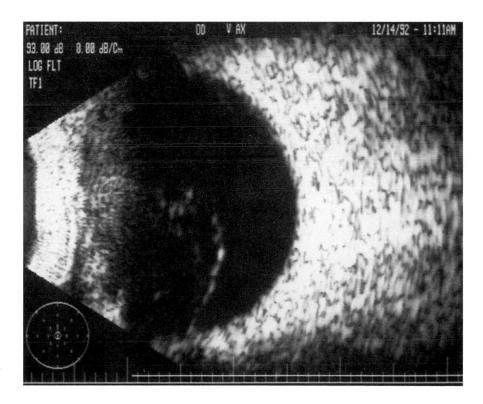

FIGURE 4-4
B-scan ultrasonogram of a PVD. Note that the vitreous body has collapsed in an anterior and inferior location.

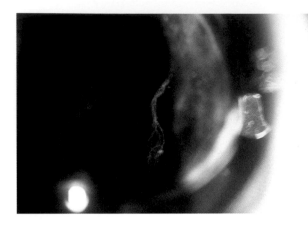

FIGURE 4-5
Vitreous strands seen in a patient with a PVD.

times, a sheetlike adhesion covers a large area of the posterior pole.[44] The gliotic ring is the attachment of the cortex to the disc margin. It surrounds the prepapillary hole and can be seen on ultrasonography (Figure 4-7). This avulsed gliotic ring can sometimes be seen as a dark object floating in the vitreous after a PVD. It typically has an annular shape (Weiss's, Vogt's, or Gartner's ring), but it may be twisted into a figure-eight or have a semicircular "open C" or linear shape when it is broken. The prepapillary gliotic ring may be perfectly round or contracted to an out-of-round collapsed shape (Figure 4-8). Sometimes part of the gliotic ring may remain attached to the margin of the optic disc and therefore have an unusual torn appearance (Figure 4-9). Because the peripapillary glial ring is close to the visual axis, it is easily seen by the patient and is often the first reported symptom of a PVD. Frequently, glial strands radiate from the glial ring onto the surrounding retinal surface; after a PVD, they may be seen as fine strands radiating from the glial ring during ophthalmoscopy. The patient may see them as spikes, threads, or a spider web next to the ring. During ophthalmoscopy through an undilated pupil, the observance of this peripapillary ring can be enhanced by having the patient move her eyes in vertical saccades so that the ring may pass behind the pupil in the ascension-descension phenomenon.[45]

cavity (Figure 4-6). This is more likely to be found in eyes with vitreous degeneration, such as highly myopic eyes.

The posterior vitreous cortex is most adherent to the inner eye wall at the vitreous base (which straddles the ora serrata), to the optic disc (prepapillary gliotic ring), and to a lesser extent to the perifoveal area, chorioretinal scars, and along superficial blood vessels; adhesion is weakest along the inner limiting membrane of the retinal surface.[43] Some-

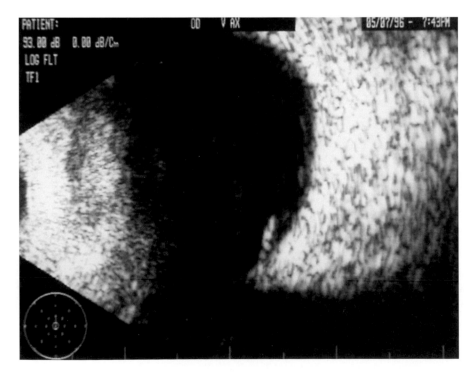

FIGURE 4-6
B-scan ultrasonogram of contracted vitreous strands and/or cortex in the inferior vitreous cavity immediately following a PVD.

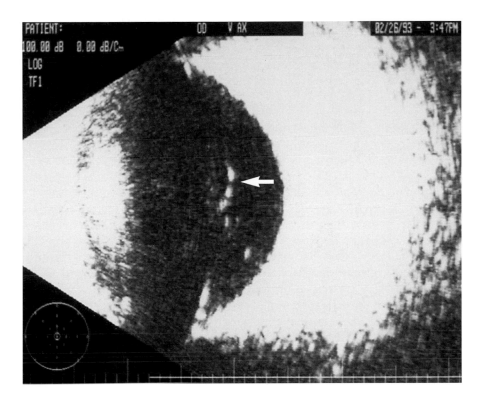

FIGURE 4-7
B-scan ultrasonogram of a PVD annulus. Note that in view is the superior glial ring (*arrow*), the prepapillary hole, and the inferior glial ring.

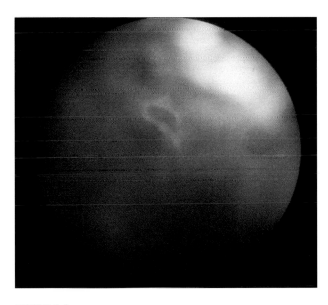

FIGURE 4-8
A partially collapsed annular glial ring of a PVD can be seen floating in the center of the vitreous cavity.

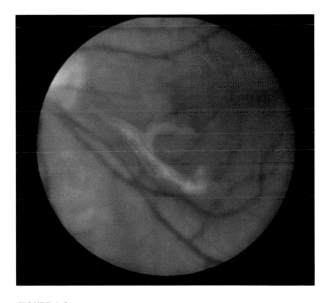

FIGURE 4-9
The annulus of a posterior vitreous detachment can be seen above the optic disc. Note that a strip of the annulus is still attached to the disc and will probably detach some time later.

An autopsy study of 320 cases of total PVDs found that 57% had glial tissue on the posterior vitreous cortex.[46] It sometimes happens that the glial ring tissue is not torn free and remains around the optic disc; thus, no annular glial ring can be seen in the vitreous cavity. Sometimes when no gliotic ring is visible the prepapillary hole (the area in the pos-

terior cortex that was over the optic disc) is visible with the ophthalmoscope or, more likely, with the precorneal condensing lens and the biomicroscope. Also, the glial ring may be so thin as to be difficult to see during ophthalmoscopy. The prepapillary hole is seen as a clear window in the center of the posterior face. Sometimes its detection is enhanced by movement of the posterior cortex on eye flicks. Rarely, a small gliotic annulus from the macula can be seen floating in the vitreous temporal to the larger annulus that originated from the optic disc.

It is well recognized that PVD begins in the region over the posterior pole,[1, 42, 47, 48] and it may well be that the liquefaction of the vitreous in the posterior pole is the result of light toxicity because most of the light is focused in this region of the vitreous body.[1] It has been proposed that liquefaction may start in this region due to the toxic metabolic waste products released by the high density of metabolically active neurons found in the macula.[10] Both light irradiation and metabolic waste products can generate free radicals that have the ability to disrupt the HA-collagen structure, thus leading to liquefaction.[49, 50] A postmortem study of 61 eyes discovered that the concentration of HA was lower in eyes with a PVD.[31] Another study found a significant decrease in the concentration of HA in aphakic eyes,[51] and another postmortem study of highly myopic eyes with an axial length over 26 mm found the HA and collagen concentration lower than in emmetropic eyes.[52] All these studies suggest that HA plays a critical role as a stabilizer of the collagen gel and that this biochemical change may lead to liquefaction of the vitreous and PVD formation. It is also possible that the free radicals may affect the cortex–basal lamina adhesive bonds and contribute to the formation of PVDs.[10] The liquefaction of the vitreous over the posterior pole leads to the formation of lacunae;[47, 48] with time they become large enough to be seen with the biomicroscope.[53]

Synchysis and syneresis result in the vitreous becoming more mobile and slowly shrinking. After a PVD, the characteristics of the vitreous change. Ultrasonographic Doppler studies have found that the vitreous becomes less "stiff."[54] Eventually, the tractional force of the moving vitreous becomes great enough to begin the separation of the vitreous cortex from the retinal surface. Synchysis is strongly associated with PVD formation.[55] Two studies, of 4,492 and 61 autopsied eyes, found a significant correlation of the degree of synchysis and the incidence of PVD.[1, 31] Another possible contributor to the etiology of a PVD is that the internal limiting membrane (ILM), or basal lamina, thickens with age (the result of continued synthesis by the Müller cells).[19, 56] This increase in thickness of the ILM may cause weakness in overall vitreoretinal adhesion by adversely affecting the ability of the Müller cells to synthesize and maintain the elements of the extracellular substance at the interface of the ILM and cortex; this may weaken the natural bond and thus lead to the development of a PVD.[44] Once liquid forms in the vitreous, there is a decrease in the stabilizing effects of HA on the collagen fibril network and there can be collapse (syneresis) of the vitreous body. With the breakdown of the posterior vitreous cortex–basal lamina interface adhesion, liquefied vitreous may be able to reach the retrovitreous space through the prepapillary hole and the premacular vitreous cortex.[12, 42, 57, 58] The loss of fluid from the vitreous body also leads to syneresis (contraction).

Fluid in the retrovitreous space can cause separation of the posterior cortex either by hydrating the adhesion bond at the cortex–basal lamina interface or by mechanically dissecting the cortex on eye movements. The latter possibility may be the result of the retrovitreous fluid being lighter than the vitreous gel and therefore being set in motion sooner than the vitreous gel, which may act as a fluid wedge to separate the vitreous cortex from the retinal surface.[59] The degenerating vitreous fibrils spanning the vitreous cavity may contract the vitreous body and pull the posterior vitreous forward.[47, 60]

To initiate a PVD, there must be enough vitreous traction or loss of bonding strength of the vitreous cortex to the retinal surface, or both, to allow for separation from the optic disc and macular area. The tearing of the cortical face in the macular area is considered the precipitating event in the formation of a PVD.[12, 58] Once the cortex is separated from the optic disc, a fairly continuous separation from the disc anteriorly to the posterior margin or the vitreous base occurs due to the strong vitreoretinal attachment at the base; it does not become involved in the vitreous separation.[61] At first, there may be only a partial or incomplete separation of the vitreous from a localized region over the posterior retina, but with time, the tractional forces will be great enough to pull the vitreous from the area of greatest adherence in the posterior region, which is the optic disc. Usually, a partial PVD rapidly progresses to a total separation, and the incidence of complete separations increases with age.[1, 6] This separation can be halted temporarily by areas of strong vitreoretinal adhesion, and continuing traction on these vitreoretinal adhesive sites can result in photopsia. The anterior displacement of the vitreous causes angular anterior-directed tractional forces on any existing vitreoretinal adhesions, the posterior margin, or the vitreous base, which may result in retinal tears. Lesions that are known to have unusually strong vitreoretinal adhesions include the enclosed ora bay, meridional fold, cystic retinal tuft, zonular traction tuft, and lattice degeneration.

The symptoms of a PVD are floaters, photopsia, blurred vision, glare, and, rarely, metamorphopsia. In many patients, however, the symptoms may be so subtle that they are not noticed and therefore not reported. Blurred vision may result from large vitreous floaters obscuring the patient's vision, vitreous hemorrhage, or cystoid macular edema (resulting from persistent vitreous strands tugging on the macula). The latter condition may also produce metamorphopsia. Glare may be produced by light scatter from the dense collagen fibril network in the detached posterior vitreous cortex.[18]

Floaters are the most common symptom of a PVD.[7] Patients often complain of vitreous debris as "cobwebs," "strings," or a "hairnet." In a study of 902 consecutive symptomatic eyes, 342 eyes had floaters only, and a PVD was found in 40% of the eyes, as compared to a control group with 20% PVD.[62] Floaters come in many shapes and sizes and are usually the result of condensation of vitreous fibrils within the vitreous cortex, glial tissue torn from the epipapillary region, or intravitreal blood from superficial retinal vessels.[63] These tiny opacities formed in the collapsing vitreous move about freely with the detached vitreous. Another form of floaters is observable only by the clinician: white cells or pigment cells floating in the anterior vitreous.[64, 65] The symptom of one or two isolated floaters that have been seen for months or years probably signifies the existence of vitreous condensation or a PVD annulus and are generally a benign symptom that do not carry a significant risk.[66] The sudden onset of such floaters should not be taken casually, however, and a dilated fundus examination should be performed. Among patients over age 50, the symptom of the sudden onset of floaters is associated with a PVD in 95% of cases.[67] The finding of a single floater may indicate a PVD annulus, with a small possibility of an asymptomatic retinal tear or detachment. Byer[7] found in a prospective study of unreferred patients with a PVD that 46% (163 in 350) complained of one or two floaters (with or without photopsia) as the presenting symptom: 7.2% of these patients (12) had a secondary retinal tear, nine had tears only, and three had tears and a retinal detachment. The acute onset of many floaters may be due to a vitreous hemorrhage and requires an immediate comprehensive eye examination.[67] The tiny floaters seen by the patient in a vitreous hemorrhage often results from the rupture of a retinal vessel during a PVD; these tend to move across the visual field as the red blood cells (RBCs) spread out in the retrovitreal fluid space of the PVD. The floaters are originally seen in the peripheral visual field from a torn anterior blood vessel, then move centrally and finally disappear as the RBCs degenerate.

On ultrasonography studies, I have found that many small areas of vitreous condensation are actually located on the posterior cortex. Because they can be found immediately after a PVD (Figure 4-10), I have surmised that they were there before the PVD was produced. These pre-existing floaters on the attached posterior cortex are small and transparent and remain stationary over the retina; therefore, they were not noticed, just as retinal vessels are not perceived due to their stationary location over the photoreceptors. Once the vitreous condensations become mobile just anterior to the retinal surface, they can be seen as transparent dark objects that move rapidly in the visual field. Also on ultrasonography, more anterior vitreous floaters tend to move in a more anterior-posterior direction rather than tangentially with small eye movements. This happens because the detached vitreous is only attached anteriorly at the ora serrata region, which would allow mostly anterior-posterior movements of the anteriorly hinged vitreous. This would also explain the observation that floaters from PVDs seem to come and go so quickly, for as the floater approaches the retina it is perceived and disappears from view as it rapidly returns to an anterior location in the vitreous cavity. Floaters that occur in the retrovitreous space may disappear from view due to gravitational migration into the inferior fundus, whereas those on the detached vitreous face cortex may persist for years.

Another form of PVD is what I call a "prominent posterior cortex" PVD; it results from the formation of a rather thick posterior cortex in the posterior pole. Some patients have an area of posterior cortex many times thicker than normal, and this can be seen on ultrasonography (Figure 4-11). When the posterior cortex separates, an obvious and large diaphanous membrane can be seen floating above the posterior pole. If the membrane floats close to the visual axis, the patient sees a rather annoying translucent membrane or complains of a slight visual annoyance, "like looking through smudged glass." The patient may find that this visual disturbance moves on eye movements. These patients are characteristically symptomatic of a PVD.

Photopsia (flashing lights) is a frequent symptom of a PVD; it results from mechanical stimulation of the retina by the traction produced by the detaching vitreous cortex. The light flash is usually bright white in appearance but occasionally may be colored.[68] Generally, photopsia occurs only when sig-

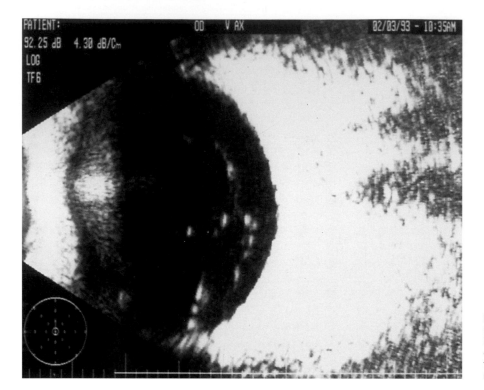

FIGURE 4-10
B-scan ultrasonogram of a PVD. Note that there are condensed areas of vitreous (*floaters*) both in the vitreous gel and on the posterior vitreous cortex.

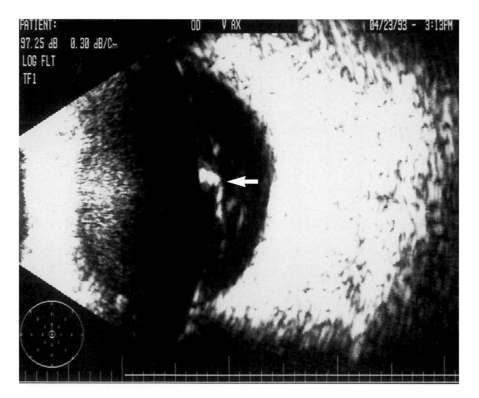

FIGURE 4-11
B-scan of "prominent" PVD showing that the posterior vitreous cortex is much thicker (*arrow*), and it may cause visual disturbances if it moves into the visual axis.

nificant traction is applied to the retina, usually during fast eye movements. Some have proposed that photopsis is caused by the actual impact of the moving vitreous on the retinal surface,[69] but it is more likely due to vitreous traction. Because the retina has no pain receptors, mechanical stimulation of the underlying photoreceptors can only result in the symptom of photopsia. It is seen by patients approximately 23–66% of the time.[7, 12, 25, 27–29, 70–73] Photopsia without floaters has been reported to occur in only 9% and 18% of eyes.[29] In a study of 902 consecutive symptomatic eyes, 203 had photopsia only and 240 had photopsia and floaters; a PVD was found in 89% of the former and 67% of the latter, compared to a control group with only 20% PVD.[62] Females report a higher incidence of photopsia than males.[68]

Photopsia usually occurs during the active process of the PVD and only persists if areas of vitreoretinal attachment remain. The photopsia from these remaining vitreoretinal attachments only ceases if the vitreous cortex ultimately separates from the retina or if the retinal tissue at the site of attachment is pulled free into the vitreous. Traction on the anterior attachment of the vitreous to the posterior vitreous base may result in the flashing arc of light characteristically seen by patients after a PVD. It is important to understand that a localized area of vitreous traction on the retina may result in photopsia that resembles a flashbulb going off or a lightning bolt in a small area of the visual field of the involved eye. It is important to examine the retina with and without scleral depression 180 degrees from the observed location of the flash for a possible retinal tear. When a patient sees a vertical arc of light in the far visual field (usually temporal), however, it is the result of significant traction on the vitreous base during eye movements and does not indicate isolated vitreoretinal traction but rather a broad band of vitreous traction. After a PVD the vitreous loses its "stiffness"[54] and becomes more mobile, making it better able to cause significant traction on the vitreous base and produce arcing flashes of light. No matter what the shape or location of the flash of light, all such patients should have a dilated fundus examination to investigate its source.

The normal aging process is thought to be the usual mechanism in the production of a PVD; however, trauma can also be responsible. This is more likely to be seen in patients who are aphakic, are myopic, have vitreoretinal degeneration, or have a history of severe ocular trauma or uveitis. The pathogenesis of a spontaneous PVD appears to be synchysis and syneresis producing liquefaction of the vitreous gel and contraction of the fibrous vitreous over the vitreous base. The contraction of collagen fibers over the vitreous base produces anterior traction on the vitreous that pulls the posterior cortex off the retina. Liquefaction of the vitreous body allows the vitreous to collapse in an anterior and inferior direction due to gravity. This process is enhanced by head trauma, so that even a slight bump on the head may initiate a PVD in older patients.

Another form of vitreoretinal separation that mimics a PVD is a forward displacement of a portion of the anterior vitreous cortex that leaves the posterior cortex layer still attached to the ILM; this is called *vitreoschisis*.[74, 75] This condition results in a prominent liquefaction with cavitation in the posterior vitreous with the outer cortical layer still attached to the ILM. It is usually seen in highly myopic eyes.[10] It differs from PVD in that it does not show ascension-descension movements on vertical saccades. Vitreoschisis may occur in eyes with proliferative diabetic retinopathy and vitreous hemorrhage.[76] One study of 140 eyes with proliferative diabetic retinopathy showed echographic evidence of vitreoschisis in 20% of cases.[77]

There is a question in my mind that the posterior vitreous cortex may play a role in the formation of the foveal light reflex. It may well be that the posterior cortex is partially or mostly responsible for the light reflex by forming a smooth concave surface as it bows posterior to cover the foveal depression. I have seen the loss of the foveal reflex immediately after a PVD and thought that it may have been the result of losing the smooth concave lining of the foveal depression with disruption of the vitreous–ILM interface or due to development of macular edema secondary to the cortical separation. Because the loss of the foveal reflex occurred within a few hours of the PVD symptoms, I am inclined to believe that it is more often due to the former. The loss of the foveal reflex has been known to increase with age,[78, 79] and generally, it seems to disappear after age 50; after age 80, it is conspicuously absent.[77, 80–82] Of interest, the age of foveal light reflex loss is almost identical to the age when partial or complete PVD occurs. The loss of the foveal reflex may indicate some disease of the macula and so its loss in younger people should alert the clinician to perform a careful macular examination.[83, 84] However, the loss of the foveal reflex in younger patients has been documented without observable maculopathy.[80, 83]

Clinical Significance

Retinal, preretinal, disc, and vitreous hemorrhages can occur after a PVD.[25, 85] Any of these hemorrhages can result from the tractional rupture of a retinal or disc vessel during a PVD or from the tearing of a vessel crossing a retinal tear caused by a PVD. The posterior vitreous cortex has perivascular attachments sometimes known as vitreoretinovascular bands that pass through tiny openings in the ILM.[19, 43, 86–89] Foos[90] found that the ILM was thinned over retinal vessels and hypothesized that this was the result of areas where vitreous fibrils passed through to develop adhesions to the underlying vessels. Also, there seems to be an absence of Müller cells in these retinal locations, which may make these vessels more susceptible to vitreous traction. These exaggerated attachments are not visible when the vitreous is in direct contact with the retinal surface.[43, 91] Tractional forces may rupture these superficial retinal vessels as the vitreous cortex pulls away from the retina. The release of RBCs that float next to the retinal surface in the retrovitreous space results in the sudden onset of numerous tiny black floaters. The patient more easily sees them as many black specks against a bright background or as a reddish tinge over the visual field. Retinal hemorrhages secondary to a PVD are usually found along the vitreous base,[63, 92] but they have also been found in the peripapillary and macular areas.[63, 93] Any peripheral punctate retinal hemorrhages should be watched carefully because they indicate areas of strong vitreoretinal traction that may later be the site of a retinal tear.[25, 27] All these areas are probable sites of strong vitreoretinal adhesions. Retinal tears are associated with 13% of the eyes with paravascular vitreoretinal attachments, and they are frequently associated with a vitreous hemorrhage.[41, 89]

Ophthalmoscopically, vitreous hemorrhages appear as tiny black specks ("black pepper") against the orange fundus reflex with the direct ophthalmoscope or during biomicroscopy with the precorneal fundus lens. They may also be seen during binocular indirect ophthalmoscopy as a faint plume of reddish "smoke" billowing into the vitreous. Vitreous hemorrhages from a PVD are generally small and self-limiting. Vitreal and retrovitreal hemorrhages tend to gravitate downward with time, and it is not unusual to find a thin line of blood along the inferior retina, which is the result of blood behind the PVD layered along the posterior border of the vitreous base or an incomplete PVD. There may be free-floating blood clots in the inferior fundus along with streaks of blood in the vitreous gel behind the posterior cortical face. With time, the RBCs balloon and finally rupture, leading to resolution of the hemorrhage, but the degenerating

hemoglobin, which is toxic to the vitreous, may initiate scarring. A small hemorrhage resolves, leaving little or no evidence of this scarring, but larger or recurrent hemorrhages usually result in some degree of scarring. The blood that gravitates inferior is usually found as small round or teardrop-shaped blood clots; these shapes are usually retained as they form small fibrotic vitreous scars. Because most vitreous bleeds from a PVD are small, there is usually no residua. If the vitreous hemorrhage obscures the fundus, then it is advisable to perform ultrasonography to determine whether the retina is detached or torn.

Studies have found some degree of vitreous hemorrhage in 6–19% of all eyes with PVD.[7, 12, 25–29, 66, 67, 85, 94] In another study, 53–86% of spontaneous vitreous hemorrhage in nondiabetics were caused by a PVD.[95–97] Studies found that 20–100% of patients with PVD and a retinal break had a vitreous hemorrhage.[7, 12, 13, 25–29, 64, 67] Vitreous blood is significant for the possible existence of a retinal tear.[65, 95–97] The incidence of tear formation is relatively high in eyes with an acute PVD and vitreous hemorrhage (8.9–47%) of cases compared to just 2–4% in eyes with an acute PVD without a vitreous hemorrhage.[25, 28, 64, 72] It must be remembered that a vitreous hemorrhage associated with a PVD does not necessarily mean that a retinal tear is present.[7, 12, 25–29, 62, 67] Peripheral retinal hemorrhages are a sign of significant vitreous traction, and their sites may be the sites of future retinal breaks.[7, 25, 27]

The forward displacement of the vitreous body is caused by the retrovitreous space filling with liquefied vitreous, mostly through the prepapillary hole in the posterior cortex (the opening in the posterior cortex surrounded by the peripapillary glial ring) and through small fractures in the posterior cortex. Aqueous can flow backward from the ciliary body to aid in filling this space. The retrovitreous space can become even larger than that occupied by the collapsing vitreous body. A large reservoir of liquefied vitreous and aqueous is thus made available to pass into any retinal break and possibly cause a retinal detachment. Liquefied vitreous and aqueous are not viscous; thus, movement of these fluid bodies is considerable during eye movements.

The forward collapsing motion and the rotational motion of the vitreous body on eye movements can exert substantial tractional forces on isolated areas of increased vitreoretinal adhesion, possibly resulting in retinal tears (Figure 4-12).[7, 12, 25, 26, 29, 59, 98–102] The posterior vitreous cortex is most adherent to the inner eye wall at the vitreous base, the optic disc, and to a lesser extent to the perifoveal area, chorioretinal scars, along superficial blood vessels, and, even more tenuously, along the ILM of the retinal surface.[41, 91, 103] There are developmental peripheral vitreoretinal interface adhesions that are known as cystic retinal tufts, rosettes, spicula, tubulus, and verruca.[104] Strong vitreoretinal adhesions are found with cystic retinal tufts, rosettes, spicula, and verruca and therefore may be associated with retinal tears. Tubuli do not have strong adhesion and probably are not associated with retinal tear formation. These particular abnormalities are very subtle and have only been found in microscopic studies. Increased vitreoretinal adhesions are found at a number of peripheral retinal developmental variations, including meridional folds, meridional complexes, retinal excavations, enclosed ora bays, zonular traction tufts, lattice degeneration, paravascular vitreoretinal attachments, and exaggerated vitreoretinal attachments adjacent to the posterior vitreous base. In an autopsy study of 252 eyes, strong vitreoretinal adhesions over retinal vessels caused a paravascular retinal tear in 11% of eyes.[43] In eyes with full-thickness tears, 29% had a PVD, and 46% of eyes with full- or partial-thickness tears (retinal pits) had a PVD.[43] Retinal tears associated with firm vitreoretinal adhesions around superficial blood vessels occur in about 13% of eyes with a PVD and are frequently accompanied by a vitreous hemorrhage from a vessel tear.[105]

As the vitreous body detaches, the potential motion forces become greater the more anterior the separation because the more vitreous is freed from the inner eye wall, the greater is the ability of the vitreous to move on eye movements. Therefore, any peripheral areas of increased vitreoretinal adhesions in the periphery are subject to more sudden and strong "whiplike" anterior-posterior actions applied by the collapsed vitreous on eye movements. Another cause for the sudden actions of the vitreous on the retina is that the vitreous gel is heavier than the retrovitreous fluid, so that after the eye makes a sudden stop during a saccade, the gel continues to move for a short period of time rather than start to recover in the other direction on a saccade in the opposite direction. This motion is akin to water in a washing machine following the agitator blades. I have demonstrated these actions on ultrasonograms, and they can produce considerable traction on the underlying retina. Areas of increased vitreoretinal adhesions in the posterior pole are subject to much milder vitreous motion forces. This may explain why retinal tears in the posterior pole are so rare, because vitreous traction that is less sudden and strong during eye movements may allow the

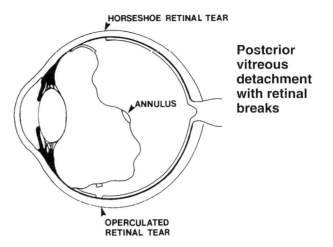

Posterior vitreous detachment with retinal breaks

FIGURE 4-12
The vitreous has moved forward and collapsed downward, producing traction at sites of increased vitreoretinal adhesion that resulted in retinal tears.

vitreous cortex to pull away from the retinal surface without causing a tear.

Syneresis and PVD are the two most important factors in the cause of retinal tears. In one study of 23 eyes with peripheral breaks, 21 demonstrated more syneresis than 21 age-matched controls.[55] Most tears occur anterior to the equator. The frequency of secondary retinal breaks in eyes with a PVD has been reported to be 8–46%.[5, 7, 12, 25–29, 55, 62, 64, 67, 72, 83, 92, 106, 107] Lindner[12] found 16 tears in 106 patients with a PVD. One study found a PVD in 80% of eyes with retinal tears,[70] but it appears that a more accurate frequency is likely to be 11–15%.[7] As many as half of these patients will have more than one retinal tear.[108] One study found that myopes over 3.00 diopters had a very significant association with PVD,[7] and in the presence of myopia over 6 diopters, retinal breaks were associated with PVD in 11.1%.[25] In high myopes who underwent uncomplicated cataract extraction, 16.2% had breaks associated with PVD.[106] However, another study found that myopes over 4.00 diopters had no retinal tears,[28] and yet another found that myopes over 6.00 diopters have the same risk of tear formation as of other refractive errors.[64] Aphakic eyes have a greater risk of retinal tear after PVD (33%, or seven of 21 eyes).[7] There is a preponderance of secondary tears in males,[12, 29, 69] and the odds ratio is 2.33:1.[7]

Some believe that symptomatic PVDs pose a greater risk of developing a retinal tear. Boldrey[64] correlated the risk of a tear secondary to a PVD based on the severity of the symptoms and showed a notably increased risk if the patient described the floaters as "like diffuse dots," if there were two or more cells in the anterior vitreous, or if there was grossly visible vitreous blood. Although photopsia is a symptom of vitreoretinal traction, patients with photopsia have no higher incidence of retinal tears than those without the symptom.[12, 27, 29, 109] Other authors have reported that the risk of a tear was essentially the same if there were flashes only, floaters only, or both flashes and floaters.[28] The largest subgroup of associated symptoms with retinal tears have both floaters and photopsia.[7] The presence of a significant vitreous hemorrhage or pigment cells in the vitreous greatly enhances the possibility of a retinal tear.[110] One study found that pigment cells in the vitreous ("tobacco dust," or Shafer's sign) was found in 14.1% of 106 eyes, all of which had an operculated or flap tear.[65] Very few eyes with an asymptomatic PVD have gone on to produce a retinal tear.[12, 111]

Tractional forces due to a PVD are often more apparent in the far peripheral retina and are most likely the result of the anterior displacement of the vitreous and the firm adhesion of the vitreous cortex to the posterior region of the vitreous base.[18, 112] These areas of increased vitreoretinal adhesion can sometimes be seen during indirect ophthalmoscopy with dynamic scleral depression in which wispy strands of vitreous may be detected in relief over the induced roll. These areas of increased adhesions can be very difficult to find, which is exemplified by the fact that most secondary tears occur in normal-appearing areas of the retina.[12, 27] Byer[7] reported that this occurred in 70% of eyes with tears and 72% of eyes with breaks. The symptoms of a retinal tear are generally the symptoms of the associated PVD. Almost all retinal breaks secondary to a PVD are discovered at the initial examination,[25–29] even if the symptoms are very brief in duration. In a study by Byer,[7] out of 42 eyes presenting with breaks at the time of the first examination, 59% (25) reported symptoms of 1 week or less, 76% (32) had symptoms of 2 weeks or less. However, there may be quite a time delay before breaks appear (3–27% of cases),[7, 25–29] and the time period may range from 2 weeks to 10 years after the initial symptoms.[7] The location of secondary tears is predominantly the superior half of the retina (70–100% of cases),[12, 25, 26, 28, 29] which is most likely due to the fact that in the upright position, the PVD has greater gravitational force on the upper half of the retina.

The retinal tears caused by a PVD may be U-shaped, L-shaped, linear, or irregularly round, and there may be an associated flap or free operculum. Because of the anterior displacement of the vitreous,

the operculum in an operculated tear is generally found anterior to the round tear. An operculated retinal tear has a far better prognosis because vitreous traction has been released from its edges. The vitreous cortex usually remains attached to the flap of a horseshoe tear (see Figure 4-12) and the anterior margin of a linear tear. If a small amount of cortex is still attached to the posterior margins of a horseshoe or linear tear, the edges may become rolled due to contraction. The continued vitreous traction on the flap of a retinal tear greatly enhances the chances for the production of a retinal detachment due to the continuous physical pulling on the sensory retina. The physical traction around a retinal tear is probably more significant in the production of a retinal detachment than is the reservoir of fluid in the retrovitreal space. Even giant retinal tears have been the result of PVD.[26]

Because the vitreous base is not involved in a PVD, the occurrence of tears within the base are very rare; if they do occur, they are usually associated with intrabasal focal traction, such as zonular traction tufts attached within the base. Also, the vitreous gel's firm structure over the base decreases the incidence of liquefaction in this area and greatly lessens the amount of fluid able to pass into a trophic hole to cause a retinal detachment.[113] After a PVD, however, considerable traction may be placed on the posterior base margin and the retina just posterior to the base. This area of the retina is commonly involved in tear formation after a PVD.[12]

Retinal detachment is another consideration in the sequela of PVD and is almost always rhegmatogenous in nature.[7, 12, 25, 26, 29] Retinal detachment is the natural aftermath of retinal tear formation in patients with PVD. Primary retinal detachments are almost always preceded by a PVD; one study found syneresis and PVD in 90% of cases of retinal detachment.[2] Almost all patients with a retinal detachment have a PVD, but half of these patients present with visual field loss or decreased vision rather than flashes or floaters.[73, 114] Fifty-eight percent of these types of detachments occur in eyes that do not display any visible predisposing retinal lesions.[115] It is estimated that 3–5% of eyes with a symptomatic PVD will develop a retinal detachment and that very few eyes with an asymptomatic PVD would ever have a detachment.[116, 117] There is a high risk of retinal detachment in aphakic eyes with a retinal tear after a PVD (85%, or 6 of 7 eyes), which may occur within days to more than a year as compared to (18%, or 8 of 43 eyes) in phakic eyes.[7]

Vitreous strands are attached to the margins of lattice degeneration (see Lattice Degeneration,

Chapter 3), and a linear tear often occurs along the posterior and lateral margins, rarely along the anterior margin of lattice degeneration after a PVD. Another retinal finding associated with a PVD is white-with- or -without-pressure, which is the result of vitreous traction[118] (see the section on White-With- or -Without-Pressure in Chapter 3).

Another possible finding is edema of the macula and optic disc, which is also produced by vitreous traction.[13, 119, 120] In the macula the ILM is thin and there are purported to be attachment plaques to the vitreous cortex,[44] which may explain the predilection of this area for traction-induced changes.[13, 57, 93, 121–123] The edema may disappear if vitreoretinal adhesions are broken, but if the traction exists for a prolonged period of time, irreversible damage may result. Macular hole formation has been suggested as a consequence of PVD,[124–129] and an operculum may be found above the hole. The pathogenesis of macular holes is multiple, but the group of macular hole disorders can be categorized on the presence or absence of an operculum, PVD, or premacular membrane.[130] A rare finding is the occurrence of a disc hemorrhage with a PVD.[131] Also, it is possible to have a PVD following panretinal photocoagulation regardless of the severity of existing diabetic retinopathy.[132]

Premacular membranes are also cited as a consequence of PVD. Clinically, premacular membranes are found in 3.5% of the population and are unilateral 80% of the time.[133] A PVD is present in 80–95% of the cases of premacular membranes.[133, 134] In one prospective study of 34 eyes with an acute PVD, only 9% demonstrated epiretinal membranes, but after 18 months, 41% of the eyes developed membranes.[135] This finding suggests that when the vitreous cortex separates from the retina, some protective influence seems to be lost. It appears that premacular membranes generally begin at an area close to the optic disc and advance toward the fovea. Abnormal proliferation of tissue at the disc has been found in half of normal human eyes at autopsy.[134] The reason for such a prevalence of cellular proliferation at the disc margin is likely due to the absence of the ILM and vitreous cortex at the optic disc, both of which may have an inhibitory influence on such cellular proliferation. Histologic studies found that this membrane is composed of astrocytes, macrophages, fibrocytes, hyalocytes, and pigment epithelial cells.[136, 137]

There are currently two theories about the production of these premacular membranes. One is that, during a PVD, transient traction is produced by the separating vitreous on the optic disc and juxtapapillary retina, which can lead to dehiscence on the surface of these structures that may allow the migration and proliferation of fibrous astrocytes onto the surface of the ILM.[38, 135] These fibrous astrocytes can organize into a membrane that can develop myofibroblast characteristics and therefore contract and cause folds to form in the superficial retina.[138] Because the strongest vitreoretinal adhesions in the posterior pole occur at the optic disc, the macula, and along superficial blood vessels, the breaks in the ILM are more likely to occur in these areas. Because there are more blood vessels in the posterior pole, it is more likely that epiretinal membranes are located in this area of the fundus.

The other likely reason for this clinical finding is that the premacular membranes may derive from hyalocytes located in the vitreous cortex. Indeed, when the vitreous cortex separates from the ILM in a PVD, the cortex may split (vitreoschisis) and leave behind remnants of the cortex.[75, 90] An autopsy study of 59 normal eyes with spontaneous PVD found that 44% had cortex remnants at the fovea.[139] Proliferation, migration, and fibrous metaplasia of these leftover hyalocytes can form a macular membrane with contractile properties.[140–143] Biomicroscopy has shown that sometimes a break in the premacular cortex can be discerned with herniation of vitreous gel, which would indicate a tear in the cortex with remnants probably on the macular surface. Given that one study found that 75% of eyes with premacular membranes did not show signs of cortical vitreous, this is only one possible way that this condition develops.[144]

Premacular membranes are capable of reducing vision by causing surface wrinkling and cystoid macular edema or angiographically proven macular edema. This was demonstrated in a study of 250 cases of premacular membrane and partial PVD.[145] There were very few cases of such maculopathy when no PVD or complete PVD was present. Therefore, a partial PVD may produce continuous traction on the posterior pole, which may lead to tiny breaks in the ILM; whereas with a complete PVD, tractional forces are usually terminated and breaks in the ILM are less likely to occur. When a complete PVD occurs in cases of premacular membranes, the membrane may peel free of the macula, with resolution of the symptoms.[146] In surgical membrane peels, the membranes formed from hyalocytes are more easily peeled off; whereas those formed by proliferating fibrous astrocytes are more difficult to peel due to their firm connection to the underlying retina.[18]

When a patient calls the office with complaints of recent onset of visual floaters or light flashes, it is best to see him in 1–2 days. Presently, there is no known way of safely or reliably preventing PVD.[101] Patients with an acute symptomatic PVD should be followed every 3–4 weeks until the condition becomes asymptomatic and no retinal tears are found. Others have suggested follow-up ranges from 2 to 6 months.[12, 25, 27, 28] Routine examinations should be performed for the first 6 months, but after 6 months, the chances for development of a retinal detachment is unlikely.[7, 28] Because the time delay between the initial symptom of a PVD and the occurrence of a break or retinal detachment can be from months to years, the choosing of any particular time for follow-up is strictly arbitrary. The best way to follow such patients is to instruct them carefully on the symptoms of a retinal tear or detachment and tell them to return immediately if they should occur.[7, 28, 29, 64] These symptoms include a sudden onset of tiny black specks, increase in photopsia, or a curtain, either during the acute phase or any time afterward. More frequent examinations are required if there is a vitreous hemorrhage,[25] especially if no retinal tear is seen,[28] and more frequent examinations are suggested if symptoms increase.[28, 29, 64] It is suggested that the examination be every 2 weeks if there is a significant vitreous hemorrhage that obscures the peripheral retina and then timely visits thereafter when a view of the periphery is possible.

Retinal tears that occur at the time of a symptomatic PVD should be treated with prophylactic retinopexy because continuing traction on these tears may result in a retinal detachment. Therefore, the prompt diagnosis and treatment of retinal tears in eyes with acute PVD (even with minimal symptoms) is the best time to apply effective preventative treatment and emphasizes the concept of treating new tears to prevent retinal detachment.[7] Recurrent vitreous bleeds from avulsed retinal tissue (operculated and flap tears) with retinal vessels still attached have occurred after a PVD.[147, 148] If the PVD causing a flap tear is not complete at the time of retinopexy, further anterior progression by the PVD may lead to extension of the tear and a possible retinal detachment.

References

1. Heller MD, Straatsma BR, et al. Detachment of the posterior vitreous in phakic and aphakic eyes. Mod Probl Ophthalmol 1972;10:23.
2. Foos RY, Wheeler NC. Vitreoretinal juncture: Synchysis senilis and posterior vitreous detachment. Ophthalmology 1982;89:1502–1512.
3. Pischel DK. Detachment of the vitreous as seen with slit-lamp examination. Am J Ophthalmol 1953;36:1497–1507.
4. Tolentino FI, Schepens CL, et al. Vitreoretinal disorders: Diagnosis and Management. Philadelphia: Saunders, 1976;130–190.
5. Foos RY. Posterior vitreous detachment. Trans Am Acad Ophthalmol Otolaryngol 1972;76:480–497.
6. Osterlin S. Vitreous Changes after Cataract Extraction. In HM Freeman, T Hirose, CL Schepens (eds), Vitreous Surgery and Advances in Fundus Diagnosis and Treatment. New York: Appleton-Century-Crofts, 1977;15–21.
7. Byer NE. Natural history of posterior vitreous detachment with early management as the premier line of defense against retinal detachment. Ophthalmology 1994;101: 1503–1514.
8. Perichon JY, Brasseur G, et al. Ultrasonographic study of posterior vitreous detachment in emmetropic eyes. J Fr Ophtalmol 1993;16:538–544.
9. Rieger H. Über die bedeutung der aderhautveranderungen fur die entstehung der glaskorperabhebung. Graefes Arch Ophthalmol 1937;136:118–165.
10. Sebag J. Vitreous Pathology. In W Tasman, EA Jaeger EA (eds), Clinical Ophthalmology. Vol. 3. Philadelphia: Harper & Row, 1992;39:1–26.
11. Yonemoto J, Ideta H, et al. The age of onset of posterior vitreous detachment. Graefes Arch Clin Exp Ophthalmol 1994;232:67–70.
12. Lindner B. Acute posterior vitreous detachment and its retinal complications. A clinical biomicroscopic study. Acta Ophthalmol Scand Supp 1966;87:1–108.
13. Jaffe NS. Vitreous traction at the posterior pole of the fundus due to alterations in the posterior vitreous. Trans Am Acad Ophthalmol Otolaryngol 1967;71:642–652.
14. Akiba J. Prevalence of posterior vitreous detachment in high myopia. Ophthalmology 1993;100:1384–1388.
15. Morita H, Funata M, et al. A clinical study of the development of posterior vitreous detachment in high myopes. Retina 1995;15:117–124.
16. Singh A, Paul SD, et al. A clinical study of vitreous body (in emmetropia and refractive errors). Orient Arch Ophthal 1970;8:11–17.
17. Pierro I, Camesasa FI, et al. Peripheral retinal changes and axial myopia. Retina 1992;12:12–17.
18. Hyams SW, Neumann E, et al. Myopia-aphakia. II. Vitreous and peripheral retina. Br J Ophthalmol 1975; 59:483–485.
19. Sebag J. The Vitreous: Structure, Function and Pathology. New York: Springer-Verlag, 1989;47–55.
20. Pruett RC, Albert DM. Vitreous Degeneration in Myopia and Retinitis Pigmentosa. In CL Schepens, A Neetens (eds), The Vitreous and Vitreoretinal Interface. New York: Springer-Verlag, 1987;211–228.
21. Grossniklaus HE, Green WR. Pathological findings in pathologic myopia. Retina 1992;12:127–133.
22. Brandt HP. Liedloff H. Biomicroscopie der glasskorpers bei kindlicher myopie. Klin Monatsbl Augenheilkd 1970;156:340–348.
23. Smith TJ. Dexamethasone regulation of glycosaminoglycan synthesis in cultured human skin fibroblasts: Similar effects of glucocorticoid and thyroid hormones. J Clin Invest 1984;74:2157–2163.
24. Sirek OV, Sirek A, et al. The effect of sex hormones on glycosaminoglycan content of canine aorta and coronary arteries. Atherosclerosis 1977;27:227–233.
25. Tasman WE. Posterior vitreous detachment and periph-

eral retinal breaks. Trans Am Acad Ophthalmol Otolaryngol 1968;72:217–224.

26. Jaffe NS. Complications of acute posterior vitreous detachment. Arch Ophthalmol 1968;79:368–371.

27. Kanski JJ. Complications of acute posterior detachment. Am J Ophthalmol 1975;80:44–46.

28. Tabotabo MM, Karp LA, et al. Posterior vitreous detachment. Ann Ophthalmol 1980;12:59–61.

29. Novak MA, Welch RB. Complications of acute symptomatic posterior vitreous detachment. Am J Ophthalmol 1984;97:308–314.

30. Balazs EA. The vitreous. Int Ophthalmol Clin 1973; 13:169–187.

31. Larsson L, Osterlin S. Posterior vitreous detachment: A combined clinical and physiochemical study. Graefes Arch Clin Exp Ophthalmol 1985;223:92–95.

32. Takahashi M. Posterior vitreous detachment as an aging process: Analysis of 1077 normal eyes [in Japan]. Rinsho Ganka 1982;36:1137–1141.

33. Wedrich A, Velikay M, et al. Ocular findings in asymptomatic amateur boxers. Retina 1993;13:114–119.

34. Lindner BJ. Posterior vitreous detachment: A possible complication of noncontact tonometry. Ann Ophthalmol 1993;25:54–55.

35. Takahashi M, Jalkh A, et al. Biomicroscopic evaluation and photography of liquid vitreous in some vitreoretinal disorders. Arch Ophthal 1981;99:1555–1559.

36. Takahashi M, Schepens CL, et al. Biomicroscopic evaluation and photography of posterior vitreous detachment. Arch Ophthalmol 1980;98:665–669.

37. Kakehashi A, Akiba J, et al. Vitreous photography with a +90-diopter double aspheric preset lens vs. El Bayadi–Kajiura preset lens. Arch Ophthalmol 1991;109: 962–965.

38. Kakehashi A, Tremple CL. A comprehensive approach to biomicroscopic vitreous examination. Ann Ophthalmol 1993;25:24–28.

39. Kakehashi A, Akiba J, et al. Vitreous photography with a wide-angle funduscopic lens. Retina 1993;13:142–144.

40. Hikichi T, Akiba Jun, et al. Vitreous observation using a CCD camera and a computerized unit for image processing and storage. Retina 1995;15:505–512.

41. Kakehashi A, Kado M, et al. Biomicroscopic vitreous videography. Retina 1995;15:508–512.

42. Sebag J, Balazs EA. Morphology and ultrastructure of human vitreous fibers. Invest Ophthalmol Vis Sci 1989;30:1867–1871.

43. Spencer LM, Foos RY. Paravascular vitreoretinal attachment: Role in retinal tears. Invest Ophthalmol 1970; 84:557–564.

44. Sebag J. Age-related differences in the human vitreo-retinal interface. Arch Ophthalmol 1991;109:966–971.

45. Schepens CL. Methods of Examination. In Retinal Detachment and Allied Diseases. Philadelphia: Saunders, 1983;126–133.

46. Foos RY, Roth AM. Surface structure of the optic nerve head. II. Vitreopapillary attachments and posterior vitreous detachment. Am J Ophthalmol 1973;76:662–671.

47. Sebag J. Age-related changes in human vitreous structure. Graefes Arch Clin Exp Ophthalmol 1987;225:89–93.

48. Kishis S, Shimizu K. Posterior precortical vitreous pocket. Arch Ophthalmol 1990;108:979–982.

49. Uneo N, Sebag J, et al. Effects of visible-light irradiation on vitreous structure in the presence of a photosensitizer. Exp Eye Res 1987;44:863–870.

50. Kakehashi A, Uneo N, et al. Molecular mechanisms of photochemically induced posterior vitreous detachment. Ophthalmic Res 1994;26:51–59.

51. Osterlin S. On the molecular biology of the vitreous in the aphakic eye. Acta Ophthalmol Scand Supp 1977;55:353–361.

52. Berman ER, Michaelson IC. The chemical composition of the human vitreous body as related to age and myopia. Exp Eye Res 1964;3:9–15.

53. Goldmann H. The diagnostic value of biomicroscopy of the posterior parts of the eye. Br J Ophthalmol 1961; 45:449–460.

54. Wong D, Restori M. Ultrasonic Doppler studies of the vitreous. Eye 1988;2:87–91.

55. O'Malley P. The Pattern of Vitreous Syneresis: A Study of 800 Autopsy Eyes. In AR Irvine, P O'Malley (eds), Advances in Vitreous Surgery. Springfield, IL: Thomas, 1976:17–33.

56. Hogan MJ, Alavardo JA, et al. Histology of the Human Eye: An Atlas and Textbook. Philadelphia: Saunders, 1971;607.

57. Sebag J. Vitreo-Retinal Interface and the Role of Vitreous in Macular Disease. In R Brancato, G Coscas, B Lumbroso (eds), Proceedings of the Retina Workshop. Amsterdam: Kugler & Ghedini, 1987;3–6.

58. Eisner G. Biomicroscopy of the Peripheral Fundus. New York: Springer-Verlag, 1973.

59. Rosengren B, Osterlin S. Hydrodynamic events in the vitreous space accompanying eye movements: Significance for the pathogenesis of retinal detachment. Ophthalmologica 1976;173:513–524.

60. Sebag J. Aging of the vitreous. Eye 1987;1:254–262.

61. RG Michels, CP Wilkinson, TA Rice (eds). Retinal Detachment: Diagnosis and Management. St. Louis: Mosby, 1990.

62. Hikichi T, Trempe CL. Relationship between floaters, light flashes, or both, and complications of posterior vitreous detachment. Am J Ophthalmol 1994;117:593–598.

63. Cibis GE, Watzke RC, et al. Retinal hemorrhages in posterior vitreous detachment. Am J Ophthalmol 1975; 80:1043–1046.

64. Boldrey EE. Risk of retinal tears in patients with vitreous floaters. Am J Ophthalmol 1983;96:783–787.

65. Brod RD, Lightman DA, et al. Correlation between vitreous pigment granules and retinal breaks in eyes with acute posterior vitreous detachment. Ophthalmology 1991;98:1366–1369.

66. Diamond JP. When are simple flashes and floaters ocular emergencies? Eye 1992;6:102–104.

67. Murakami K, Jalkh AE, et al. Vitreous floaters. Ophthalmology 1983;90:1271–1276.

68. Benson WE. Retinal Detachment. Diagnosis and Management (2nd ed). Philadephia: Lippincott, 1988.

69. Verhoeff FH. Are Moore's lightning streaks of serious portent? Am J Ophthalmol 1956;41:837–840.

70. Moore RF. Subjective "lightning streaks." Br J Ophthalmol 1935;19:545–547

71. Wise GN. Relationship of idiopathic preretinal macular fibrosis to posterior vitreous detachment. Am J Ophthalmol 1975;79:358–362.

72. Lindner B. Acute posterior vitreous detachment. Am J Ophthalmol 1975;80:44–50.

73. Morse PH, Scheie HG, et al. Light flashes as a clue to retinal disease. Arch Ophthalmol 1974;91:179–180.

74. Balazs EA. Fine structure of the developing vitreous. Int Ophthalmol Clin 1973;15:53–63.

75. Kakehashi A, Schepens CL, et al. Biomicroscopic findings of posterior vitreoschisis. Ophthalmic Surg 1993;24:846–850.

76. Green RL, Byrne SF. Diagnostic Ophthalmic Ultrasound. In SJ Ryan (ed), Retinal Disease. St. Louis: Mosby, 1985;17.

77. Chu TG, Green RL, et al. Schisis of the posterior vitreous cortex: An ultrasonographic finding in diabetic retinopathy (ARVO abstract). Invest Ophthalmol Vis Sci 1991;32:1028.

78. Newcomb RD, Potter JW. Clinical investigation of the foveal light reflex. Am J Opt Physiol Optics 1981;58:1110–1119.

79. Johnson GL. Observations on the macula lutea. Arch Ophthalmol 1982;21:1–21.

80. Ballantyne AJ. The reflexes of the fundus oculi. Proc R Soc Med 1940;34:19–42.

81. Wick RE, Wick B. Clinical recording of fundus features. Am J Optom Physiol Optics 1974;51:214–219.

82. Gass JDM. Pathogenesis of disciform detachment of the neuroepithelium. III. Senile disciform macular degeneration. Am J Ophthalmol 1967;63:617–659.

83. Ballantyne AJ, Michaelson. Textbook of the Fundus of the Eye (2nd ed). Baltimore: Williams & Wilkins, 1970;61–63.

84. Yanoff M. The Macula. In LA Yanuzzi, KA Gitter, H Schatz (eds), A Text and Atlas. Baltimore: Williams & Wilkins, 1979;3–13.

85. DeVries S. Retinal hemorrhages in posterior vitreous detachment. Ophthalmologica (Basel) 1951;122:245–248.

86. Kuwabara T, Cogan DG. Studies of retinal vascular pattern. I. Normal architecture. Arch Ophthalmol 1960;64:904–911.

87. Pedler C. The inner limiting membrane of the retina. Br J Ophthalmol 1961;45:423–426.

88. Wolter JR. Pores in the internal limiting membrane of the human retina. Acta Ophthalmol 1964;42:971–974.

89. Mutlu F, Leopold IH. Structure of the human retinal vascular system. Arch Ophthalmol 1964;71:93–101.

90. Foos RY. Vitreoretinal juncture, epiretinal membranes and vitreous. Invest Ophthalmol Vis Sci 1977;16:416–422.

91. Foos RY. Vitreous Base, Retinal Tufts, and Retinal Tears: Pathogenic relationships. In RC Pruett, CDJ Regan (eds), Retina Congress. New York: Appleton-Century-Crofts, 1972;259–280.

92. Teng CC, Chi HH. Vitreous changes and the mechanism of retinal detachment. Am J Ophthalmol 1957;44:335–356.

93. Schachat AP, Sommer A. Macular hemorrhages associated with posterior vitreous detachment. Am J Ophthalmol 1986;102:647–649.

94. Dana MR, Werner MS, et al. Spontaneous and traumatic vitreous hemorrhage. Ophthalmology 1993;100:1377–1387.

95. Lincoff H, Kreissig I, et al. Acute vitreous hemorrhage: A clinical report. Br J Ophthalmol 1976;60:454–458.

96. Morse PH, Aminlari A, et al. Spontaneous vitreous hemorrhage. Arch Ophthalmol 1974;92:297–298.

97. Winslow RL, Taylor BC. Spontaneous vitreous hemorrhage: Etiology and management. South Med J 1980;73:1450–1452.

98. Linder K. Aur Klinik des Gaskorpers. III. Glaskorper und netzhautabhebung. Albecht Von Graefes Arch Ophthalmol 1937;137:157–160.

99. Schepens CL. Retinal Detachment and Allied Diseases. Philadelphia: Saunders, 1983.

100. Byer NE. Cystic retinal tufts and their relationship to retinal detachment. Arch Ophthalmol 1981;99:1788–1790.

101. Daicker B. Anatomie und Pathologie der nemschlichen retino-ziliaren. Fundusperipherie. Ein Atlas und Textbuch. Munich: Karger, 1972;99–121.

102. Foos RY. Zonular traction tufts of the peripheral retina in cadaver eyes. Arch Ophthalmol 1969;82:620–632.

103. Dunker S, Glinz J, Faulborn J. Morphologic studies of the peripheral vitreoretinal interface in humans reveal structures implicated in the pathogenesis of retinal tears. Retina 1997;17:124–130.

104. Foos RY. Postoral peripheral retinal tears. Ann Ophthalmol 1974;6:679–687.

105. Lewis H, Kreiger AE. Rhegmatogenous Retinal Detachment. In TD Duane, EA Jaeger (eds), Clinical Ophthalmology. Vol. 3. Philadelphia: Harper & Row, 1993;26:1–30.

106. Hyams SW, Neumann E. Peripheral retina in myopia with particular reference to retinal breaks. Br J Ophthalmol 1969;53:300–306.

107. Jaffe NS. Vitreous Detachments. In The Vitreous in Clinical Ophthalmology. St. Louis: Mosby, 1969;83–98.

108. Morse PH, Scheie HG. Prophylactic cryotherapy of retinal breaks. Arch Ophthalmol 1974;92:204–207.

109. McPherson A, O'Malley R, et al. Management of the fellow eyes of patients with rhegmatogenous retinal detachment. Ophthalmology 1981;88:922–934.

110. Lean JS. Diagnosis and Treatment of Peripheral Retinal Lesions. In WR Freeman (ed), Practical Atlas of Retinal Disease and Therapy. New York: Raven, 1993;12:211–220.

111. Colyear BH Jr. A Clinical Comparison of Partially Penetrating Diathermy and Xenon-Arc Photocoagulation. In A McPherson (ed), New and Controversial Aspects of Retinal Detachment. New York: Hoeber, 1968;176–185.

112. Sigelman J. Vitreous base classification of retinal tears: Clinical application. Surv Ophthalmol 1980;25:59–70.

113. Delaney WV Jr, Oates PR. Retinal detachment in the second eye. Arch Ophthalmol 1978;96:629–634.

114. Byer NE. Rethinking Prophylactic Treatment of Retinal Detachment. In M Stirpe (ed), Advances in Vitreoretinal Surgery. Acta of the Third International Congress on Vitreoretinal Surgery. New York: Ophthalmic Communications Society, 1991;399–411.

115. Colyear BH, Pischel DK. Clinical tears in the retina without detachment. Am J Ophthalmol 1956;41:773–792.

116. Davis MD. Natural history of retinal breaks without detachment. Arch Ophthalmol 1974;92:183–194.

117. Wadsworth JAC. Symposium: Retinal detachment. Etiology and pathology. Trans Am Acad Ophthalmol Otolaryngol 1952;56:370–397.

118. Straatsma BR, Foos RY, et al. Rhegmatogenous Retinal Detachment. In TD Duane, EA Jaeger (eds), Clinical Ophthalmology. Vol. 3. Philadelphia: Harper & Row, 1980;27:1–10.

119. Schepens CL. Clinical aspects of pathological changes in the vitreous body. Am J Ophthalmol 1954;38:8–21.

120. Tolentino F, Schepens CL. Edema of posterior pole after cataract extraction. Arch Ophthalmol 1965;74:781–786.

121. Sebag J, Balazs EA. Pathogenesis of cystoid macular edema: Anatomic consideration of vitreo-retinal adhesions. Surv Ophthalmol (Suppl) 1984;28:493–498.

122. Jaffe NS. Macular retinopathy after separation of vitreoretinal adherence. Arch Ophthalmol 1967;78:585–591.

123. Foos RY. Vitreoretinal juncture: Topographical variations. Invest Ophthalmol 1972;11:801–808.

124. Morgan CM, Schatz H. Involutional macular thinning: A pre-macular hole condition. Ophthalmology 1986;93:153–161.

125. McDonald PJ, Patel A, et al. Comparison of intracapsular and extracapsular cataract surgery: Histopathologic study

of eyes obtained postmortem. Ophthalmology 1985;92: 1208–1225.

126. Frangieh GT, Green WR, et al. A histopathologic study of macular cysts and holes. Retina 1981;1:311–336.

127. Margherio RR, Schepens CL. Macular breaks. I. Diagnosis, etiology, and observations. Am J Ophthalmol 1972;74:233–240.

128. Akiba J, Quiroz MA, et al. Role of posterior vitreous detachment in idiopathic macular holes. Ophthalmology 1990;97:1610–1613.

129. Hikichi T, Akiba J, et al. Effect of the vitreous on the prognosis of full thickness idiopathic macular hole. Am J Ophthalmol 1993;116:273–278.

130. Sebag J, DeBustros S, et al. Disorders at the Vitreomacular Interface. In CE Margo, RN Mames, L Hamed (eds), Diagnostic Problems in Clinical Ophthalmology. Philadelphia: Saunders, 1992.

131. Roberts TV, Gregory-Roberts JC. Optic disc hemorrhages in posterior vitreous detachment. Aust N Z J Ophthalmol 1991;19:61–63.

132. Sebag J, Buzney SM, et al. Posterior vitreous detachment following panretinal laser photocoagulation. Graefes Arch Clin Exp Ophthalmol 1990;228:5–8.

133. Wise G. Clinical features of idiopathic preretinal macular fibrosis. Am J Ophthalmol 1975;79:349–357.

134. Roth AM, Foos RY. Surface structure of the optic nerve head. I. Epipapillary membranes. Am J Ophthalmol 1972;74:977–985.

135. Wiznia RA. Posterior vitreous detachment and idiopathic preretinal macular gliosis. Am J Ophthalmol 1986;102:196–198.

136. Kampik A, Kenyon KR, et al. Epiretinal and vitreous membranes: Comprehensive study of 56 cases. Arch Ophthalmol 1981, 99;1445–1454.

137. Smiddy WE, Maguire AM, et al. Idiopathic epiretinal membranes: Ultrastructural characteristics and clinicopathologic correlation. Ophthalmology 1989;96:811–821.

138. Wallow IHL, Stevens TS, et al. Actin filaments in contraction preretinal membranes. Arch Ophthalmol 1984; 102:1370–1375.

139. Kishi S, Demaria C, et al. Vitreous cortex remnants at the fovea after spontaneous vitreous detachment. Int Ophthalmol 1986;9:253–260.

140. Gass JDM. Vitreous Maculopathies. In JDM Gass (ed), Stereoscopic Atlas of Macular Diseases. St. Louis: Mosby, 1987;676–713.

141. Bellhorn MB, Friedman AH, et al. Ultrastructure and clinicopathologic correlation of idiopathic preretinal macular fibrosis. Am J Ophthalmol 1975;79:366–373.

142. Rentsch FJ. The ultrastructure of preretinal macular fibrosis. Graefes Arch Clin Exp Ophthalmol 1977;203:321–337.

143. Trese M, Chandler DB, et al. Macular pucker. II. Ultrastructure. Graefes Arch Clin Exp Ophthalmol 1983;221:16–26.

144. Hikichi T, Takahashi T, et al. Relationship between premacular cortical vitreous defects and idiopathic premacular fibrosis. Retina 1995;15:413–416.

145. Hirokawa H, Jalkh AE, et al. Role of vitreous in idiopathic preretinal macular fibrosis. Am J Ophthalmol 1986;101: 166–169.

146. Messner KH. Spontaneous separation of preretinal macular fibrosis. Am J Ophthalmol 1977;83:9–11.

147. Theodossiadis GP, Koutsandrea CN. Avulsed retinal vessels with and without retinal breaks. Trans Ophthalmol Soc UK 1985;104:887–892.

148. Robertson DM, Curtin VT, et al. Avulsed retinal vessels with retinal breaks: A cause of recurrent vitreous hemorrhage. Arch Ophthalmol 1971;85:669–672.

Vitreous Floaters

A vitreous floater is any area of vitreous that is dense enough to be detected by the patient (symptom) or to be seen during ophthalmoscopy by the clinician (sign). Floaters generally derive from material naturally found within the eye but may come from external sources, such as intravitreal foreign bodies. Vitreous floaters can be the result of vitreous degeneration, such as that of the natural synchysis, syneresis, and PVD caused by aging; from hereditary vitreoretinal degenerations; secondary to vitreous inflammation, as in cases of vitritis, pars planitis, retinochoroiditis, and scarring due to inflammation and trauma (such as vitreous foreign bodies) (Figure 4-13). Floaters are the most common entopic phenomenon reported by patients.

Vitreous floaters come in many different sizes, varying from many disc diameters to just perceptible. Floaters may appear spherical, discoid, in thin linear or curvilinear strands, as broken pieces of strands, as rings, cysts, and many other forms. In young eyes the vitreous is gelatinous and floaters tend to move very little on eye movements, but in older eyes with PVD, their motion can be considerable. Floaters can be found in any area of the vitreous cavity but are more likely to be found above the posterior pole and above the far peripheral retina. The most common color is transparent to grayish, but they may appear whitish secondary to postinflammatory scarring, reddish in red blood cells,

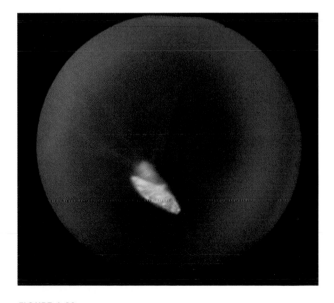

FIGURE 4-13
A piece of windshield glass is seen entrapped in the vitreous with faint white strands attached to it.

brown in melanocytes and melanin granules, and occasionally blackish.

Clinical Significance

Vitreous floaters behind the lens may be vitreous strands, RBCs, white blood cells (WBCs), pigment cells, and asteroid hyalosis. The vitreous strands become more apparent following a PVD due to the contraction that occurs after anterior vitreous collapse because of their easy movement in the detached vitreous. Because the strands move quite readily, they tend to intertwine and form a twisted mass within the vitreous. The RBCs are the result of a vitreous bleed and look like tiny red dots in the anterior vitreous. WBCs are seen as tiny white specks dispersed throughout the anterior vitreous and are usually the result of an iridocyclitis. The pigment specks seen behind the lens may result from release of pigment granules or from iris melanocytes secondary to trauma or anterior segment surgery, an occasional finding in diabetics. Pigment cells in this location, known as tobacco dust or Shafer's sign, may result from a rhegmatogenous retinal detachment. This occurs when retinal pigment epithelium cells beneath a retinal detachment migrate into the subretinal space, through the retinal break, and then disperse throughout the vitreous cavity or when the pigment epithelial cells exposed in a break migrate into the vitreous cavity. The finding of pigment cells in the anterior vitreous behind the iris or the lens indicates the possibility of a rhegmatogenous detachment and requires a careful dilated fundus examination.[1-3] One study of 106 consecutive phakic eyes with acute PVD found pigment cells in the vitreous in 14.1% of the eyes, all of which had an operculated or flap tear.[4] On rare occasions, metastatic malignant melanomas may cause pigment floaters in the anterior vitreous and anterior chamber.[5] It is possible that an erroneous diagnosis of an anterior iridocyclitis may be made if the clinician does not notice that the cells behind the lens are pigmented, not white.

Posteriorly located vitreous floaters seen during ophthalmoscopy are often the result of posterior vitreous condensation, vitreous strands, RBCs, blood clots, pars planitis, retinochoroiditis, and PVD. Synchysis causes areas of the vitreous to degenerate and undergo condensation, which leads to small, rather transparent floaters in the vitreous gel or deposits on the posterior cortex. We often refer to these as typical vitreous floaters. Some floaters are the result of vitreous strands that intertwine and become visible during ophthalmoscopy. RBCs from

a rupture of a retinal vessel may spread out in the vitreous or float above the retinal surface in the retrovitreal space of a PVD. They are seen as tiny, just perceptible opacities with a possible faint reddish tinge. In more extensive vitreous bleeds, the blood may be compartmentalized in vitreous pockets and thus undergo clotting and be seen as round red floaters. Pars planitis can produce "fluffy" white floaters above areas of peripheral inflammation. Sometimes retinochoroiditis can be so severe that the overlying vitreous becomes involved in the inflammatory process, which may lead to postinflammatory vitreous condensation above old chorioretinal scars. When the margins of the scar have overlying condensed vitreous, a ring floater may be found over the chorioretinal scar after separation during a partial or complete PVD.

Asteroid hyalosis can produce vitreous floaters that may number in the hundreds. These small, whitish to yellowish spheroids are seen in the vitreous gel. When only a few asteroids are present, they are most often found in the anterior vitreous above the far periphery of the retina; when numerous, they are found in all areas of the vitreous gel. In the past, asteroid hyalosis spheres were thought to be composed of calcium soaps, but more recent studies have determined that they are made of many compounds. Electron diffraction studies have demonstrated the presence of calcium oxalate monohydrate and calcium hydroxyphosphate, and another study found calcium hydroxyapatite and other forms of calcium phosphate crystals.[6, 7] An ultrastructural study found intertwined ribbons of multilaminar membranes characteristic of lipids (especially phospholipids).[7] In all these studies, energy-dispersion x-ray analysis showed that calcium and phosphorus were the main elements in asteroid bodies.[8] The exact etiology of asteroid hyalosis is not known, but some propose that it is related to aging collagen,[9] and others have suggested that it is preceded by depolymerization of HA.[10] The condition has been associated with diabetes mellitus,[11, 12] but others dispute this association.[13, 14]

Almost all patients with asteroid hyalosis have no floater symptoms, with a few exceptions.[15, 16] Vision is not generally affected because floaters are small and scattered through the vitreous; therefore, light can pass around these tiny opacities and still be focused well onto the retina. Because these asteroid bodies are very small, they generally cannot cast a shadow significant enough to be detected by the photoreceptors at such a distance from the retinal surface and therefore are not seen as floaters. The

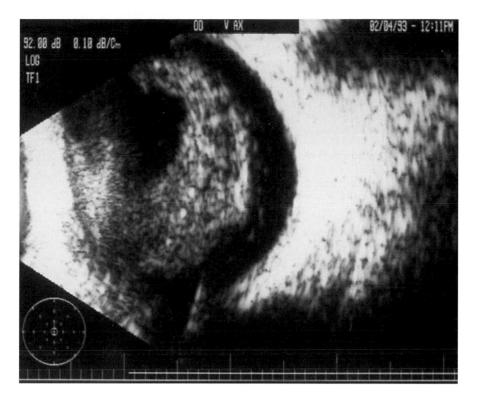

FIGURE 4-14
B-scan ultrasonogram of a PVD in a case of asteroid hyalosis. Note that the vitreous is filled with asteroid bodies and the lacuna in the anterior-superior region of the vitreous body. Also note that the vitreous body has moved anteriorly away from the inner eye wall.

exception may be that in some eyes the spheroid bodies are closer than normal to the retinal surface and may be perceived by the patient.[16] Ultrasonogram studies that I have performed demonstrate that the asteroid bodies are mostly in the center region of the vitreous gel and are often separated from the retinal surface by a normal area of vitreous that is approximately one-fourth of the vitreous cavity in length; this finding has been seen by others.[17] However, I have seen cases of asteroid hyalosis bodies found just above the retinal surface. In the case of a PVD, advanced asteroid hyalosis allows for superb imaging of the extent of the PVD (Figure 4-14). In cases of PVD with asteroid hyalosis, the vitreous body does not seem to collapse nearly to the extent seen in typical PVD, and it may be that the vitreous with this condition has greater structure.

Synchysis scintillans (sometimes called cholesterosis bulbi) results in tiny vitreous floaters composed of cholesterol crystals.[18] The appearance is that of flat, refractile, golden brown bodies. With eye movements, the cholesterol bodies move freely in the vitreous cavity due to liquefaction of the vitreous;[19] thus, they are stirred up like the particles in a glass-enclosed winter snow scene. After the eye movement, the tiny refractile bodies tend to gravitate to the inferior vitreous and rest along the retinal surface. They seem to be related to chronic vitreous

bleeds and are present when no vitreous hemorrhage is present.[8]

Other disease conditions that cause vitreous floaters include amyloidosis[7,19]; vitreoretinal degenerations, such as Wagner's and Stickler's diseases; and neoplasms, such as retinoblastoma, reticulum cell sarcoma, choroidal melanoma, and metastatic carcinoma.[20] Retinoblastoma tumors can fragment and seed to vitreous, causing fluffy white floaters.[21] Reticulum cell sarcoma is a malignant histiocytic lymphoma in which the infiltrative cells first pass through the optic nerve and retina to coat the posterior vitreous cortex but later can spread throughout the vitreous in massive amounts.[22, 23] Aggressive choroidal or ciliary body melanomas can seed into the vitreous after the choroidal tumors break through the basal lamina (Bruch's membrane).[24] After choroidal melanomas seed the vitreous (see Figure 3-22A), they can be associated with intraocular hemorrhage and melanomalytic glaucoma.[25]

References

1. Hamilton AM, Taylor W. Significance of pigment granules in the vitreous. Br J Ophthalmol 1972;56:700–702.
2. Shafer DM. Comment. In CL Schepens, CDJ Regan (eds), Controversial Aspects of Management of Retinal Detachment. Boston: Little, Brown, 1965;51.

3. Stafford T. Comment. In CL Schepens, CDJ Regan (eds), Controversial Aspects of Management of Retinal Detachment. Boston: Little, Brown, 1965;51.

4. Brod RD, Lightman DA, et al. Correlation between vitreous pigment granules and retinal breaks in eyes with acute posterior vitreous detachment. Ophthalmology 1991;98:1366–1369.

5. Bowman CB, Guber D, et al. Cutaneous malignant melanoma with diffuse intraocular metastases. Arch Ophthalmol 1994;112:1213–1216.

6. March WF, Shoch D. Electron diffraction study of asteroid bodies. Invest Ophthalmol 1975;14:399–400.

7. Streeten BA. Disorders of the Vitreous. In A Gardner, GK Klintworth (eds), Pathology of Ocular Disease: A Dynamic Approach. Part B. New York/Basel: Marcel, 1982;1381–1419.

8. Sebag J. Vitreous Pathology. In W Tasman, EA Jaeger (eds), Clinical Ophthalmology. Vol. 3. Philadelphia: Harper & Row, 1992;39:1–26.

9. Yu SY, Blumenthal HT. The Calcification of Elastic Tissue. In BM Wagner, DE Smith (eds), The Connective Tissue. Baltimore: Williams & Wilkins, 1967;17–49.

10. Lamba PA, Shukla KM. Experimental asteroid hyalopathy. Br J Ophthalmol 1971;55:279–283.

11. Smith JL. Asteroid hyalitis: Incidence of diabetes mellitus and hypercholesterolemia. JAMA 1958;168:891–893.

12. Cockburn DM. Are vitreous asteroid bodies associated with diabetes mellitus? Am J Optom Physiol Opt 1985;62:40–44.

13. Hatfield RE, Gastineau CF, et al. Asteroid bodies in the vitreous: Relationship to diabetes and hypercholesterolemia. Mayo Clin Proc 1962;37:513–514.

14. Luxemberg M, Sime D. Relationship of asteroid hyalosis to diabetes mellitus and plasma lipid levels. Am J Ophthalmol 1969;67:406–413.

15. Potter JW, Jones WL, et al. Vision symptoms with asteroid bodies in the vitreous. J Am Optom Assoc 55:419–422, 1984.

16. Noda S, Hayasaka S, et al. Patients with asteroid hyalosis and visible floaters. Jpn J Ophthalmol 1993;37:452–455.

17. Coleman DJ, Silverman RH, et al. Ultrasonic Evaluation of Vitreous and Retina. In W Tasman, EA Jaeger (eds), Clinical Ophthalmology. Vol. 3. Philadelphia: Harper & Row, 1992;39:5.

18. Andrews JS, Lynn C, et al. Cholesterosis bulbi: Case report with modern chemical identification of the ubiquitous crystals. Br J Ophthalmol 1973;57:838–844.

19. Spencer WH. Vitreous. In WH Spencer (ed), Ophthalmic Pathology: An Atlas and Text. Vol. 2. Philadelphia: Saunders, 1985;548–588.

20. Jones WL. A case in point: Intraocular metastatic disease to the eye. J Am Optom Assoc 1981;52:741–744.

21. Ellsworth RM, Boxrud CA. Retinoblastoma. In W Tasman, EA Jaeger (eds), Clinical Ophthalmology. Vol. 3. Philadelphia: Harper & Row, 1991;39:6–8.

22. Vogel MH, Font RL, et al. Reticulum cell sarcoma of the retina and uvea. Am J Ophthalmol 1968;66:205–215.

23. Chess J Sebag J, et al. Pathologic processing of vitrectomy specimens: A comparison of pathologic findings with celloidin bag and cytocentrifigation preparation of 102 vitrectomy specimens. Ophthalmology 1983;90:1560–1564.

24. Halverson KD, Ruder AJ, et al. Intraocular melanoma. Clin Eye Vision Care 1994;6:146–148.

25. El Baba F, Hagler WS, et al. Choroidal melanoma with pigment dispersion in vitreous and melanomalytic glaucoma. Ophthalmology 1988;95:370–377.

Vitreous Hemorrhage

The symptom of a vitreous bleed is the sudden onset of numerous tiny black floaters—the "swarm of gnats" or "black pepper specks"—that are best seen against a bright background, such as the blue sky or a white wall. They are the result of the shadow cast by RBCs close to the retinal surface. The RBCs are very small and must be positioned just above the retinal surface to cast a shadow significant enough to be detected by the photoreceptors. Because the retrovitreal space is filled with a fluid media, the RBCs can float next to the surface of the retina and therefore be seen as numerous small floaters moving across the visual field. The patient may complain of blurry or smoky vision with a red tinge if a substantial amount of blood is found in the visual axis of the vitreous body (Figure 4-15). Ultrasonography can also be used to judge the extent of vitreous hemorrhage, especially if the view of the vitreous is poor (Figure 4-16). If there is a large vitreous hemorrhage, the patient may complain of very poor vision. Vitreous hemorrhage may occur as the result of trauma, a retinal tear, or from any type of hemorrhagic retinopathy (especially diabetes). One study of the records of 253 consecutive patients with newly diagnosed vitreous hemorrhage found that spontaneous vitreous hemorrhages occurred in diabetic retinopathy (35.2%), trauma (18.3%), retinal vein occlusion (7.4%), retinal tear without detachment (7.0%), PVD (6.5%), proliferative sickle cell retinopa-

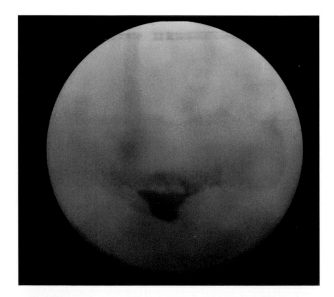

FIGURE 4-15
A vitreous hemorrhage is found in the center of the photograph and light plumes of red blood cells can be seen spreading away from the central blood clot. Symptoms would be the sudden onset of many tiny black floaters.

thy (6.5%), retinal tear with a detachment (4.8%), subretinal neovascularization from age-related macular degeneration (2.2%), hypertensive retinopathy (1.7%), unknown (2.5%), and other causes (8.7%).[1]

The blood that spreads into the vitreous from a ruptured retinal vessel passes through channels and usually compartmentalizes in small vitreous lacuna. Therefore, it is common to see multiple blood clots in the vitreous during ophthalmoscopy or ultrasonography. Most of the blood in the vitreous settles inferiorly, where it clots and loses its red pigmentation over several weeks. The areas of clotted blood become yellowish white, round or teardrop-shaped vitreous scars with time and remain stationary in the attached formed vitreous (Figures 4-17). The clinical finding of yellowish white strands with blood clots intermixed within them is indicative of a rather recent vitreal bleed.

It may not be possible to see the fundus during a large vitreous bleed, even with the brightest power setting of the binocular indirect ophthalmoscope. Ultrasonography can be used to obtain a view of the vitreous cavity and the posterior structures and is done to determine whether a retinal tear, retinal detachment, or vitreoretinal mass is present.[2, 3] The patient is instructed to watch TV while sitting in a chair and to sleep with two pillows; this facilitates the gravitation of blood to the inferior vitreous cavity (Figure 4-18). The patient is told not to become involved in strenuous or rapid physical activity that may mix the settling blood higher up in the vitreous. Sometimes patients are placed on strict bedrest and bilateral eye patching to reduce head and eye movements to facilitate the gravitational effect further. The patient is instructed to return in a week for an evaluation to see if the vitreous blood has degenerated and settled enough to obtain a view of the fundus.

A pseudomembrane of the vitreous can result from the sheetlike formation of hazy vitreous gel secondary to vitreous hemorrhage. This pseudomembrane can be mistaken for a retinal detachment; unlike a retinal detachment, however, the pseudomembrane does not have blood vessels. Small, fresh blood clots in the vitreous close to the retina are bright red and can be mistaken for a retinal break, except that they tend to move a little on eye movements. These two entities are usually differentiated on careful examination by binocular indirect ophthalmoscopy with and without scleral depression or with a precorneal condensing lens or three-mirror lens.

Vitreous hemorrhages in infants is rare and has been reported to occur in birth trauma, shaken-baby syndrome, protein C deficiency, disseminated intravascular coagulation disorder, inflammation, Terson's syndrome, retinopathy of prematurity, and *Toxocara* infection.[4, 5–8] Because the vitreous in infants is more formed and gelatinous, hemorrhages tend to remain concentrated and take longer to disperse than in adults. Vitreous hemorrhages can take as long as 2–13 weeks to dissipate in infants.[7, 9] A residual finding in vitreous hemorrhages in infants

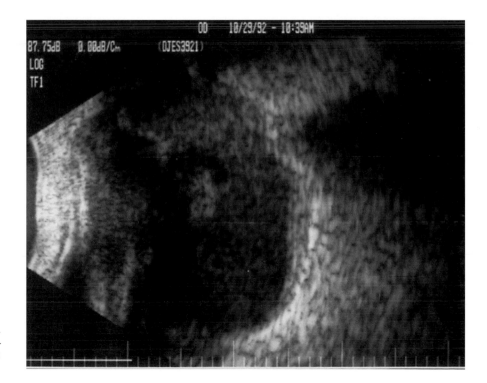

FIGURE 4-16
B-scan ultrasonogram of diffuse vitreous bleed. Dark area in the superior region of the vitreous bleed is a lacuna.

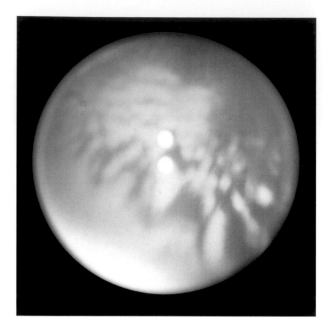

FIGURE 4-17
Old vitreous blood in the inferior vitreous is seen as whitish deposits in the indirect condensing lens.

is the development of a pigmentary retinopathy after such a bleed.[4, 10]

Clinical Significance

A vitreous hemorrhage can lead to vitreous gel degeneration, which is believed to be the result of the effects of the breakdown of hemoglobin from degenerating RBCs on the HA present in the vitreous. The by-products of degenerating hemoglobin are toxic to the vitreous, and the result is extensive loss of water from the vitreous gel. Lysis of red blood cells in the vitreous may result in the formation of scarring and vitreous membranes. Both these degenerative changes can produce substantial tractional forces that may result in a retinal break or detachment.[11, 12] Repeated vitreous hemorrhaging can produce extensive vitreous scarring, which can often result in vision restricted to hand motion and light perception. Treatment for scarred vitreous is vitrectomy with irrigation and infusion. A complication of this surgical procedure is retinal tears.

In infants the complications following a vitreous hemorrhage are amblyopia ex anopsia, anisometropia, epiretinal membranes, and retinal tear and detachment.[4, 6, 7, 9, 10, 13] Due to the length of time necessary for vitreous hemorrhage to disperse in infants (2–13 weeks), the lack of visual sensory input may lead to amblyopia. It is estimated that in infants, occlusion amblyopia can develop as early as 6–8 weeks after monocular occlusion.[14, 15] Anisometropia following a vitreous hemorrhage is possible after 6 months of visual occlusion. One study found that occlusion effects 3 months and 6 weeks after a vitreous hemorrhage in infants resulted in a unilateral myopic shift in refraction of 7.50 and 9.25 diopters, respectively.[7]

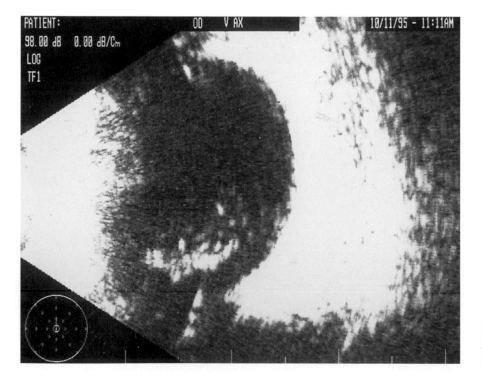

FIGURE 4-18
B-scan ultrasonogram of a rather fresh hemorrhage with gravitational movement into the inferior vitreous.

References

1. Dana MR, Werner MS, et al. Spontaneous and traumatic vitreous hemorrhage. Ophthalmology 1993;100:1377–1387.
2. Green RL, Byrne SF. Diagnostic Ophthalmic Ultrasound. In SJ Ryan (ed), Retinal Diseases. St. Louis: Mosby, 1989;116–120.
3. DiBernnardo C, Blodi B, et al. Echographic evaluation of retinal tears in patients with spontaneous vitreous hemorrhage. Arch Ophthalmol 1992;110:511–514.
4. Ferrone PJ, de Juan E Jr. Vitreous hemorrhage in infants. Arch Ophthalmol 1994;112:1185–1189.
5. Butner RW, McPherson AR. Spontaneous vitreous hemorrhage. Ann Ophthalmol 1982;14:268–270.
6. Puido JS, Lingua RW, et al. Protein C deficiency associated with vitreous hemorrhage in a neonate. Am J Ophthalmol 1987;104:546–547.
7. Miller-Meeks MJ, Bennett SR, et al. Myopia-induced vitreous hemorrhage in a neonate. Am J Ophthalmol 1990; 109:199–203.
8. Wiznia RA, Price J. Vitreous hemorrhages and disseminated intravascular coagulation in the newborn. Am J Ophthalmol 1976;82:222–226.
9. Braendstrup P. Vitreous hemorrhage in the newborn: A rare type of neonatal intraocular hemorrhage. Acta Ophthalmol 1969;47:502–513.
10. Billotte C, Lecoq PJ, et al. A propos du syndrome de Terson et d'un cas post-traumatique chez le nourisson. Bull Soc Ophthalmol Fr 1988;88:111–114.
11. Tolentino FT, Schepens CL, et al. Vitreoretinal Disorders: Diagnosis and Management. Philadelphia: Saunders, 1976.
12. Pischel DK. Retinal detachment: A manual. Trans Am Acad Ophthalmol Otolaryngol 1965;77.
13. Gauthier L, Fristch E, et al. Le syndrome de Terson—a partie de 2 cas. Bull Soc Ophthalmol Fr 1988;88:253–255.
14. Birch EE, Stager DR. Prevalence of good visual acuity following neonatal surgery for congenital monocular cataract. Arch Ophthalmol 1988;106:40–43.
15. Beller DR, Hoyt CS, et al. Good visual function after neonatal surgery for congenital monocular cataracts. Am J Ophthalmol 1981;91:559–565.

Vitreous Bands and Membranes

Vitreous bands and membranes appear to be different physical manifestations of the same degenerative process of the vitreous. They are usually the result of condensation of vitreous gel into strands of sheetlike structures that vary in length, width, thickness, and location. They can be fairly transparent or opaque (Figure 4-19). The membranes can become dense enough to markedly decrease vision. Generally, the membranes consist of an acellular hyaline layer coated with cells that often resemble fibrocytes. [1, 2] Vitreous membranes rarely have blood vessels; thus, the absence of blood vessels is a sign that differentiates these membranes from a retinal detachment. High-resolution color-flow Doppler can differentiate vitreous membranes from a retinal detachment by detecting the blood flow in the detached retina. [3]

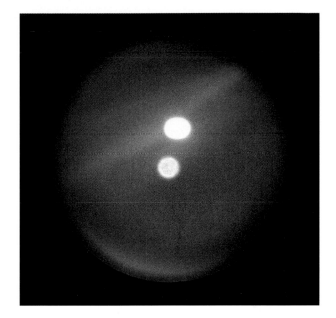

FIGURE 4-19
A vitreous strand above the peripheral retina can be seen through the indirect condensing lens.

Vitreous membranes are usually found over the vitreous base but they can criss-cross the vitreous body in any direction. They can float freely in the liquefied vitreous with each end terminating in the vitreous, or one end may be attached to the retina or pars plana; rarely, both ends are attached to the inner surface of the eye. They are more frequently found in myopes and aphakes and in eyes with vitreoretinal degeneration. Their etiology may be congenital[4] or acquired, as in cases of blunt or penetrating ocular trauma; vitreous hemorrhage; postinflammatory chorioretinitis; PVD; and after retinal reattachment, photocoagulation, cryotherapy, and, occasionally, retinal neovascularization.[5, 6] Entities associated with peripheral vitreous membranes include Wagner's syndrome, Stickler's syndrome, Goldmann-Favre syndrome, familial exudative vitreoretinopathy, and juvenile X-linked retinoschisis (see Hereditary Vitreoretinopathies).

Clinical Significance

Vitreous membranes that have a broad attachment to the retina usually do not produce a retinal break unless considerable force is applied. If such a force occurs, as with ocular trauma, a giant retinal tear may develop. A small area of vitreous attachment requires much less force to produce a retinal break, which usually takes the form of a linear, horseshoe, or operculated tear.[7] Vitreous membranes or bands that result in isolated retinal traction can produce a small area of pigment epithelial hyperplasia (pigment clumping) by physically stimulating the retina through years of periodic traction. A sign of traction is taut membranes that may display stress lines. Other signs suggesting tractional forces are vitreous gel shrinkage and hemorrhage. Some membranes attached to the retina may appear to be lax and gently sway in the vitreous cavity. These may give a false impression of their tractional forces because on eye movements, there may be a sudden stretching and abrupt tugging on the underlying retina.

Vitreous membranes may be attached to retinal tufts and meridional folds, and traction may result in avulsed pieces of these structures being pulled up into the vitreous. Lattice degeneration, chorioretinal scars, and pigment clumps typically have associated vitreous membranes, and traction may lead to the production of a retinal break (see the section on Lattice Degeneration, Chorioretinal Scar, and Hyperplasia and Retinal Pigment Epithelium Clumping in Chapter 3). Other signs of exaggerated tractional forces being applied by vitreous membranes or bands are large meridional retinal folds, retinoschisis, and retinal detachment. There can also be a deepening of the anterior chamber from membranes secondary to proliferative vitreoretinopathy on the iris and ciliary body.[8]

Vitreous membrane attachment to the macula and optic disc can result in edema of the involved tissue. This is secondary to continual traction applied by the membrane. The edema can sometimes be resolved with a vitrectomy to release tractional forces. Extensive vitreous band and membrane formation may require a vitrectomy, in which microscissors or a vitreous nibbler is inserted to cut away and remove these membranes.

References

1. Smith T. Importance of the Vitreous Body in Retina Surgery with Special Emphasis on Reoperations. In CL Schepens (ed), Pathologic Findings after Retina Surgery. St. Louis: Mosby, 1960;61–93.
2. Constable T, Tolentino FT, et al. Clinico-Pathological Correlation of Vitreous Membranes. In RC Pruett, CD Regan (eds), Retina Congress Infirmary. New York: Appleton-Century-Crofts, 1972;245–257.
3. Wong AD, Cooperberg PL, et al. Differentiation of detached retina and vitreous membrane with color-flow Doppler. Radiology 1991;178:429–431.
4. Jones WL. Developmental retrovitreous opacities. J Am Optom Assoc 1978;49:1197–1198.
5. Tolentino FI, Lee PF, et al. Biomicroscopic study of vitreous cavity in diabetic retinopathy. Arch Ophthalmol 1966;75:238–246.
6. Apple DJ, Rabb MF. Ocular Pathology: Clinical Applications and Self-Assessment (3rd ed). St Louis: Mosby, 1985.
7. Marren SE. Idiopathic peripheral vitreous membranes. Optom Vis Sci 1996;73:562–568.
8. Tolentino FI, Schepens CL, et al. Vitreoretinal Disorders: Diagnosis and Management. Philadelphia: Saunders, 1976;7:130–190.

Avulsion of Vitreous Base

The vitreous base is a condensation of cortical vitreous that adheres firmly to the peripheral retina and pars plana on either side of the ora serrata.[1] The base extends 1.5–2 mm anterior to the ora serrata, 1–3 mm posterior to the ora serrata,[2] and several millimeters into the vitreous body.[3] After very severe ocular contusion, the base may become disinserted from the oral region. Avulsion of the vitreous base occurs when it is torn away from its anchorage to the base area (Figure 4-20). An avulsed vitreous base appears as a whitish translucent band floating in the vitreous cavity and is frequently twisted like a garland[4] (Figure 4-21) or may have a bucket-handle appearance (Figure 4-22). It may or may not be associated with a retinal dialysis or peripheral retinal breaks and is most frequently seen superonasally, which is the same region in which traumatic retinal dialyses usually occur. It commonly occurs in young people. Inner retinal layers may be stripped away and adhere to the avulsed vitreous base.

Clinical Significance

The existence of an avulsed vitreous base confirms prior trauma. It has no clinical significance except as a cause of symptomatic floaters. Its clinical significance is in its association with blunt trauma and therefore may be seen in conjunction with vitreous hemorrhage, retinal tears, or retinal detachment. Simultaneous retinal dialysis and avulsion of the vitreous base are found in about 25% of patients with retinal detachment secondary to ocular contusion.[5] Ocular trauma that is not severe enough to produce a retinal tear or avulsion of the vitreous base may result in a tenting-up of the peripheral retina and epithelium of the pars plana. Treatment is not necessary for an avulsed vitreous base without a concomitant retinal tear or detachment.

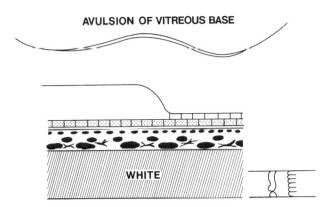

AVULSION OF VITREOUS BASE

WHITE

FIGURE 4-20
Avulsed vitreous base has been torn free from the region of the ora serrata and is floating in the vitreous. It is common to find twists in the avulsed band that give it a garland appearance.

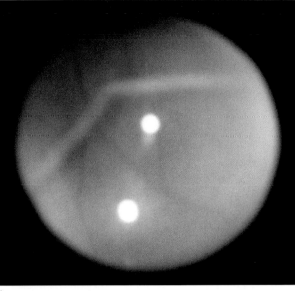

A

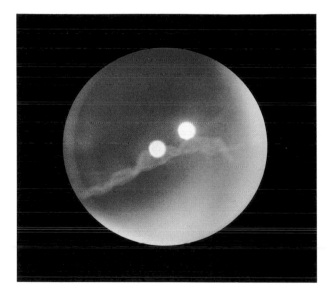

FIGURE 4-21
Avulsed vitreous base is a white "garland" floating in the vitreous above the inferior peripheral retina. This was caused by severe trauma to this 60-year-old patient when he was a child. No retinal tear was found in the region of the vitreous base. View is through the indirect condensing lens.

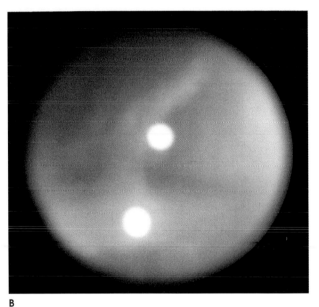

B

FIGURE 4-22
A. Avulsed vitreous base is seen as a yellow-white ribbon "bucket handle" floating in the vitreous above the inferior peripheral retina. This was caused by severe ocular trauma. No retinal tear was found in the region of the vitreous base avulsion. The view is through the indirect condensing lens.
B. The avulsed vitreous base can be followed back to its attachment at the ora serrata. The view is through the indirect condensing lens during scleral depression.

References

1. Teng CC, Chi HH. Vitreous changes and the mechanism of retinal detachment. Am J Ophthalmol 1957;44:335–356.
2. Hogan MJ. The vitreous: Its structure in relation to the ciliary body and retina. Invest Ophthalmol 1963;2:418–445.
3. Resser FH, Aaberg T. Vitreous Humor. In PE Records (ed), Physiology of the Human Eye and Visual System. Hagerstown, MD: Harper & Row, 1979;1–31.
4. Tasman W. The Vitreous. In TD Duane, EA Jaeger (eds), Clinical Ophthalmology. Vol. 3. Philadelphia: Harper & Row, 1976;38:14–16.
5. Schepens CL. Retinal Detachment and Allied Diseases. Philadelphia: Saunders 1983;5:73.

Chapter 5

Peripheral Retinal Breaks

Clinical Description

A retinal break is a full-thickness break in the retina (loss of the sensory retina) and is classified as either a hole or a tear. An incomplete break that involves the inner retinal layers is called a partial or lamellar break, retinal excavation, pit, or erosion. Most retinal breaks are less than 0.25 disc diameter; in one study, 67% of breaks were less than 0.25 disc diameter.[1] In general, the prevalence of retinal breaks ranges from 0.59% to 14%.[2–10] Autopsy studies have shown a prevalence of 3.3–18.3%.[1,3, 8, 11–14] Byer[1] performed a routine examination with dilation in 1,700 patients and found that 98 (5.8%) had one or more full-thickness breaks. Of the 3,400 eyes, 111 (3.3%) had a break, the majority being single. Nearly all were asymptomatic (two complained of flashing lights or floaters). Altogether, 156 breaks were discovered: 120 were holes, 20 were operculated tears, and 16 were horseshoe or flap tears. Davis[15] found that most (>90%) retinal breaks are holes and few are flap tears. Most retinal breaks are found as solitary lesions, but there could be as many as 18 breaks in one eye.[7] Full-thickness tears are found in 3.3% of patients.[16] Retinal breaks are more commonly found in the temporal half of the fundus and are often superotemporal. Asymptomatic breaks were seen in 5–6% of patients.[1, 13, 17, 18] Davis[15] found most asymptomatic breaks in the inferotemporal fundus between the ora serrata and equator.

Myopes have a higher incidence of retinal breaks due to their higher incidence of posterior vitreous detachment (PVD) and their thin peripheral retina, which is more susceptible to breaks.[19, 20] In myopes over 6.00 diopters, peripheral retinal breaks occur at the rate of 11.1–18%.[21–23] In myopes who underwent cataract surgery, the prevalence of retinal breaks after PVD was as high as 16.2%.[24] In another study, the prevalence of retinal breaks in myopic eyes over 24 mm in axial length was 12.1%.[22]

An atrophic retinal hole is a break that is not caused by traction. It is most likely produced by an atrophic process and is generally thought to be the result of underlying vascular disease insufficiency of the choroid and choriocapillaris. Retinal tears are caused by degeneration of the inner retinal layers, overlying vitreous degeneration, and traction. These tears may be round, linear, or horseshoe-shaped, depending on the particular characteristics of the retina and vitreous traction that produced them.

Retinal holes and tears appear red because of the absence of retinal tissue that normally mutes the choroidal reflex. Therefore, breaks appear more red (relative increase in redness) compared to the surrounding fundus color. They may be pink, clear, or light gray in a detached retina. Retroillumination of a break in a detached retina results in a glowing defect (retinal transillumination), whereas a retinal hemorrhage appears darker. Often it is necessary to differentiate between a break and a hemorrhage, which is done by rolling the suspected area with a scleral depressor. A break tends to change color (from dark red to gray) during depression due to compression of the underlying choroidal vasculature, whereas a hemorrhage does not change color during scleral depression. Also, the edges of a retinal break can be seen during scleral depression and a shadow may be visible at the posterior margin due to a localized retinal detachment; a hemorrhage rolls evenly without displaying elevated edges. Last, small retinal breaks usually have smooth, regular borders, but hemorrhages commonly display irregular borders that often have a feathered appearance on a magnified view with a mirror contact lens or a 90-diopter precorneal lens evaluation.

Retinal tears are nearly always found in the peripheral retina due to the strong vitreoretinal adhesion in this region. If there are no areas of such adhesions, it is unlikely that a retinal tear will occur. Juxtabasal tears pose a higher risk due to the degree of vitreous traction associated with the tears. The posterior pole rarely has retinal tears because of the lack of strong vitreoretinal adhesions and a thicker retina supported by numerous large retinal vessels and nerve fibers. However, occasionally a tear can be found in the posterior retina (see Figures 5-9 and 5-14). Retinal tears are often referred to as equatorial or oral, based on their physical location in the fundus. Equatorial tears are prevalent in older patients and are usually the result of traction on sites of increased vitreoretinal adhesion. Areas of strong peripheral vitreoretinal adhesions exist perivascularly,[25, 26] at posterior extensions of the vitreous base or retinal tufts,[27, 28] at pigment clumps,[15] and in meridional folds,[29] enclosed ora bays,[30] and lattice degeneration.[31, 32] However, there are some other developmental vitreoretinal areas of adhesion that may lead to retinal tear formation and they are known as rosette, spicula, tubulus, and verruca. These abnormalities are very subtle and have only been found on microscopic studies.[33] Ora breaks are more frequently seen in younger patients and are often the result of ocular trauma. Full-thickness retinal tears, excluding those at the ora serrata, have been found in 1.9% of autopsied eyes and were bilateral in 11.2% of patients; they were generally located temporally (58%) and inferiorly (54%) and 95% of most tears were juxtabasal or extrabasal (basal refers to the vitreous base).[34] Another study found that they occurred in the superior fundus in over 94% of the cases.[35, 36] In phakic eyes, breaks are usually superotemporal, as are phakic retinal detachments, and in aphakes the incidence of superonasal breaks is somewhat more frequent than aphakic detachments.[37–39]

Retinal infections can lead to the formation of retinal breaks due to destruction of the retina. This may be seen in cases of cytomegalovirus retinal infection in acquired immunodeficiency syndrome (AIDS).[40, 41]

Symptoms of a retinal tear include photopsia from vitreous traction, which results from mechanical stimulation to the retina, and the sudden onset of numerous tiny black floaters, which result from a vitreous bleed. Patients with these symptoms have been reported to have retinal breaks in 10–15% of cases.[24, 35] The flash of light is perceived in the visual field of the involved eye 180 degrees from the internal location of the physical stimulation on the retina. The flashing lights may be a transient event at the time of the actual formation of the break or continual and episodic due to remaining traction on the intact retina. Also, phophopsia may persist if there is remaining vitreous adhesion and traction to a

torn retinal flap or the edges of a tear (see Figure 5-14A and C). Flashing lights do not necessarily indicate the production of a retinal break but may be the result of vitreous traction that is not sufficient to produce a break, or they may occur because the vitreoretinal adhesions were not strong and vitreous cortical separation occurred without tearing the retina. All these mechanisms are most frequently associated with advanced vitreous degeneration and PVD. An autopsy study of the relationship of PVD to retinal tears found that it was present in 14.3% of all cases of eyes with tears.[42] Clinical studies found tears in 8–15% of eyes with acute symptomatic PVDs.[24, 25, 43] A fresh or acute retinal tear is described either as symptomatic (photopsia), having a retinal hemorrhage at the edge of the tear, or found in an area of the retina where no tear was found on prior examination; and it is produced by a PVD or ongoing traction.[44] Therefore, in the presence of a PVD, the clinician should look for a free operculum, projecting retinal flap, hemorrhage, or localized retinal pigment epithelium alternations.[4] It is estimated that 3–5% of eyes with a symptomatic PVD will develop a retinal detachment (see Chapter 4).[15, 45]

Another symptom of a retinal tear is the sudden onset of numerous tiny black floaters, sometimes referred to as a swarm of gnats. These are most noticeable when the patient looks at blue sky or a blank white wall. The floaters generally originate in one region of the visual field and slowly spread over most other areas of vision; because most tears occur in the peripheral retina, the floaters often seem to originate in the peripheral visual field and migrate across the central visual field. They are the result of a small vitreous hemorrhage caused by the rupturing of a retinal blood vessel during the formation of the retinal tear[46] (see Figures 3-80, 4-15, 4-16, and 5-14A) or secondary to vitreous traction on a superficial retinal vessel during a PVD. As long as there is no recurrent bleeding, the hemorrhage will slowly disappear over a few days to weeks (depending on volume of extravasated blood) due to the degeneration of red blood cells in the vitreous. This symptom is not to be confused with the patient's complaint of a floater that has been seen for months or years and moves in the same direction as the eye moves. This is a typical floater that is usually formed from small areas of condensed vitreous (Figure 5-1). A massive vitreous hemorrhage can obscure a retinal tear. In such cases, B-scan ultrasonography may be able to detect a large retinal tear, but small tears are generally not detectable (see Chapter 4).

Any patient who complains of symptoms of photopsia or sudden onset of numerous dark floaters should have a retinal examination with a binocular indirect ophthalmoscope through a dilated pupil. If a retinal break is discovered, the fundus examination should be continued to identify additional breaks, because it is not uncommon to find more than one in an eye. There have been as many as 29 retinal breaks in one eye.[47] If no retinal break is discovered but a PVD is present, a follow-up retinal examination is advisable in 3–4 weeks to check for the possible subsequent formation of a retinal break. After the patient becomes asymptomatic and no retinal tear is found, a follow-up visit should be scheduled for 6 months to determine if any breaks develop in the near future.

Histopathology

The retinal break shows full-thickness loss of sensory retina, leaving the pigment epithelium in place. A torn section of sensory retina may be associated with the break, possibly located above the break attached to the detached vitreous cortex, or the torn tissue may be attached to the edge of the break (usually the anterior edge). Surrounding the break may be an accumulation of liquefied vitreous and aqueous in the subneural space, resulting in a localized or subclinical retinal detachment.

Clinical Significance

In eyes with silent breaks, a single break was found in 87.5%. Half of silent breaks in normal eyes occur in patients less than 40 years old. Yet over 75% of unilateral nontraumatic retinal detachments occur in patients over age 40; therefore, it is generally safe to watch a single round hole in the far peripheral retina in patients under 40.[46] One study of 111 asymptomatic retinal breaks found that only 5% progressed to a detachment.[15] Byer[17] found that no asymptomatic breaks without subretinal fluid displayed any progression. A retinal break accompanied by symptoms is almost always produced by vitreous traction and has a 30–40% chance of developing a retinal detachment.[15, 17] Davis[15] states that the single most important factor in predicting the progression of a retinal break is the presence of symptoms. In his study of 31 eyes with symptomatic breaks, 11 (35%) had some degree of retinal detachment. Vitreous hemorrhage and photopsia are the most important symptoms in the possible development of a retinal detachment.[15]

Retinal breaks may lead to a retinal detachment, and even though it is essential for a break to occur to produce a detachment, clinical and autopsy studies have demonstrated that the prevalence of retinal

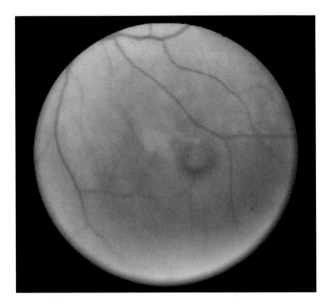

FIGURE 5-1
Typical vitreous floater casting a shadow on the underlying retinal surface. It would cause the symptom of a single floater that moves in the same direction as the eye moves and probably has been noticed for months to years.

breaks and their precursors far exceeds that of retinal detachment in the general population.[1, 3, 4, 6, 10, 17, 18, 42, 48–50] It has been reported that only about 1 of 70 retinal breaks develops a detachment.[3, 17, 51] The reason that so few retinal detachments occur is probably that the forces maintaining the sensory retina in apposition to the pigment epithelium are greater than those trying to separate it through the break. The forces acting to detach the retina are passage of liquefied vitreous and aqueous through the break, fluid currents along the retinal surface threatening to raise the edges of the break, and vitreous traction.[35, 51–57] In most cases it is probably a combination of forces that result in a majority of rhegmatogenous detachments, but I believe that vitreous traction is the most important factor.

Traction on the retina has the most influence on separating the sensory retina and therefore is most frequently associated with retinal detachments. The best way to evaluate the presence of vitreous traction and to quantify the magnitude of the traction is unknown.[58] One suggested method is to observe the area in question with binocular indirect ophthalmoscopy during dynamic scleral depression and look for a wispy strand of vitreous as the area rolls over the tip of the depressor. The longer a break exists without producing a detachment, the less likely it is that a detachment will result. This is probably due to the fact that the pigment epithelium around the break is able to keep the surrounding retina in place against the forces trying to separate it; however, a detachment is still possible in the future, especially if significant vitreous traction occurs. Tears often occur in normal-looking areas of the retina,[35, 59] and one study found that this occurred in 70% of the 350 eyes.[60] Therefore, peripheral retinal abnormalities are not essential in the formation of retinal tears, and abnormal areas of vitreoretinal adhesion occur in areas of ophthalmoscopically normal-appearing retina.

PVD is the most significant entity in the development of vitreous traction and is therefore very instrumental in the production of retinal tears. Almost all tears occur at the time of the initial diagnosis of a PVD.[21, 59, 61–63] Byer[60] found that 76% of the eyes he studied had a tear within 2 weeks of PVD symptoms. However, tears may develop much later, from 2 weeks to 6 months in 11–27% of eyes.[21, 59–63] Retinal tears have been reported in 8–46% of patients with a PVD,[21, 53, 61–65] and in studies that consisted of patients seen initially by the authors, the incidence was 11–15%.[21, 53, 61, 62] An autopsy study of 250 eyes by Foos[42] found that 14.8% had a PVD with a secondary retinal tear. The presence of a vitreous hemorrhage in eyes with a PVD greatly increases the chances of a retinal break (38–91%).[21, 53, 55, 59, 61–65] Vitreous hemorrhage indicates significant localized vitreoretinal traction on a superficial retinal vessel, causing the vessel to rupture. Traction of this magnitude may result in the formation of a retinal tear. However, the finding of a vitreous hemorrhage does not mean that a vitreous tear is present or will develop, and the percentage of eyes with a hemorrhage that did not result in a tear has been reported to range from 8.9% to 62%.[21, 53, 56, 59, 62–65] Aphakic eyes with a PVD have a higher frequency of retinal tears (36.8%, which is 3.8 times that of phakic eyes).[60] The incidence of secondary breaks in males with a PVD is greater than in females;[53, 61, 63] in one study, 2.33 that of females.[60] These secondary breaks are in the superior half of the retina 70–100% of the time.[21, 53, 55, 59, 61, 63]

Retinal tears pose a greater risk for a detachment than an atrophic hole. Approximately half of full-thickness retinal tears are associated with a localized retinal detachment, more commonly if the tear is located in the superior half of the retina.[66] In the past, it was accepted that superior breaks were more dangerous because gravitational forces would facilitate the fluid in a subclinical detachment to dissect downward and result in a clinically significant detachment. More recent studies seem to indicate, however, that there is no greater incidence of clinically significant detachment formation from superior breaks than from inferior ones.[15, 17, 45, 67]

Retinal tears secondary to vitreous traction along the posterior margin to the vitreous base are the most common cause of clinically significant rhegmatogenous detachments that are not associated with cystic retinal tufts or lattice degeneration.[26, 28] A rhegmatogenous detachment occurs in 28–50% of cases of symptomatic retinal tears. Many authorities believe that 30–40% of rhegmatogenous detachments are associated with lattice degeneration with retinal tears, and approximately 20% are caused by atrophic retinal holes and retinal dialysis.[68–70] Even though highly myopic eyes have an increased risk for retinal detachment, two studies of myopic eyes determined that asymptomatic breaks are unlikely to cause a subsequent detachment[23, 44] and that most of these breaks do not require treatment.[71] A study by Byer[60] found that aphakes have a risk of retinal tears that is 3.8 times greater than that of phakic eyes and that tears in aphakic eyes have an 85% chance of progressing to a detachment, compared to 18% in phakic eyes.

Patients with a history of a retinal detachment in one eye have a greater frequency of retinal break formation in the fellow eye (25–40%).[72–76] These breaks often (10–31%) develop a subsequent retinal detachment over a rather short period of time in the fellow eye.[74–80] Folk et al.[81] found that phakic fellow eyes with lattice degeneration had a 2.5 times greater incidence of new retinal tear or detachment than prophylactically treated eyes over a 7-year period. Prophylactic treatment of vitreoretinal abnormalities in the fellow eye has proved to be beneficial,[62, 82–84] and in Israel, the prophylactic treatment of fellow eyes reduced the incidence of retinal detachment to in those eyes from 11% to 3%.[74, 79] However, another study suggests that prophylactic treatment may be unnecessary[85] and that because retinal detachment development is such a rare event, it would require that a large number of patients receive prophylactic treatment to prevent a small number of detachments.

Aphakia and pseudophakia have an increased risk of retinal detachment (pseudophakic eyes have a slightly lower risk),[20, 86] which is probably due to the free-moving vitreous in a large vitreous cavity caused by the absence of the lens.[87] One study found that untreated breaks in aphakic eyes progressed to retinal detachment in 50% of cases compared to 9% in phakic eyes.[88] Others found that 33% of aphakic eyes developed a retinal tear or detachment.[60] Several studies of asymptomatic tears and holes in aphakic eyes state that such breaks can be safely followed without treatment, but some experts believe that flap tears may warrant treatment if the tears are large or posteriorly located.[23, 85, 88] The incidence of retinal detachment in aphakic fellow eyes is reported to be 21–36%.[75, 89, 90] It is therefore very beneficial to perform prophylactic treatment on all breaks, lattice degeneration, and vitreoretinal tags.[89, 91] In this country, neodymium-yttrium-aluminum-garnet laser capsulotomy for posterior capsular opacification with or without intraocular lens implantation increases the risk of retinal break or detachment by a factor of 4.[92]

In years past, the finding of a retinal break usually resulted in treatment, which may have been justified on the misconception that most breaks developed into a subsequent retinal detachment. Studies in the 1950s and 1960s of untreated retinal breaks found that 28–33% resulted in a detachment over a period of months to years.[15, 45, 67] This fact, coupled with the lower success rate of retinal detachment surgery at that time, probably encouraged retinal specialists to favor prophylactic treatment. With the advent of binocular indirect ophthalmoscopy with scleral depression in the 1950s, more peripheral retinal lesions that could potentially cause a retinal detachment were discovered and studied.[93] Some studies show a reduction in the rate of retinal detachment after prophylactic treatment of peripheral retinal lesions,[94, 95] but they may lack solid statistical foundation.[96]

The need for treatment of asymptomatic retinal breaks has always been controversial, and many authors agree that those found on routine examination should rarely be treated.[15, 96] Some state that they should not be treated in phakic eyes unless the breaks are unusually large, very posteriorly located, or associated with a progressing adjacent retinal detachment.[17] Even such asymptomatic breaks in pseudophakic eyes do not necessarily require prophylactic treatment, but they do require close monitoring.[74] Fresh, symptomatic breaks, however, probably should be treated due to a higher associated risk of progressing to a retinal detachment because they have a 30–40% chance of developing a retinal detachment.[15, 17] In one study, all symptomatic retinal breaks and retinal tears progressed to a retinal detachment within 6 weeks from the onset of symptoms.[15] It has been suggested that an eye with one or more flap tears that fail to undergo progression after this period lowers the chances of subsequent detachment from 30–50% down to 10%.[15] There is a risk of new breaks and retinal detachment after treatment. The incidence of retinal detachment after prophylactically treated breaks without regard to the type of break ranges from 1% to 13.7%.[87, 94, 97–100] Davis[15] found a higher incidence (18%), but with the exclu-

sion of aphakia, symptomatic eyes, and subclinical detachments, the incidence was reduced to 5%. The overall success rate of preventing subsequent retinal detachment with prophylactic treatment is estimated to be about 95%.[77, 101]

In the case of atrophic holes and operculated tears, there is an insignificant improvement in the outcome based on prophylactic treatment; however, treatment does significantly reduce the progression to a retinal detachment in eyes with flap tears. It is best to keep in mind that retinal tears in the fellow eye of a patient with a retinal detachment indicates the chronology of the vitreoretinal disease process rather than an early stage of development, which is important when considering the necessity of treatment.[15] Because most retinal breaks do not progress to a retinal detachment, only certain cases require treatment.[44]

The goal of prophylactic treatment is to gain the maximum effective preventative and minimize the complications or adverse reactions. Including the patient in a discussion of the risks and benefits of performing prophylactic treatment is more likely to result in a cooperative and relaxed patient. The treatment of retinal breaks usually involves using laser, photocoagulation, or cryotherapy (freezing) to form a chorioretinal scar that makes the retina adhere to the underlying pigment epithelium and choroid or scleral buckling, which reduces transvitreal traction and enhances chorioretinal scarring to the detached retina. The suffix -pexy, used in laser-pexy and cryopexy, means "to affix." Diathermy, an older treatment method that is only occasionally used today, scars the sensory retina to the underlying pigment epithelium and choroid. In several studies, the retinal adhesions produced by cryopexy were found to be stronger than the normal adhesion between the retina and the pigment epithelium.[102–106] The strength of the adhesion seemed to be independent of the intensity of the application.[102] However, one report showed that the normal retina had a stronger adhesive quality to the pigment epithelium than does a chorioretinal scar, and therefore the primary function of such a scar may be to inhibit the ingress of fluid through the retinal break.[107] Both cryopexy and laser retinopexy scars begin to heal within days, forming an adherent scar in 1–2 weeks.[108] It is best to avoid treating the pigment epithelium at the base of the break because this may cause a release of pigment epithelial cells into the vitreous and may enhance the development of proliferative vitreoretinopathy (PVR).[109] One report stated that the incidence of PVR after the treatment of tears was at least 7%.[110] A newer form of treatment is biological chorioretinal glue, one form of which is transforming growth factor beta. It has been shown to stimulate proliferation of fibroblasts and osteoblasts and to inhibit the proliferation of epithelial, endothelial, and embryonic fibroblast cells and lymphocytes; it is also chemotactic for fibroblasts.[111–113] The biological glue is introduced into the eye with a needle and a bead is placed under the localized detachment surrounding the break. It is hoped that this approach is less likely to overstimulate the RPE cells and thus cause fewer incidences of PVR.

Cryotherapy is the preferred treatment for anterior breaks because it is easier to apply treatment between the break and the ora serrata. Photocoagulation is used to treat posterior breaks due to its ease of application compared to cryotherapy: The photocoagulation beam does not easily penetrate a cataract or vitreous blood. If cryotherapy is required for posterior breaks, then "cutting" cryotherapy may be necessary. This treatment involves making a small incision in the conjunctiva and Tenon's capsule to allow posterior passage of the cryoprobe.[50] If extensive cryotherapy is required, it is best to divide the treatments into a number of sessions to reduce the incidence of macular pucker and macular edema.[109]

No matter what form of treatment is chosen, it is imperative that the entire region around the break be adequately treated, for the most common reason for subsequent retinal detachment is failure to apply adequate treatment anterior to a flap tear.[114–116] The most frequent cause of subsequent retinal detachment is inadequate treatment anterior to a flap tear.[89, 114, 115] Thus, continued vitreous traction on the flap may result in anterior extension of the tear and allow fluid greater access to the tear. Sometimes the PVD that forms a flap tear is incomplete, and further separation may enlarge the tear even after prophylactic treatment, but if treatment has been properly applied anterior to the tear, it is likely to remain sealed.[109] The use of a scleral buckle for prophylactic reasons is usually reserved for high-risk circumstances or those with numerous risk factors.

Patients who receive prophylactic treatment should be watched closely and instructed to return immediately if significant symptoms occur, such as photopsia, new floaters, loss of visual field, or loss of vision. It is common to have the patient back in 1 week and again in 3–6 weeks after treatment.[44]

It is important to follow the patient closely because 7% of treated patients have developed additional breaks, 95% of which were detected within the first 3 months.[116] A study of 100 patients followed for 6 months to 6 years after prophylactic treatment found that only two patients developed a subsequent retinal detachment; no other complications were discovered.[86] In another study, subsequent rhegmatogenous detachments occurred in 6% of eyes receiving prophylactic treatment, 8% developed new retinal tears, and macular abnormalities were suspected in 2% of the cases. The development of retinal detachments after prophylactic treatment is often the result of new tears at what appeared to be normal areas of retina (25% of cases) or at the edge of treated areas; this may be the result of areas of exaggerated vitreoretinal adhesions.[96] These new tears can rapidly progress to a clinically significant detachment.[60, 107] Even without treatment, new tears most often occur in areas of normal-appearing retina.[58, 60, 62] The finding of new tears in normal-looking retina should temper the decision to administer prophylactic treatment because such treatment may initiate tear production in unsuspected locations. In aphakic eyes, prophylactic treatment is not as successful, which may be due to tiny retinal breaks in the far periphery typically found in these eyes and the more significant degree of vitreous traction found in aphakic eyes.[117] It is also important to follow the patient closely at first because initial application of the treatment weakens the normal adhesion of the sensory retina to the underlying pigment epithelium and may cause a retinal detachment.[50] It is fairly common to find retinal breaks at the border of a cryoscar, which is likely due to the fact that the scar is a site for anchoring the retina and that traction produced by the retina on the edge of the scar during eye movements or from vitreous traction may lead to a break.[118]

Complications of treatment include corneal lesions, macular pucker, macular edema, and retinal tear and detachment. Macular pucker after peripheral retinal photocoagulation or cryopexy occurs at a 0–3% rate.[68, 96, 119] Macular pucker from cryoptherapy is less than 1%.[77, 115, 120] Epiretinal macular membranes can occur in treated and untreated eyes (spontaneous macular pucker formation has been documented).[114] It is not clear whether they are the direct result of treatment or are spontaneously formed membranes associated with a PVD or a retinal tear.[50, 107] A macular pucker is likely to occur after treatment, especially if the treatment is extensive.[72] Prophylactic treatment has been known to induce new tears, perhaps due to inadequate treatment of the anterior margin of lattice degeneration with flap tears[89] or due to vitreous shrinkage secondary to treatment. New breaks are not a common sequel of proper treatment but may be the result of overzealous application of photocoagulation or cryotherapy. Excessive treatment can lead to retinal break formation due to retinal necrosis. In one study, new breaks occurred in 5% of treated cases.[119] Iatrogenic retinal detachment is also a rare complication of treatment.[107]

References

1. Byer NE. Clinical study of retinal breaks. Trans Am Acad Ophthalmol Otolaryngol 1967;71:461–472.
2. Adams ST. Retinal breaks in eye bank eyes. Arch Ophthalmol 1956;55:254–260.
3. Okun E. Gross and microscopic pathology in autopsied eyes. III. Retinal breaks without detachment. Am J Ophthalmol 1961;51:369–391.
4. Rutnin U, Schepens CL. Fundus appearance in normal eyes. IV. Retinal breaks and other findings. Am J Ophthalmol 1967;64:1063–1078.
5. Barisak YR, Stein R. Retinal breaks without retinal detachment in autopsied eyes. Acta Ophthalmol Scand Suppl 1972;50:147–158.
6. Foos RY. Pastoral peripheral retinal tears. Ann Ophthalmol 1977;6:679–687.
7. Halpern JL. Routine screening of the retinal periphery. Am J Ophthalmol 1966;62:99–102.
8. Green WR. Vitreoretinal Juncture. In SJ Ryan (ed), Retinal Disease. St. Louis: Mosby, 1989;13–69.
9. Straatsma BR, Zeegan PD, et al. Lattice degeneration of the retina. Edward Jackson Memorial Lecture. Am J Ophthalmol 1974;77:619–649.
10. Rutnin U, Schepens CL. Fundus appearance in normal eyes. III. Peripheral degenerations. Am J Ophthalmol 1967;64:1040–1062.
11. Foos RY, Simons KB, et al. Comparison of lesions predisposing to rhegmatogenous retinal detachment by race of subjects. Am J Ophthalmol 1983;96:644–649.
12. Teng CC, Katzin HM. An anatomic study of the periphery of the retina. I. Nonpigmented epithelial cell proliferation and hole formation. Am J Ophthalmol 1951;34:1237–1248.
13. Boniuk M, Butler FC. An Autopsy Study of Lattice Degeneration, Retinal Breaks and Retinal Pits. In A McPherson (ed), New and Controversial Aspects of Retinal Detachment. New York: Hoeber, 1968;59–75.
14. Foos RY, Allen RA. Retinal tears and lesser lesions of the peripheral retina in autopsy eyes. Am J Ophthalmol 1967;64:643–655.
15. Davis MD. Natural history of retinal breaks without detachment. Arch Ophthalmol 1974;92:183–194.
16. Straatsma BR, Foos RY, et al. Degenerative Diseases of the Peripheral Retina. In TD Duane, EA Jaeger (eds), Clinical Ophthalmology. Philadelphia: Harper & Row, 1976;1–30.
17. Byer NE. Prognosis of asymptomatic retinal breaks. Arch Ophthalmol 1974;92:208–210.
18. Byer NE. The natural history of asymptomatic retinal breaks. Ophthalmology 1982;89:1033–1039.
19. Jaffe NS. Vitreous Detachments. In The Vitreous in Clinical Ophthalmology. St. Louis: Mosby, 1969;83–98.
20. Benson WE. Retinal Detachment. Diagnosis and Management (2nd ed). Philadephia: Lippincott, 1988;33–52.
21. Tasman WS. Posterior vitreous detachment and peripheral retinal breaks. Trans Am Acad Ophthalmol 1968;72:217–224.
22. Pierro I, Camesasa FI, et al. Peripheral retinal changes and axial myopia. Retina 1992;12:12–17.
23. Hyams SW, Neumann E, et al. Myopia–aphakia. II. Vitreous and peripheral retina. Br J Ophthalmol 1975;59:483–485.
24. Hyams SW, Neumann E. Peripheral retina in myopia with particular references to retinal breaks. Br J Ophthalmol 1969;53:300–306.
25. Benson WE, Tasman WS. Rhegmatogenous retinal detach-
ments caused by paravascular vitreoretinal traction. Arch Ophthalmol 1984;102:669–670.
26. Spencer LM, Foos RY, et al. Paravascular vitreoretinal attachments. Role in retinal tears. Arch Ophthalmol 1970;84:557–564.
27. Byer NE. Cystic retinal tufts and their relationship to retinal detachment. Arch Ophthalmol 1981;99:1788–1790.
28. Foos RY. Vitreous Base, Retinal Tufts, and Retinal Tears: Pathogenic Relationships. In RC Pruett, CDJ Regan (eds), Retina Congress. New York: Appleton-Century-Crofts, 1972;259–280.
29. Spencer LM, Foos RY, et al. Meridional folds, meridional complexes and associate abnormalities of the peripheral retina. Am J Ophthalmol 1970;70:697–718.
30. Spencer LM, Foos RY, et al. Enclosed bays of the ora serrata. Arch Ophthalmol 1970;83:421–425.
31. Straatsma BR, Zeegen PD, et al. Lattice degeneration of the retina. Trans Am Acad Ophthalmol Otolaryngol 1974;77:619–649.
32. Yanoff M, Fine BS. Ocular Pathology: A Text and Atlas. Philadelphia: Harper & Row, 1982;455–462.
33. Dunker S, Glinz J, Faulborn J. Morphologic studies of the peripheral vitreoretinal interface in humans reveal structures implicated in the pathogenesis of retinal tears. Retina 1997;17:124–130.
34. Straatsma BR, Foos RY, et al. Degenerative Diseases of the Peripheral Retina. In TD Duane, EA Jaeger (eds), Clinical Ophthalmology. Philadelphia: Harper & Row, 1980;26:1–30.
35. Lindner B. Acute posterior vitreous detachment and its retinal complications. Acta Ophthalmol Scand Suppl 1966;87:65–68.
36. Jaffe NS. Vitreous traction at the posterior pole of the fundus due to alterations in the posterior vitreous. Trans Am Acad Ophthalmol Otolaryngol 1967;71:642–652.
37. Everett WG, Katzin D. Meridional distribution of retinal breaks in aphakic retinal detachment. Am J Ophthalmol 1968;66:928–932.
38. Norton EWD. Retinal detachment in aphakia. Trans Am Ophthalmol Soc 1973;61:770–779.
39. Phelps CI. Distribution of breaks in aphakic and "senile" eyes with retinal aphakic detachment. Br J Ophthalmol 1963;47:744–751.
40. Jabs DA, Enger C, et al. Retinal detachments in patients with cytomegalic retinitis. Arch Ophthalmol 1911;109:794–799.
41. Freeman WR, Qicerno JI, et al. Surgical repair of rhegmatogenous retinal detachment with cytomegalic retinitis. Ophthalmology 1992;99:466–474.
42. Foos RY. Posterior vitreous detachment. Trans Am Acad Ophthalmol Otolaryngol 1972;76:480–497.
43. Teng CC, Chi HH. Vitreous changes and the mechanism of retinal detachment. Am J Ophthalmol 1957;44:335–356.
44. Schachat A, Beauchamp G, et al. Retinal Detachment: Preferred Practice Pattern. San Francisco: American Academy of Ophthalmology, 1990.
45. Colyear BH, Pischel DK. Clinical tears in the retina without detachment. Am J Ophthalmol 1956;41:773–792.
46. Schepens CL. Retinal Detachment and Allied Diseases. Philadelphia: Saunders, 1983;668–672.
47. Pischel DK. Retinal Detachment. A Manual. Am Acad Ophthalmol Otolaryngol 1965;73.
48. Foos RY. Retinal holes. Am J Ophthalmol 1978;86:354–358.
49. Byer NE. Clinical study of lattice degeneration of the retina. Trans Am Acad Ophthalmol Otolaryngol 1965;69:1064–1081.

50. Benson WE. Retinal Detachment: Diagnosis and Management (2nd ed). Philadephia: Lippincott, 1988;193–207.
51. Machemer R. The importance of fluid absorption, traction, intraocular currents, and chorioretinal scars in the therapy of rhegmatogenous retinal detachments. Am J Ophthalmol 1984;98:681–693.
52. Gonin J. Le traitemint de decollement retinien. Ann Oculist 1921;158:175.
53. Leber T. Über die Entstehung der Netzhautablosung. Berl Vers Ophthalmol Ges 1882;14:18.
54. Eisner T. Biomicroscopy of the Peripheral Retina. New York: Springer-Verlag, 1973.
55. Avila MP, Jalkh AE, et al. Biomicroscopic study of the vit reous in macular breaks. Ophthalmology 1983;90:1277–1283.
56. Lindner K. Über die Herstellung von Modellen zu Modellversuchen der Netzhautavhlung. Klin Monatsbl Augenheilkd 1933;90:289–300.
57. Rosengren B, Osterlin S. Hydrodynamic events in the vitreous space accompanying eye movements. Significance to the pathogenesis of retinal detachment. Ophthalmologica 1976;173:513–524.
58. Sebag J. Vitreous Pathology. In W Tasman, EA Jaeger (eds), Clinical Ophthalmology. Vol. 3. Philadelphia: Harper & Row, 1992;39:1–26.
59. Tabotabo MM, Karp LA, et al. Posterior vitreous detachment. Ann Ophthalmol 1980;12:59–61.
60. Byer NE. Natural history of posterior vitreous detachment with early management as the premier line of defense against retinal detachment. Ophthalmology 1994;101:1503–1514.
61. Jaffe NS. Complications of acute posterior vitreous detachment. Arch Ophthalmol 1968;79:568–571.
62. Kanski JJ. Complications of acute posterior detachment. Am J Ophthalmol 1975;80:44–46.
63. Novak MA, Welch RB. Complications of acute symptomatic posterior vitreous detachment. Am J Ophthalmol 1984;97:308–314.
64. Boldrey EE. Risk of retinal tears in patients with vitreous floaters. Am J Ophthalmol 1983;96:783–787.
65. Murakami K, Jalkh AE, et al. Vitreous floaters. Ophthalmology 1983;90:1271–1276.
66. Straatsma BR, Foos RY, et al. Degenerative Diseases of the Peripheral Retina. In TD Duane, EA Jaeger (eds), Clinical Ophthalmology. Philadelphia: Harper & Row, 1993;1–30.
67. Colyear BH, Pischel DK. Preventative treatment of retinal detachment by means of light coagulation. Trans Pac Coast Ophthalmol Soc 1960;41:193–217.
68. Michels RG, Wilkinson CP, et al. Retinal Detachment: Diagnosis and Management. St. Louis: Mosby, 1990.
69. Sidman RL. Histochemical studies on photoreceptor cells. Ann NY Acad Sci 1958–1959;74:182–195.
70. Rohlich P. The interphotoreceptor matrix. Electron microscopic and histochemical observations on the vertebrate retina. Exp Eye Res 1970;10;80–86.
71. Neumann E, et al. The Natural History of Retinal Holes with Specific References to the Development of Retinal Detachment and the Time Factor Involved. In IC Michaelson, ER Berman (eds), Causes and Prevention of Blindness. New York: Academic, 1972;404–408.
72. Sigelman J. Vitreous base classification of retinal tears: Clinical application. Surv Ophthalmol 1980;25:59–74.
73. Robertson DM, Prilick IA. 360 degree prophylactic cryoretinopexy: A clinical and experimental study. Arch Ophthalmol 1979;97:21–30.
74. Merin S, Feiler V, et al. The fate of the fellow eye in retinal detachment. Am J Ophthalmol 1971;71:477–481.
75. Davis MD, Segal PP, et al. The Natural Course Followed by the Fellow Eye in Patients with Rhegmatogenous Retinal Detachment. In RC Pruett, CDJ Regan (eds), Retinal Congress. New York: Appleton-Century-Crofts, 1972:643–660.
76. Hyams SW, Meir E, et al. Chorioretinal lesions predisposing to retinal detachment. Am J Ophthalmol 1974;78:429–437.
77. Dollfus M. Le traitement previntif du decollement de la retine. XVIII Concilium Ophthalmolgicum. Vol. 1. Brussels: Imprimerie Medicale et Scientifique, 1958;988–989.
78. Haut J, Massin M, et al. Frequence des decollements de retine dans la population francaise. Pourcentage des decollements bilateraux. Arch Ophthalmol 1975;35:533–536.
79. Stein R, Feller-Ofry V, et al. The Effect of Treatment in the Prevention of Retinal Detachment. In IC Michaelson, ER Berman (eds), Causes and Prevention of Blindness. New York: Academic, 1972;409–410.
80. Tornquist R. Bilateral retinal detachment. Acta Ophthalmol Scand Suppl 1963;41:126–133.
81. Folk JC, Arrindell EL, et al. The fellow eye of patients with phakic lattice retinal detachment. Ophthalmology 1989;96:72–79.
82. Morse PH, Sheie HG. Prophylactic cryoretinopexy of retinal breaks. Arch Ophthalmol 1974; 92:204–207.
83. Okun E, Cibis PA. Photocoagulation in "Limited" Retinal Detachment and Breaks Without Detachment. In A McPherson (ed), New and Controversial Aspects of Retinal Detachment. New York: Harper & Row, 1968;164–171.
84. Pollak A, Oliver M. Argon laser photocoagulation of symptomatic flap tears and retinal breaks of fellow eyes. Br J Ophthalmol 1981;65:469–472.
85. Neumann E, Hyams S. Conservative management of retinal breaks: A follow-up study of subsequent retinal detachment. Br J Ophthalmol 1972;56:482–486.
86. Straatsma BR, Allen RA, et al. The prophylaxis of retinal detachment. Trans Pac Coast Ophthalmol Soc 1965; 46:211–236.
87. Friedman Z, Neumann E. Posterior vitreous detachment after cataract extraction in non-myopic eyes and the resulting retinal lesions. Br J Ophthalmol 1975;59:451–454.
88. Friedman Z, Neumann E, et al. Vitreous and peripheral retina in aphakia. Br J Ophthalmol 1973;57:52–57.
89. Benson WE, Morse PH, et al. Late complications following cryotherapy of lattice degeneration. Am J Ophthalmol 1977;84:514–516.
90. Campbell CJ, Rittler MC. Cataract extraction in the retinal detachment-prone patient. Am J Ophthalmol 1972;73:17–24.
91. McPherson A, O'Malley R, et al. Management of the fellow eyes of patients with rhegmatogenous retinal detachment. Ophthalmology 1981;88:922–934.
92. Javitt JC, Tielsch JM, et al. National outcomes of cataract extraction. Increased risk of retinal complications associated with Nd-YAG laser capsulotomy. Ophthalmology 1992;99:1487–1498.
93. Schepens CL. Subclinical retinal detachments. Arch Ophthalmol 1952;47:593–606.
94. Goldberg MF. Clear lens extraction for axial myopia. Ophthalmology 1987;94:571–582.
95. Luisky M, Winberger D, et al. The prevalence of retinal detachment in aphakic high myopic patients. Ophthalmic Surg 1987;18:444–445.

96. Barraquer C, Cavelier C, et al. Incidence of retinal detachment following clear-lens extraction in myopic patients. Arch Ophthalmol 1994;112:336–339.

97. Mortimer CB. The prevention of retinal detachment. Can J Ophthalmol 1966;1:206–212.

98. Colyear BH, ed. A Clinical Comparison of Partially Penetrating Diathermy and Xenon–Arc Photocoagulation: New and Controversial Aspects of Retinal Detachment. New York: Harper & Row, 1968;176–185.

99. Sollner F. Uber die prophylaktische Behandlung der Ablatio retinae durch Lichtcoagulation. Bericht Deutsche Ophthalmologische Gesellschaft 1965;66:327–336.

100. Schepens CL. The preventative treatment of idiopathic and secondary retinal detachment. Acta Concilium Ophthalmolgicum 1959;1:1019–1027.

101. Meyer-Schwickerath G, Fried M. Prophylaxis of retinal detachment. Trans Ophthalmol Soc UK 1980;100:56–65.

102. Bloch D, O'Connor P, et al. The mechanism of cryosurgical adhesions. III. Statistical analysis. Am J Ophthalmol 1971;71:666–673.

103. Zauberman H. Tensile strength of chorioretinal lesions produced by photocoagulation, diathermy and cryopexy. Br J Ophthalmol 1969;53:749–752.

104. Zauberman H. Experimental cleavage of chorioretinal scars by traction and subretinal fluid. Ann Ophthalmol 1976;8:1301–1308.

105. Lincoff H, Kreissig I. The mechanism of the cryosurgical adhesions. IV. Electron microscopy. Am J Ophthalmol 1971;71:674–689.

106. Bose M, Rassow B, et al. The strength of the retinal scar tissue after argon, xenon, and cryocoagulation. Graefes Arch Clin Exp Ophthalmol 1981;216:291–299.

107. Lewis H, Kreiger AE. Rhegmatogenous Retinal Detachment. In TD Duane, EA Jaeger (eds), Clinical Ophthalmology. Vol. 3. Philadelphia: Harper & Row, 1993;27:1–12.

108. Lincoff H, O'Connor P, et al. The cryosurgical adhesion. Part II. Trans Am Acad Ophthalmol Otolaryngol 1970; 74:98–107.

109. Lean JS. Diagnosis and Treatment of Peripheral Retinal lesions. In WR Freeman (ed), Practical Atlas of Retinal Disease and Therapy. New York: Raven, 1993;12:211–220.

110. Hilton G, Machemer R, et al. The classification of retinal detachment with proliferative vitreoretinopathy. Ophthalmology 1983;90:121–125.

111. Smiddy WE, Glaser DM, et al. Transforming growth factor beta: A biological chorioretinal glue. Arch Ophthalmol 1989;107:577–580.

112. Sporn MB, Roberts AB, et al. Some recent advances in the chemistry and biology of transforming growth factor beta. J Cell Biol 1987;105:1039–1045.

113. Smiddy WE, Glaser BM, et al. Transforming growth factor-B-2 significantly enhances the ability to flatten the rim of subretinal fluid surrounding macular holes: Preliminary anatomic results of a multicenter prospective randomized study. Retina 1993;13:296–301.

114. Delaney WV. Retinal tear extension through the cryosurgical scar. Br J Ophthalmol 1971;55:205–209.

115. Robertson DM, Norton EWD. Long-term follow-up of treated retinal breaks. Am J Ophthalmol 1973;75:395–404.

116. Goldberg RE, Boyer DS. Sequential retinal breaks following a spontaneous initial retinal break. Ophthalmology 1981;88:10–12.

117. Lean JS. Diagnosis and Treatment of Peripheral Retinal Lesions. In WR Freeman (ed), Practical Atlas of Retinal Disease and Therapy. New York: Raven, 1993;14:237–241.

118. Moisseiev J, Glaser BM. New and previously unidentified retinal breaks in eyes with recurrent retinal detachment with proliferative vitreoretinoapthy. Arch Ophthalmol 1989;107:1152–1154.

119. Benson WE. Prophylactic therapy of retinal breaks. Surv Ophthalmol 1977;22:41–47.

120. Chignell AH, Shilling J. Prophylaxis of retinal detachment. Br J Ophthalmol 1973; 57:291–298.

Atrophic Retinal Hole

An atrophic retinal hole is a retinal break that is not caused by traction and is most likely produced by an atrophic process. It is generally thought to be the result of underlying vascular insufficiency of the choroid and choriocapillaris. Even though vitreous traction may be present adjacent to a hole,[1] vitreous contraction leading to a PVD does not seem to play an important role in the formation of these breaks.[2] The resultant retinal thinning and degeneration eventually leads to a circumscribed disappearance of the retina, which clinically appears as a hole. However, often the adjacent retina looks normal and there is no reactive pigment epithelial hyperplasia. These lesions are small, round, red defects typically found in an area of thin and partially opaque retina (Figure 5-2; see also Figures 3-1 and 3-43). Their size generally varies from a pinpoint to 1.5 disc diameters.[3] Atrophic holes are more commonly found in younger people because they are not associated with a PVD.[4] Table 5-1 shows the differentiation between atrophic retinal holes and tears.

The red color is the result of the absence of the overlying retinal tissue, which allows the red choroidal reflex to appear brighter in the defect as compared to the surrounding fundus. They are pink, clear, or light gray when seen in a detached retina. Atrophic retinal holes may be differentiated from a peripheral retinal hemorrhage by the hole's perfectly smooth borders, whereas a hemorrhage has irregular margins where the blood diffuses into the adjacent retinal tissue. The red color of a retinal hole changes as it is rolled during scleral depression, which does not occur with hemorrhages. Scleral depression can also aid in the discovery of a hole that is not obvious because holes are often in an area of retinal degeneration. Even if the area of degeneration appears essentially normal in color, any area of degenerating retina becomes more whitish on depression (white-with-pressure), and thus depression enhances the subtle redness of the hole compared to the adjacent whitish retina. Retinal holes are generally confined to the region between the equator and the ora serrata. Most holes are found in the vitreous base, and there seems to be no evidence

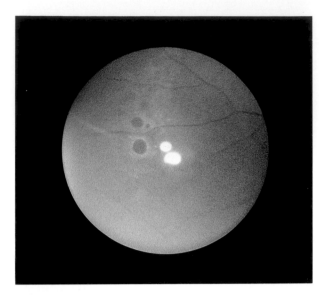

FIGURE 5-2
Three atrophic retinal holes in the nasal retina seen through the indirect condensing lens.

of quadrant predilection.[2, 5] Holes within the base do not produce a retinal detachment. Holes located posterior to the base may produce a detachment. Atrophic retinal holes are found in 0.4% of patients at autopsy.[5] One study of 156 retinal breaks found that 77% were atrophic holes.[4] Lattice degeneration has been reported to have an incidence of atrophic holes that ranges from 18.2% to 42%.[6–8] One study reported that approximately 75% of atrophic holes are found associated with lattice degeneration.[9] Myopes are more likely to develop atrophic holes. One study found that holes or tears had an incidence of 12.1% in patients with high myopia.[10]

Histopathology

A retinal hole is produced by the loss of sensory retinal tissue in a circumscribed area of thinning. The edges of the hole become rounded with time due to degeneration and contraction (Figure 5-3). There is minimal reactive gliosis and no significant changes in the adjacent pigment epithelium or vitreous.[4]

TABLE 5-1. Comparison of Atrophic Hole, Operculated Tear, and Horseshoe Tear

Atrophic Hole	Operculated Tear	Horseshoe Tear
Round to oval	Round with disc-shaped operculum floating above break attached to the separated vitreous cortex	Horseshoe-shaped with central flap
May have a white collar surrounding hole, which may represent retinal degeneration or localized detachment	May have a white collar surrounding hole, which may represent retinal degeneration or localized detachment	May have elevated surrounding white margin of a localized detachment
Red when found in attached retina but may be pink, gray, or clear in appearance in detached retina	Same	Same
No vitreous traction associated with lesion	Vitreous traction present initially in formation of break but usually absent afterward	Continuous vitreous traction is usually associated with lesion
Usually found in the far peripheral retina but may be found in the posterior pole (macular hole)	Usually found in the far to midperiphery and rarely in the posterior pole region	Usually found in the far to midperiphery and rarely in the posterior pole region
Retinal and vitreal hemorrhages not associated	Retinal and vitreal hemorrhages not frequently associated with tear formation	Retinal and vitreal hemorrhages are often associated with tear formation
Not symptomatic unless a macular hole is produced or a clinically significant detachment occurs	May be symptomatic with photopsia and vitreous floaters present during tractional phase or if a clinically significant detachment occurs	Often symptomatic with photopsia and vitreous floaters present during tractional phase or if a clinically significant detachment occurs
Lowest incidence of producing a retinal detachment	Higher incidence of producing a detachment than an atrophic hole but less than a horseshoe tear	Approximately one-third of symptomatic tears produce a clinically significant detachment
Often are not treated unless there are related significant risk factors—e.g., high myopia, vitreoretinal disease, history of retinal detachment in fellow eye	May or may not be treated depending on risk factors present, but treatment is indicated with symptoms of vitreous traction	Always treated unless patient is too debilitated to have the necessary procedure

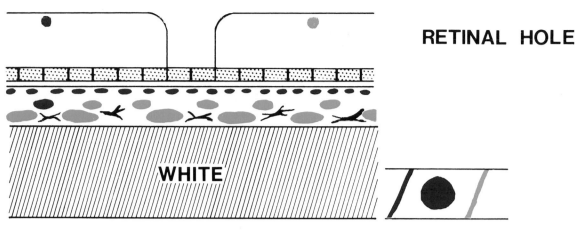

RETINAL HOLE

WHITE

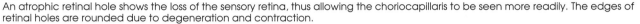

FIGURE 5-3
An atrophic retinal hole shows the loss of the sensory retina, thus allowing the choriocapillaris to be seen more readily. The edges of retinal holes are rounded due to degeneration and contraction.

Clinical Significance

Most retinal holes do not lead to a retinal detachment because no strong vitreous traction is present. They should be followed on a periodic basis, however, to rule out the formation of a localized subclinical (>1 disc diameter but <2 disc diameters posterior to the equator) or clinically significant retinal detachment. The patient should be instructed to be aware of and to measure his or her visual field and to return immediately if a loss of visual field is experienced. The diagnosis of an atrophic hole with a localized retinal detachment can be facilitated by performing scleral depression (Figure 5-4). The small surrounding detachment produces a shadow at the posterior margin of the break; this can be seen during scleral depression by placing the break on a tangential view. Most atrophic holes are not likely to progress to a clinically significant retinal detachment.[2, 11–14] One report states that an atrophic hole without subretinal fluid has only a 7% chance of progressing into a clinically significant retinal detachment, which increased to 33% for those with a subclinical detachment.[15] Atrophic holes in aphakia have a higher incidence of retinal detachment and are often associated with small breaks in the nasal periphery.[16, 17]

Atrophic holes generally do not require treatment (even in the presence of a PVD), but sometimes, if a retinal detachment occurred in the fellow eye, treatment may be considered.[2, 11–13, 18–20] Even aphakic eyes with asymptomatic holes can be safely followed without treatment.[11, 21, 22] The prevention of a retinal detachment by prophylactic treatment of atrophic holes in lattice degeneration

made an insignificant difference.[2] Follow-up after treatment is usually done in 1 week and then again in 3–6 weeks; the patient should be told to return immediately if photopsia, new floaters, or visual field loss occur.[18] Atrophic retinal holes, with or without a localized retinal detachment, may be adequately treated with cryopexy or photocoagulation. The holes should be surrounded by a 2-mm contiguous rim of cryopexy or laserpexy and the treatment extended all the way anterior so that there can be no anterior leakage of fluid through the break.[23, 24]

References

1. Okun E. Gross and microscopic pathology in autopsied eyes. III. Retinal breaks without detachment. Am J Ophthalmol 1961;51:369–391.
2. Lewis H, Kreiger AE. Rhegmatogenous Retinal Detachment. In TD Duane, EA Jaeger (eds), Clinical Ophthalmology. Philadelphia: Harper & Row, 1993;27:1–12.
3. Schepens CL. Retinal Detachment and Allied Diseases. Philadelphia: Saunders, 1983;158.
4. Byer NE. Clinical study of retinal breaks. Trans Am Acad Ophthalmol Otolaryngol 1967;71:461–472.
5. Straatsma BR, Foos RY, et al. Degenerative Diseases of the Peripheral Retina. In TD Duane, EA Jaeger (eds), Clinical Ophthalmology. Philadelphia: Harper & Row, 1980;1–30.
6. Byer NE. Lattice degeneration of the retina. Surv Ophthalmol 1979;23:213–248.
7. Byer N. Long-term natural history of lattice degeneration of the retina. Ophthalmology 1989;96:1396–1402.
8. Straatsma BR, Zeegan PD, et al. Lattice degeneration of the retina. Am J Ophthalmol 1974; 77:619–649.
9. Foos RY. Retinal holes. Am J Ophthalmol 1978;86:354–358.
10. Pierro I, Camesasa FI, et al. Peripheral retinal changes and axial myopia. Retina 1992;12:12–17.

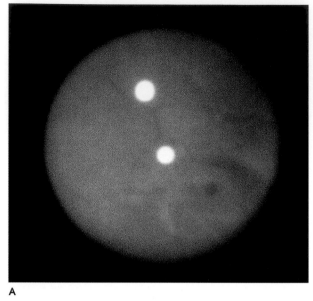

A

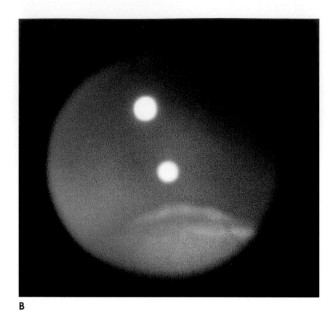

B

FIGURE 5-4
A. An atrophic retinal hole with a surrounding localized retinal detachment is seen through the indirect condensing lens. B. A further rolling of the hole now shows the localized detachment on profile; the hole is not visible now because it is at the apex of the detachment.

11. Neumann E, Hyams S. Conservative management of retinal breaks: A follow-up study of subsequent retinal detachment. Br J Ophthalmol 1972;56:482–486.
12. Byer NE. Prognosis of asymptomatic retinal breaks. Arch Ophthalmol 1974;92:208–210.
13. Byer NE. The natural history of asymptomatic retinal breaks. Ophthalmology 1982;89:1033–1039.
14. Hirose T. Acquired Retinoschisis: Observations and Treatment. In RC Pruett, CDJ Regan (eds), Retinal Congress. New York: Appleton-Century-Crofts, 1972;489–504.
15. Davis MD. Natural history of retinal breaks without detachment. Arch Ophthalmol 1974;92:183–194.
16. Ashrafzadeh MT, Schepens CL, et al. Aphakic and phakic retinal detachment. Arch Ophthalmol 1973;89:476–483.
17. Rutnin U, Schepens CL. Fundus appearance in normal eyes. II. The standard peripheral fundus developmental variations. Am J Ophthalmol 1967;64:840–852.
18. Schachat A, Beauchamp G, et al. Retinal Detachment: Preferred Practice Pattern. San Francisco: American Academy of Ophthalmology, 1990.
19. Benson WE. Retinal Detachment. Diagnosis and Management (2nd ed). Philadephia: Lippincott, 1988.
20. Hyams SW, Meir E, et al. Chorioretinal lesions predisposing to retinal detachment. Am J Ophthalmol 1974;78:429–437.
21. Friedman Z, Neumann E, Hyams S. Vitreous and peripheral retina in aphakia. Br J Ophthalmol 1973;57:52–57.
22. Hyams SW, Neumann E, et al. Myopia–aphakia. II. Vitreous and peripheral retina. Br J Ophthalmol 1975;59:483–485.
23. Benson WE, Natawan P, et al. Late complications following cryotherapy of lattice degeneration. Am J Ophthalmol 1977;84:514–16.
24. Robertson DM, Norton EWD. Long-term follow-up of treated retinal breaks. Am J Ophthalmol 1973;75:395–404.

Operculated Retinal Tear

Operculated retinal tears are round, red breaks with an avulsed round (disc-shaped) retinal plug (operculum) adherent to the detached cortical vitreous (Figures 5-5, 5-6, 5-7, and 5-8; see also Figure 3-28). The operculum floats in the vitreous cavity (see Figure 3-1) and is most frequently located anterior to the hole. This is due to the anterior displacement of the vitreous during a PVD (see Figures 4-4, 4-12, 5-7, and 5-8). However, the operculum can be found directly above the hole or in any direction from the hole, depending on the force of vitreous traction at the time of avulsion. An operculum is most likely a sudden event that occurs at the time of PVD formation and therefore in a matter of hours or weeks rather than being a slowly progressive process.[1] The operculum usually appears smaller than the retinal break due to degeneration and contraction caused by the loss of blood supply to the avulsed retinal tissue. On high magnification, it is common to find cystoid degeneration of the operculum, which gives it a honeycomb appearance. The base of the break often has a stippled and granular appearance due to degeneration of the pigment epithelium.[2] Most operculated tears are small and round, which is likely secondary to a small round area of vitreous adhesion to the surface of the retina that pulls out a small round plug of tissue. In other cases, the tear

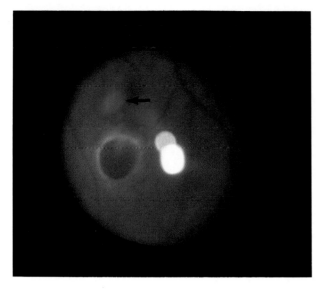

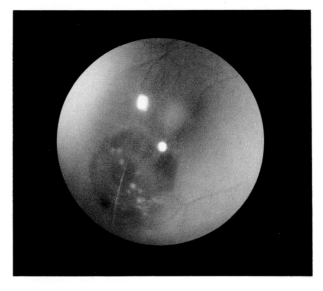

FIGURE 5-5
Operculated retinal tear with localized surrounding retinal detachment and an operculum floating above that is still attached to the detached vitreous cortex. The operculum is five times smaller than the retinal break indicating that it has been present for months to years. The white surrounding collar is fibrosis secondary to retinal degeneration. The view is through the indirect condensing lens. Note the giant drusen in the superior base of the break.

FIGURE 5-6
Operculated retinal tear with a localized retinal detachment surrounded by a surrounding pigmented demarcation line. Note the operculum above the break and the giant pathologic drusen underneath the detachment. The view is through the indirect condensing lens.

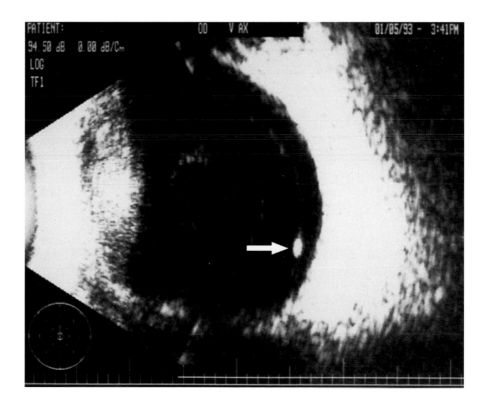

FIGURE 5-7
B-scan ultrasonogram of an inferiorly located operculum. Note that the thin posterior vitreous cortex can be seen with the operculum (*arrow*) attached to it.

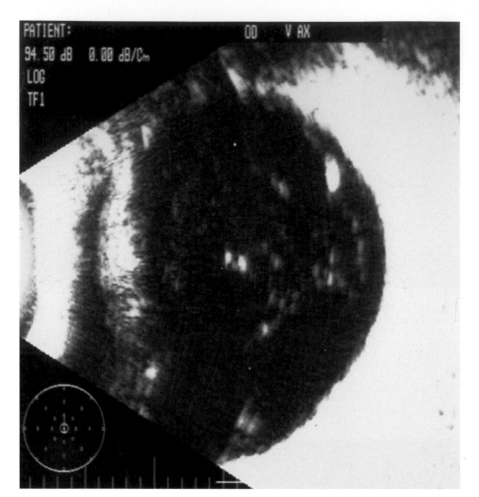

FIGURE 5-8
B-scan ultrasonogram of a superior operculum. Note that the thin posterior cortex runs through the operculum and anteriorly attaches itself to the posterior margin of the vitreous base. Also note the floaters in the vitreous body.

may be larger or irregular in shape, which is likely due to the area of vitreous adhesion being larger and having irregular margins; sometimes the tear may be a disc diameter in size. The clinician must be careful because a horseshoe tear with an avulsed flap can look like a large operculated tear (the flap being mistaken for an operculum); a correct diagnosis can be made by noting that the avulsed tissue is elongated like a flap. Differentiation between operculated tears, flap tears, and atrophic holes is found in Table 5-1.

Most operculated tears are asymptomatic; however, they may be symptomatic in the initial phase of their development due to traction on the retina. After formation of the operculum, traction is released from the retina and the patient becomes asymptomatic. However, persistent vitreous traction to the retina adjacent to the break may lead to continued photopsia. The patient would only become symptomatic again if a clinically significant retinal detachment occurs. The edges of the tear become smooth and rounded with time due to

degeneration and contraction. There appears to be no predilection for eye involved or gender in the occurrence of these tears.

The underlying cause of the operculated tear is probably a long-standing focal area of increased vitreoretinal adhesion in the peripheral retina. These adhesions most often occur around blood vessels, and their existence over years is likely to produce a localized area of cystic retinal degeneration and weakness. When a PVD occurs, the increased tractional force results in a plug of sensory retina being pulled away from the pigment epithelium. The edges of the break become rounded with time due to degeneration and contracture of the adjacent retinal tissue. The traction at the site of the increased vitreoretinal adhesion over months to years can cause reactive hyperplasia of the pigment epithelium (pigment clump), and so it is not unusual to find pigmentation adjacent to the break or on the operculum (Figure 5-9).[3] (See Acquired Hyperplasia of the Pigment Epithelium.)

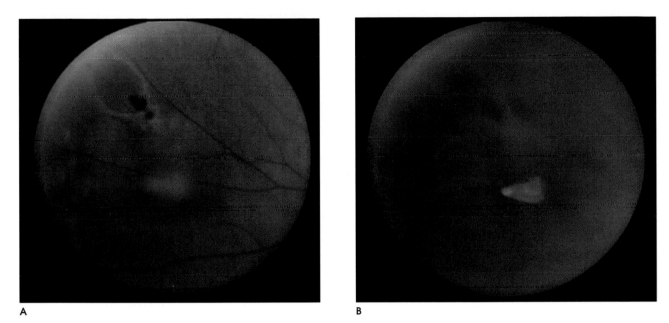

A   B

FIGURE 5-9
A. A large operculated tear in the temporal midperiphery of the retina. The pigment clump at one end of the tear indicates years of previous traction at this retinal site, which led to the formation of the break. A small round retinal atrophic hole is adjacent to the pigment clump opposite the larger retinal tear. The operculum is out of focus above and inferior to the break. B. The operculum in focus. Note the pigment clump on the operculum; it was previously located next to the pigment clump on the underlying retina.

One study reported that operculated tears were found in 13% of 156 breaks.[4] Another study of 183 eyes with asymptomatic breaks found that 30 were operculated tears (none of which progressed to a retinal detachment).[1] Operculated tears are found more frequently in older people because of the close association with PVD, and PVD is more commonly found in eyes with operculated or flap tears (even if asymptomatic) than in eyes with atrophic holes. There appears to be no predilection for eye involved or gender in the occurrence of these tears.[1, 4]

Operculated tears are usually located between the ora serrata and the equator, more often in the superior half of the fundus,[1] but they may be found in any region. They frequently occur in areas of lattice degeneration and retinal thinning. Operculated and horseshoe tears most commonly occur at the posterior border of the vitreous base, areas of lattice degeneration, pigment clumps, cystic retinal tufts, or invisible areas of vitreoretinal adhesions. Most of the breaks are less than 0.25 disc diameter.[5] The breaks may have small yellow spheroids within their borders. These are known as giant pathologic drusen (see Figures 5-5 and 5-6) and are the result of drusen formation by the pigment epithelium in response to the abnormal condition caused by the absence of overlying sensory retina and exposure to the vitreous cavity.[6]

The holes may be surrounded by white-with-or-without-pressure. Therefore, it is advisable that scleral depression be performed in an area of the fundus where a round floater is found in the vitreous. This may enhance the appearance of a retinal break that is just barely visible (see White-With-or-Without-Pressure in Chapter 3). Remember that an operculum is disc-shaped because it is a plug of sensory retina and a vitreous floater is usually spheroid. Circumscribed subretinal fluid may accumulate around the hole, producing a subclinical or localized retinal detachment (Figures 5-6 and 5-10). The white circumscribed area around the break may be (1) fibrotic tissue from local degeneration (see Figure 5-5), (2) a localized retinal detachment or (see Figure 5-6), (3) a reattached localized detachment. If the whitish area around the break is not elevated when evaluated with binocular indirect ophthalmoscopy with and without scleral depression or with higher magnification with a precorneal lens or fundus mirror contact lens, then it is likely to be 1 or 3 above. If the localized retinal detachment remains stationary for 3 months or longer, a pigmented retinal demarcation line may be produced (see Figures 5-6 and 6-24). This pigment line is produced by the proliferation of pigment epithelial cells and is believed to form a weak bond at the edge of the retinal detachment that may retard its progression (see Chapter 6).

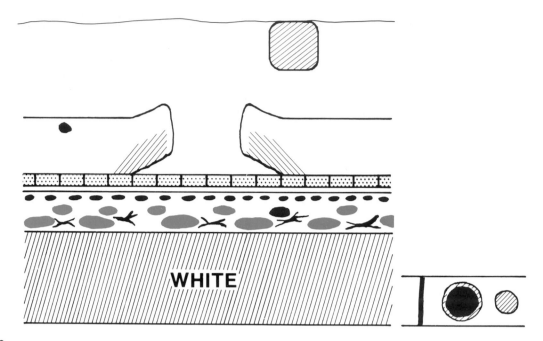

FIGURE 5-10
Operculated retinal tear with operculum still attached to the detached vitreous cortex and a localized surrounding retinal detachment, which produced the white collar around the break. The operculum is smaller than the retinal break due to degeneration and contraction, which is also responsible for the rounded edges of the break.

Histopathology

The avulsed retinal tissue that is attached to the cortical vitreous displays marked degeneration and contraction with time. The retinal hole shows full-thickness loss of sensory retina, leaving the pigment epithelium in place (see Figure 5-10). Surrounding the hole may be an accumulation of liquefied vitreous and aqueous in the subneural space, usually resulting in a localized retinal detachment.

Clinical Significance

Approximately 50% of full-thickness retinal tears have an associated localized retinal detachment; this seems to occur more frequently with superior breaks.[2] Therefore, it is quite common to find such detachments with operculated tears. It is interesting that in most cases the localized surrounding detachments are usually equally distant and very circular around the retinal break because, if the detachment is due to the ingress of fluid from the vitreous, then why is the shape not more asymmetric? Also, if the cause of the localized detachment is the ingress of fluid, why would it stop so close to the break, as it does in the vast majority of cases? It would seem reasonable that the detachment would continue to progress just as easily as it did when the initial localized detachment was produced. If it was so easy to detach the retina next to the break, then why not a number of disc diameters further away from the break? Therefore, it seems more reasonable that the localized detachment occurred at the time of the tear formation and remained stable with little to no progression. A likely scenario is that an operculated tear occurs from marked vitreous traction on the retinal surface, which results in a tenting of the retina (small, purely tractional localized detachment); with further traction, a plug of retina is torn from the center of the localized detachment. Afterward, the break in the localized retinal detachment allows for the ingress of fluid that effectively inhibits the cuff of detached retina from reattaching. The result is a small localized detachment with an operculated round tear in it that remains stable for years. This would help to explain why some operculated tears occurring after a PVD do not produce a localized detachment, because the tear occurred without the tenting (localized detachment) of the retina. The other explanation is that the fluid from the vitreous cavity enters the retinal break and dissects the adjacent sensory retina away from the pigment epithelium, but it would seem likely that the process should continue into a larger detachment.

Operculated retinal tears can lead to a clinically significant retinal detachment (Figure 5-11). The risk of retinal separation from an operculated tear is much less than the risk from a horseshoe tear because vitreous traction to the retina has usually been released. However, it is thought that operculated tears have a slightly greater frequency of retinal detachment than do atrophic holes, but there is some controversy about this increased frequency.[1] Three studies reported that no asymptomatic operculated tears without subretinal fluid progressed to a detachment.[1, 7, 8] Two small studies reported that 1 of 6 untreated fresh operculated tears will develop a detachment[1, 9] and another study found that none of 26 eyes with an operculated tear developed a detachment.[10] The presence of an associated localized detachment increases the risk of a subsequent subclinical or clinically significant retinal detachment.[1] There may be an associated vitreous hemorrhage if a retinal vessel traversing the involved area ruptures during formation of the tear, and retinal detachments produced by an operculated or flap tear are often associated with a vitreous hemorrhage.[11] There have been cases of recurrent vitreous hemorrhage due to the avulsion of a retinal vessel that was still attached to the operculum of the tear.[12, 13]

No treatment is necessary for asymptomatic operculated tears without a localized detachment. Treatment may be considered if the patient has high myopia, aphakia, extensive vitreoretinal degeneration, or family or personal history of retinal detachment, but this is decided on a case-by-case basis. Fresh operculated tears that are large, superiorly located, or associated with a vitreous hemorrhage should be referred for consideration of retinopexy.[11, 14] If vitreous traction can be detected as adherent to the edge of the tear or adjacent blood vessel, the operculated tear should be thought equivalent to a flap tear and treatment should be considered.[1, 11] Tears with no vitreous traction on the adjacent retina have not been documented to cause a detachment and do not require treatment.[14] The observance of vitreous traction can be achieved by employing scleral depression during binocular indirect ophthalmoscopy or three-mirror or 90-diopter examination with or without scleral depression. The clinician should look for the presence of vitreous strands or vitreous condensation adjacent to the break; however, these vitreous changes are often difficult to see.

Symptomatic tears, with or without a localized retinal detachment, may be adequately treated with cryopexy or photocoagulation. However, the prevention of a retinal detachment with prophylactic

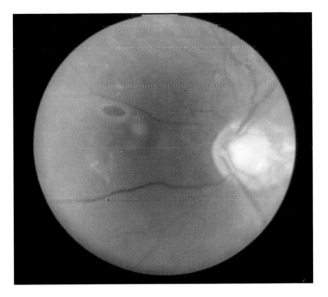

FIGURE 5-11
An operculated retinal tear in a retinal detachment extending from the nasal margin of the optic disc to the nasal equator. Notice the loss of choroidal detail underneath the retinal detachment. The operculated tear is along the superior margin of the detachment with the out-of-focus operculum adjacent to the break and toward the optic disc. The white collar around the break was a localized surrounding retinal detachment for months to years. The operculated tear was produced by a posterior vitreous detachment in this patient with diabetes mellitus. (Patient also shown in Figure 5-13.)

treatment of operculated tears in lattice degeneration made an insignificant difference.[1] Operculated tears should be surrounded by a 2-mm contiguous rim of cryopexy or laserpexy, and the treatment should be extended all the way anterior so that there can be no anterior leakage of fluid through the break.[8, 15]

References

1. Davis MD. Natural history of retinal breaks without detachment. Arch Ophthalmol 1974;92:183–194.
2. Straatsma BR, Foos RY, et al. Degenerative Diseases of the Peripheral Retina. In TD Duane, EA Jaeger (eds), Clinical Ophthalmology. Philadelphia: Harper & Row, 1993; 26:1–30.
3. Spencer LM, Straatsma BR, et al. Tractional Degenerations of the Peripheral Retina. New Orleans Academy of Ophthalmology: Symposium of the Retina and Retinal Surgery. St. Louis: Mosby, 1969.
4. Byer NE. Clinical study of retinal breaks. Trans Am Acad Ophthalmol Otolaryngol 1967;71:461–472.
5. Schepens CL, Marden D. Data on the natural history of retinal detachment: Further characterization of certain unilateral nontraumatic cases. Am J Ophthalmol 1966; 61:213–226.

6. Smiddy WE, Green RW. Retinal dialysis: Pathology and pathogenesis. Retina 1982;2:94–116.
7. Byer NE. Prognosis of asymptomatic retinal breaks. Arch Ophthalmol 1974;92:208–210.
8. Robertson DM, Norton EWD. Long-term follow-up of treated retinal breaks. Am J Ophthalmol 1973;75:395–404.
9. Colyear BH, Pischel DK. Clinical tears in the retina without detachment. Am J Ophthalmol 1956;41:773–792.
10. Davis MD, Segal PP, et al. The Natural Course Followed by the Fellow Eye in Patients with Rhegmatogenous Retinal Detachment. In RC Pruett, CDJ Regan (eds), Retinal Congress. New York: Appleton-Century-Crofts, 1972;643–660.
11. Benson WE. Retinal Detachment: Diagnosis and Management (2nd ed). Philadephia: Lippincott, 1988;5.
12. Robertson DM, Curtin VT, et al. Avulsed retinal vessels with retinal breaks: A cause of recurrent vitreous hemorrhage. Arch Ophthalmol 1971;85:669–672.
13. Theodossiadis GP, Koutsandrea Ch N. Avulsed retinal vessels with and without retinal breaks—treatment and extended follow-up. Trans Ophthalmol Soc UK 1985;104:887–892.
14. Schachat A, Beauchamp G, et al. Retinal detachment: Preferred practice pattern. San Francisco: American Academy of Ophthalmology, 1990.
15. Benson WE, Morse PH, et al. Late complications following cryotherapy of lattice degeneration. Am J Ophthalmol 1977;84:514–516.

Horseshoe or Linear Retinal Tear

A horseshoe (flap) tear or linear retinal tear is the result of vitreous traction to an area of thinned or atrophic retina (Figure 5-12). It frequently affects areas of the retina that suffer from lattice degeneration. As the vitreous separates from the retina and undergoes collapse, tractional forces are applied to areas of firm vitreoretinal adherence. If traction is sufficient, it may tear a flap of retina, leaving the anterior margin continuous with the peripheral retina. Often the tear stops at the posterior margin of the base because the vitreous base is firmly attached and retinal tears usually cannot progress through it (see Figure 4-12). However, the tear may stop short of reaching the posterior margin of the vitreous base, which is likely due to a decrease in the tractional force of the vitreous strands as the vitreous base collapses centrally. Like releasing tension on a rubber band, the less the band is stretched, the less pulling there is along its length.

As the vitreous moves forward, the flap assumes an elongated triangular shape with the apex pointing toward the posterior pole and the base of the triangle attached to the anterior margin of the break (Figures 3-1 and 5-13), much like the way wallpaper tears when one edge is grabbed with a pair of pliers. In the posterior pole, tears do not always proceed in a strict anterior direction and may have other directional orientations (Figure 5-14A, C). The attached vitreous show up as translucent strands, which may be seen more easily on scleral depression or during eye movement. Eye movement causes the vitreous strands to move, making them more apparent against the fundus background. Sometimes strands of retinal tissue can be seen bridging the break from the flap to the edge of a new tear.

One study found that 10% of breaks were horseshoe tears.[1] Davis[2] discovered that 39% of 183 asymptomatic breaks were flap tears (six had multiple tears), one of which developed a subsequent retinal detachment. Byer[3] found that 16% (30) of 113 patients with asymptomatic breaks had flap tears. Most studies have found flap tears occurring at the lower range of these percentages. Flap tears are usually less than 0.5 disc diameter.[1] Flap and operculated tears are more commonly seen in older patients, probably because of the importance of PVD in the formation of these breaks. PVD is more commonly found in eyes with flap tears or operculated tears (even if asymptomatic) than in eyes with atrophic holes.[1, 2] A horseshoe tear usually forms in a rather sudden episode over hours, days, or weeks rather than being a slowly progressive process and this is likely due to a PVD. Neither eye and neither gender is more likely to have of these tears.

Horseshoe and linear tears occur more often in the peripheral retina due to vitreous traction being more tangential in this region of the retina, which is the result of the anterior displacement of the detached vitreous. The posterior detached vitreous is anchored or hinged at the vitreous base, so the more anterior the detached vitreous, the more tangential the tractional force applied to an area of increased vitreoretinal adhesion. In comparison, when the PVD is just separating from the posterior retina, the tractional force is more anterior-posterior in nature. Movement of the flap on eye movements is common, especially if the vitreous remains attached to the flap. Rarely, vitreous traction is so strong or retinal tissue is so weak that the flap may be torn into and display a bifid appearance. Also rarely, the flap may tear free of its anterior anchorage on the break and appear as a large operculum over the break (avulsed flap).[4–6] I have seen one retinal hole in the flap of a horseshoe tear; this was probably the result of the hole occurring in an area of retinal degeneration with increased vitreoretinal adhesion. The edges of the tear become smooth and rounded with time due to degeneration and contraction.

Sometimes it is helpful to perform scleral depression to detect a subtle tear because it causes a

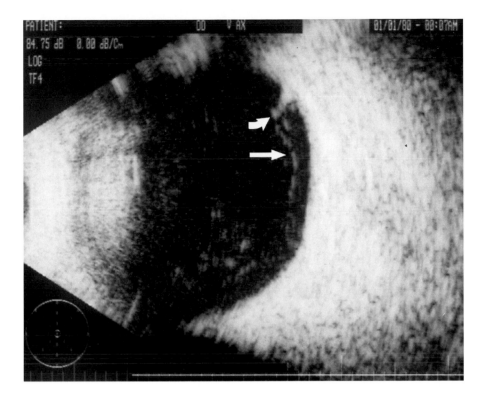

FIGURE 5-12
B-scan ultrasonogram of a vitreous strand (*straight arrow*) attached to a superior flap retinal tear (*curved arrow*).

whitening of the degenerative retinal tissue around the tear (white-with-pressure) and enhances the visible edges of the tear and the elevation of the flap. A three-mirror contact lens and precorneal 90-diopter fundus lens can be used to evaluate the lesion with a higher degree of magnification. Either lens may be used with doctor-assisted scleral depression to detect microscopic flap tears.

The break itself appears red due to the loss of retinal tissue that normally mutes the choroidal reflex; however, in a detached retina it is pink, clear, or light gray. A fresh flap appears whitish because of ischemic edema and subsequent degeneration resulting from loss of circulation to the outer retinal layers and sometimes to the inner retinal layers from the choriocapillaris and the retinal circulation, respectively. A long-standing flap is both thin and transparent due to atrophy of the retinal layers (outer greater than inner). Rarely, flap tears are very difficult to detect, the lower contrast of tear to fundus background making this much more common in blonde fundi. Premonitory symptoms are photopsia (light flashes), numerous recent floaters (vitreous bleed), and a progressive loss of peripheral vision if a retinal detachment is produced.

Over time, the flap shrinks (as little as one-fifth the size of the break and sometimes even smaller) as the tissue degenerates with subsequent contraction

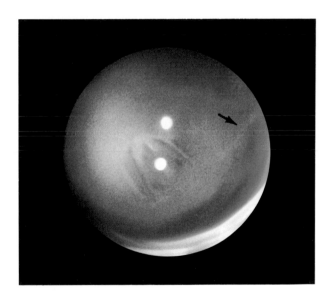

FIGURE 5-13
Horseshoe retinal tear in a retinal detachment seen through the indirect condensing lens. Note the retinal hemorrhage on either side of the base of the flap, the whitish color of the detached retina, and the loss of choroidal pattern beneath the detachment. The retinal tear stopped its anterior progress at the posterior border of the vitreous base, which is seen as a faint white line on the detached retina (*arrow*).

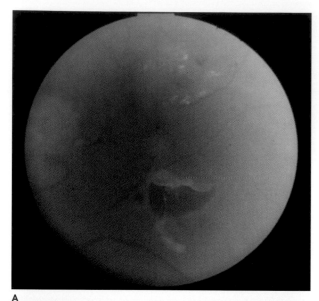

A

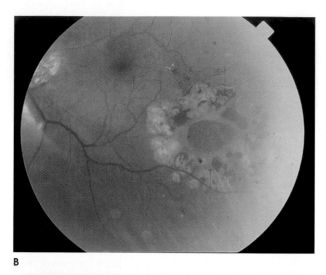

B

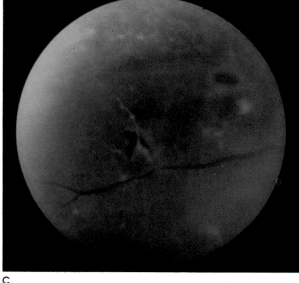

C

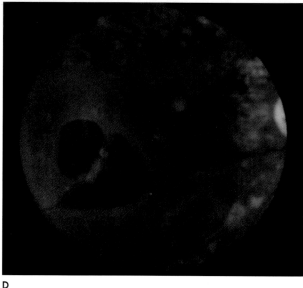

D

FIGURE 5-14

A. Flap retinal tear inferotemporal to the macula (left eye). The tear was produced by a posterior vitreous detachment; the vitreal strand is still attached to the flap. Three retinal hemorrhages at one edge of the retinal break are the result of a ruptured vessel caused by the retinal tear. This diabetic patient also shows dot hemorrhages and waxy exudates. B. Old argon laser retinopexy spots now can be seen around the break, and the flap is no longer detectable because of contraction of the surrounding retina after treatment. Note how close the tear was to the macula (above and nasal to the break). C. Persistent vitreous traction caused a flap tear on the retinal detachment months after the original rhegmatogenous detachment was found (same patient as in Figure 5-11). Note the same operculated tear in the upper right region of the retinal detachment and the newly formed flap tear with a vitreous strand extending from the tip of the flap to the overlying vitreous. The barrage of argon laser spots around the detachment were applied in an attempt to halt its progression. D. Continued vitreous traction on the flap tear enlarged the original break so that it does not resemble the initial tear. A retinal vessel is bridging the tear, which may lead to a vitreous bleed.

(Figures 3-1 and 5-15). Sometimes the retinal flap takes unusual shapes, like an hourglass or a J; this is often the result of a retinal blood vessel coursing over the flap. The retinal blood vessel gives more structural support, so there is less tissue contraction where the vessel is located on the flap. On high mag-

nification, a long-standing flap displays cystoid degeneration and has a honeycomb appearance.

Horseshoe or linear tears can be located in any part of the peripheral retina, but they may be more frequently found in the superior half of the retina. Superior tears did not progress to retinal detachment any more frequently than inferior tears.[2] Horseshoe and operculated tears most commonly occur at the posterior border of the vitreous base, in areas of lattice degeneration (see Figure 3-78), or in pigment clumps, cystic retinal tufts (see Figure 3-38), or an invisible area of vitreoretinal adhesions. These tears are sometimes associated with a chorioretinal scar. Because the tears may be associated with pigment clumping, there may be pigment on the flap, usually near the apex, which is the site of firm vitreoretinal adhesion. Flap tears frequently appear at the vitreous base,[5] where there is a sharp or irregular posterior margin; this is due to vitreous forces being applied to a small retinal area rather than to broad expanses with no posterior projections. There is some evidence to suggest that intrabasal tears pose a low risk of developing a clinical retinal detachment.[7] Blunt trauma can cause a rapid expansion of the equatorial region of the globe,[8] producing severe traction on the vitreous base and resulting in a linear tear along the posterior vitreous base.[9] The differential diagnosis of flap tears, operculated tears, atrophic holes, and retinal tears is found in Table 5-1.

Histopathology

The histopathology of a horseshoe or linear tear is similar to that of an operculated tear. It is characterized by a loss of the retinal layers, with organized vitreous strands often remaining attached to the border of the flap. There may be gliosis and degeneration adjacent to the margins of the tear and a combination of cell breakdown and hyperplasia in the underlying pigment epithelium[10] (Figure 5-16).

Clinical Significance

Horseshoe or linear tears are the leading cause of rhegmatogenous retinal detachment. Asymptomatic horseshoe tear has a 25–90% chance of progressing to a retinal detachment,[1, 2, 11–13] with most of the reports being closer to the low percentages. Even asymptomatic flap tears with associated subretinal fluid (localized detachment) have a 40% chance of progressing to retinal detachment, but in the absence of subretinal fluid in asymptomatic flap tears, only 10% progressed to retinal detachment.[2] One study of 42 patients with retinal detachments found that 7 of the phakic fellow eyes with flap tears developed a detachment.[14] Most authorities agree that the small peripheral tears that cause most detachments long after cataract surgery are produced by chronic vitreous traction at the vitreous base rather than by an acute PVD.[7] The frequency of

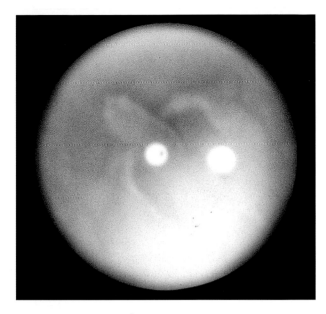

FIGURE 5-15
A large tear with a narrow flap seen during scleral depression through the indirect condensing lens in the superotemporal fundus. The shadow at the far end of the tear denotes the shallow, detached edge of the posterior region of the tear on the posterior aspect of the scleral roll. Note the pigment clump close to the end of the flap.

these tears increases with age, suggesting that they are degenerative in nature.

Retinal tears are commonly associated with a PVD. Sometimes there is a small localized retinal detachment around the edges of the flap tear that may be stable for months to years (Figures 5-17 and 5-18). It would seem reasonable that the localized detachment occurred at the time of the tear formation and then remained stable with little to no progression. A likely scenario is that a flap tear occurs from marked vitreous traction on the retinal surface, which initially results in a tenting of the retina (small, purely tractional localized detachment). With further traction, a progressive zippering tear in the central area of detached retina occurs anteriorly. Afterward, the break in the localized retinal detachment allows for the ingress of fluid, which effectively inhibits the cuff of detached retina from reattaching. The result is a small localized detachment along the edges of the tear that remains stable for a considerable period of time. Another possible explanation is that during the physical process of tearing, the retina adjacent to the tear also pulls away, leading to the formation of a localized detachment. Yet another possibility is that continued traction on the anterior edge of the break is transmitted along the margins of the tear in a posterior direction, which leads to the formation of a

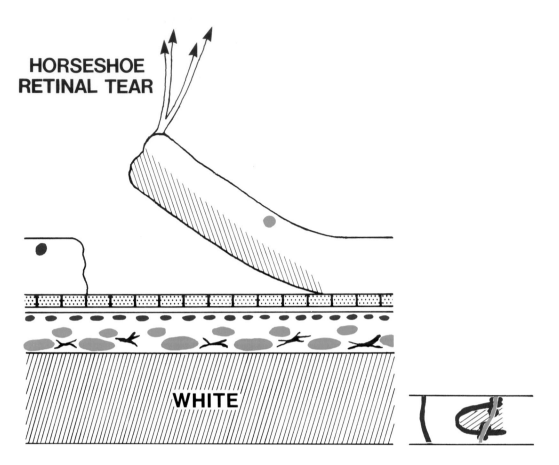

FIGURE 5-16
Flap retinal tear with vitreous traction. The shearing of a retinal venule has resulted in vitreous and retinal hemorrhage. The flap appears whitish due to degeneration from the loss of apposition to the choriocapillaris. The flap is a little smaller than the break due to degeneration and contraction, which is also responsible for the rounded edges of the break.

localized detachment. Or, it may be that after the tear, the fluid from the vitreous cavity effectively separates the sensory retina from the pigment epithelium. It seems logical, however, that if it were so easy to separate the retina around the break, the break would easily continue on to a clinically significant retinal detachment.

One of these explanations may account for localized retinal detachments, or the cause may be a combination of these processes. A lack of significant vitreous traction or reduced ability of the intravitreal fluid to enter the break may result in a localized detachment, but if significant traction remains around the break, then it is possible to create a clinically significant detachment. The first two explanations would help to explain why some flap tears after a PVD do not produce a clinically significant detachment, for the localized detachment occurred at the time of the tearing process and little or no vitreous traction forces remained to advance the detachment.

Therefore, continued tractional forces applied to the flap greatly increase the chance of a retinal detachment.[3, 5] During eye movements, there is considerable action of detached vitreous. The most likely scenario is that the vitreous traction pulls on the flap and starts to separate the sensory retina from the pigment epithelium around the anterior margin of the break. Once the retina is separated, fluid from the vitreal cavity can leak in and keep the photoreceptors apart from the pigment epithelium. This vicious cycle continues, and a clinically significant detachment may ensue. The best way of evaluating the presence of vitreous traction and quantifying the magnitude of the traction is currently not known.[15] Of 10 eyes followed without treatment, 40% (4 eyes) developed a clinically significant detachment. Large flap tears may develop lateral tears at the base of the tear due to continued traction on the flap. With time, the lateral tears may enlarge into a giant tear and detachment, which is more difficult to repair due to the size of the break. Therefore, horseshoe tears are more likely to present with a subclinical retinal detachment. Of 71 eyes with one or more such tears, 13 had an associated subclinical detachment.[2]

Vitreous hemorrhage is a frequent concomitant finding and is the result of tearing of a retinal vessel that is incorporated in the tear. Retinal detachments caused by a flap or operculated tear often have an associated vitreous bleed[4] (see Figures 4-15 and 4-16). (See Vitreous Hemorrhage, Chapter 4.) Because retinal vessels that approach the ora serrata turn and travel parallel to the ora, they are sometimes involved in a flap tear in the far periphery. The vitreous hemorrhage is responsible for the symptoms of the sudden onset of numerous tiny black floaters moving across the patient's visual field. The existence of a retinal vessel bridging the retinal break of the tear (from the flap to the surrounding retina) greatly enhances the chances of a vitreous bleed and possible rebleeds.[16] This is due to the continued traction on the vessel by the vitreous, which can produce

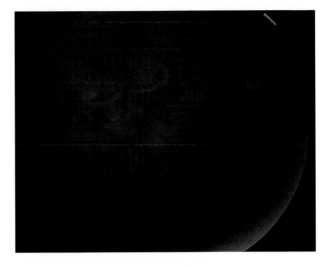

FIGURE 5-17
An asymptomatic bilobed flap tear along a retinal vessel with a light gray localized surrounding retinal detachment. The tear is in the midperiphery as seen through a fundus camera.

tugging sufficient to rupture the vessel. Some authors believe that, due to the increased risk of a vitreous hemorrhage from a bridging blood vessel, it is necessary to treat the eye with photocoagulation or scleral buckling.[5, 17] Others believe that a bridging blood vessel may result in a vitreous bleed with or

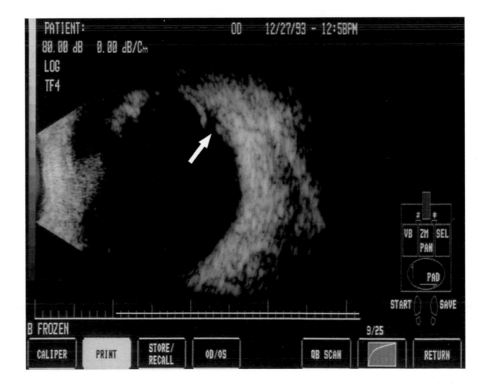

FIGURE 5-18
B-scan ultrasonogram of a superior flap tear with a localized surrounding retinal detachment (*arrow*).

without treatment.[18, 19] Some authors actually suggest that the bridging vessel itself be treated.[20]

Asymptomatic flap tears have a low propensity to progress to a retinal detachment and therefore can usually be followed without treatment, especially if the vitreous traction has been freed from the involved area.[3, 13, 21–23] In a study by Davis,[2] of 222 eyes followed for 10 years, 58 had asymptomatic flap tears, 11 (two aphakic) developed a retinal detachment, and two of these were subclinical detachments with no further progression during follow-up periods of 6 and 3 years. The period between diagnosis and time of progression was 6 months to 9 years. Of the remaining 46 eyes with asymptomatic horseshoe tears without retinal detachment, one eye developed a detachment over the study period, but five of the eyes developed additional breaks. However, symptomatic tears in patients with aphakia, pseudophakia, high myopia, or vitreoretinal degeneration and in those who are active in contact sports or have a personal or family history of retinal detachment should be referred to a retinal specialist for retinopexy treatment consideration. Asymptomatic flap tears in high myopes, aphakes, and pseudophakes are sometimes treated,[20] but several studies have stated that asymptomatic round holes and tears in myopes and aphakes can be followed without treatment, unless the breaks are large or posteriorly located.[13, 20, 24, 25] Some believe that tears in aphakes or pseudophakes should be treated, especially if the tears are large or posteriorly located.[13, 24–27] Flap tears in asymptomatic fellow eyes of patients with a retinal detachment are frequently treated. Eyes with asymptomatic flap tears being considered for cataract surgery should have treatment due to the increased risk of retinal detachment formation after such surgery.[20] In reality, flap and linear tears look dangerous and intimidating; therefore, most clinicians refer such cases to a retinal specialist.

Symptomatic tears with or without subretinal fluid (localized detachment) should be referred to a retinal specialist for retinopexy treatment due to the high risk of developing a retinal detachment. Symptomatic flap tears are frequently treated.[20] Studies have found that 25–90% of these types of tears have resulted in a retinal detachment, with most reports falling between 25% and 55%.[2, 12, 13, 28, 29] In one study, all eyes with a fresh symptomatic horseshoe tear that progressed to a retinal detachment did so within 6 weeks, which indicates how much risk is involved in these types of tears. If such a tear extends beyond this 6-week period, then the risk of a retinal detachment decreases to a lower value of 30–50%.[2]

The prophylactic treatment of a symptomatic tear decreases the chance of a subsequent retinal detachment to approximately 0–19%,[12, 29, 30–37] and it is more commonly stated at the lower percentages. Therefore, treatment is well justified.[2] It is important to be sure that treatment is well applied anterior to the break all the way to the ora serrata, because the most common cause of a subsequent retinal detachment is inadequate treatment anterior to the flap tear.[18, 31, 38] Continued traction may cause the tear to extend anteriorly, thus allowing fluid to reach the subretinal space, giving rise to a detachment. Cryotherapy is preferred for anterior breaks because it is easy to treat peripheral retina as far anterior as the ora serrata. The finding of horseshoe tears in the fellow eye of a patient with a fresh rhegmatogenous detachment more likely indicates the chronicity of the condition rather than an earlier stage of development; this is a factor in determining the need for prophylactic treatment of that eye.[2] The patient should be told that the risk in treatment outweighs the nontreatment risk of a possible retinal detachment. It is important to involve the patient in the decision process of whether or not to treat retinal breaks, for it makes for a patient who is more relaxed and cooperative.[6]

The prognosis for symptomatic horseshoe or linear tears is guarded because of the high probability of progression to retinal detachment. After prophylactic treatment, most eye doctors see the patient in 1 week and again in 3–6 weeks; even in patients with successful treatment, follow-up examinations every 6 months to 1 year are essential.[20] From 2.1% to 7% of such patients develop additional breaks, 95% of the breaks occurring in the first 3 months, and the chance of a subsequent retinal detachment is 1.8–6.2%.[29, 39] Sometimes a significant amount of subretinal fluid may accumulate beneath a tear and prevent the formation of an adequate chorioretinal scar, so these need to be followed closely at first to determine the established of a firm adhesion.[20] Patients with untreated asymptomatic horseshoe or linear retinal tears who decline referral for consideration of treatment should have routine eye examinations every 6 months. Any patient, treated or untreated, who develops such symptoms as photopsia, new floaters, or visual field loss should be told to return immediately.

References

1. Byer NE. Clinical study of retinal breaks. Trans Am Acad Ophthalmol Otolaryngol 1967;71:461–472.

2. Davis MD. Natural history of retinal breaks without detachment. Arch Ophthalmol 1974;92:183–194.

3. Byer NE. Prognosis of asymptomatic retinal breaks. Arch Ophthalmol 1974;92:208–210.

4. Benson WE. Retinal Detachment: Diagnosis and Management (2nd ed). Philadelphia: Lippincott, 1988.

5. Straatsma BR, Foos RY, et al. Degenerative Diseases of the Peripheral Retina. In TD Duane, EA Jaeger (eds), Clinical Ophthalmology: Vol. 3. Philadelphia: Harper & Row, 1993: 1–30.

6. Lewis H, Kreiger AE. Rhegmatogenous Retinal Detachment. In TD Duane, EA Jaeger (eds), Clinical Ophthalmology. Vol. 3. Philadelphia: Harper & Row, 1993:1–12.

7. Sigelman J. Vitreous base classification of retinal tears: Clinical application. Surv Ophthalmol 1980;25:59–74.

8. Weidenthal DT, Schepens CL. Peripheral fundus changes associated with ocular contusion. Am J Ophthalmol 1966;62:465–477.

9. Cox MS, Schepens CL, et al. Retinal detachment due to ocular contusion. Arch Ophthalmol 1966;76:678–685.

10. Spencer LM, Straatsma RA, et al. Tractional Degenerations of the Peripheral Retina. New Orleans Academy of Ophthalmology: Symposium of the Retina and Retinal Surgery. St. Louis: Mosby, 1969.

11. Straatsma BR, Zeegen PD, et al. Lattice degeneration of the retina. Trans Am Acad Ophthalmol Otolaryngol 1974; 78:87–113.

12. Colyear BIIJ, Pischell DK. Preventative treatment of retinal detachment by means of light coagulation. Trans Pac Coast Otolaryngol Ophthalmol Soc 1960;41:193–217.

13. Neumann E, Hyams S. Conservative management of retinal breaks. A follow-up study of subsequent retinal detachment. Br J Ophthalmol 1972;56:482–486.

14. Davis MD, Segal PP, et al. The Natural Course Followed by the Fellow Eye in Patients with Rhegmatogenous Retinal Detachment. In RC Pruett, CDJ Regan (eds), Retina Congress. New York: Appleton-Century-Crofts, 1972; 643–660.

15. Sebag J. Vitreous Pathology. In W Tasman, EA Jaeger (eds), Clinical Ophthalmology. Vol. 3. Philadelphia: Harper & Row, 1992;1–26.

16. Robertson DM, Norton EWD. Long-term follow-up of treated retinal breaks. Am J Ophthalmol 1973;75:395–404.

17. Theodossiadis GP, Koutsandrea Ch N. Avulsed retinal vessels with and without retinal breaks—treatment and extended follow-up. Trans Ophthalmol Soc UK 1985; 104:887–892.

18. de Bustros S, Welsch RB. The avulsed retinal vessel syndrome and its variants. Ophthalmology 1984;91:86–88.

19. Robertson DM, Curtin VT, et al. Avulsed retinal vessels with retinal breaks: A cause of recurrent vitreous hemorrhage. Arch Ophthalmol 1971;85:669–672.

20. Schachat A, Beauchamp G, et al. Retinal Detachment: Preferred Practice Pattern. San Francisco: American Academy of Ophthalmology, 1990.

21. Hirose T. Acquired Retinoschisis: Observations and Treatment. In RC Pruett, CDJ Regan (eds), Retina Congress. New York: Appleton-Century-Crofts, 1972;489–504.

22. Byer NE. The natural history of asymptomatic retinal breaks. Ophthalmology 1982;89:1033–1039.

23. Hyams SW, Meir E, et al. Chorioretinal lesions predisposing to retinal detachment. Am J Ophthalmol 1974;78: 429–437.

24. Friedman Z, Neumann E, et al. Vitreous and peripheral retina in aphakia. Br J Ophthalmol 1973;57:52–57.

25. Hyams SW, Neumann E, et al. Myopia–aphakia. II. Vitreous and peripheral retina. Br J Ophthalmol 1975; 59:483–485.

26. McPherson A, O'Malley R, et al. Management of the fellow eyes of patients with rhegmatogenous retinal detachment. Ophthalmology 1981;88:922–934.

27. Benson WE, Grand MG, et al. Aphakic retinal detachment. Arch Ophthalmol 1975;93:245–249.

28. Colyear BH, Pischel DK. Clinical tears in the retina without detachment. Am J Ophthalmol 1956;41:773–792.

29. Michels RG, Wilkinson CP, et al. Retinal Detachment: Diagnosis and Management. St. Louis: Mosby, 1990.

30. Morse PH, Sheie HG. Prophylactic cryoretinopexy of retinal breaks. Arch Ophthalmol 1974;92:204–207.

31. Robertson DM, Norton EWD. Long-term follow-up of treated retinal breaks. Am J Ophthalmol 1973;75:395–404.

32. Chignell AH, Shilling J. Prophylaxis of retinal detachment. Br J Ophthalmol 1973;57:291–298.

33. Nadel AJ, Gieser RG. The treatment of acute horseshoe retinal tears by transconjunctival cryopexy. Ann Ophthalmol 1975;7:1568–1574.

34. Pollak A, Oliver M. Argon laser photocoagulation of symptomatic flap tears and retinal breaks of fellow eyes. Br J Ophthalmol 1981;65:469–472.

35. Sollner F. Über die prophylaktische Behandlung der Ablatio retinae durch Lichtcoagulation. Bericht Deutsche Ophthalmologische Gesellschaft 1965;66:327–336.

36. Tasman W, Jaegers KR. A retrospective study of xenon photocoagulation and cryotherapy in the treatment of retinal breaks. In RC Pruett, CDJ Regan (eds), Retina Congress. New York: Appleton-Century-Crofts, 1972;557–564.

37. Meyer-Schwickerath G, Fried M. Prophylaxis of retinal detachment. Trans Ophthalmol Soc UK 1980;100:56–65.

38. Benson WE, Morse PH, et al. Late complications following cryotherapy of lattice degeneration. Am J Ophthalmol 1977;84:514–516.

39. Goldberg RE, Boyer DS. Sequential retinal breaks following a spontaneous initial retinal break. Ophthalmology 1981;88:10–12.

Retinal Dialysis

Retinal dialysis (disinsertion) was first described by Leber[1] in the 1800s, but it was Anderson[2] who coined the term *dialysis*, *dia* meaning "apart" and *lysis* meaning "dissolution." A retinal dialysis is a retinal tear that occurs at the ora serrata and is concentric with the ora (Figure 5-19). Most tears are less than 90 degrees, and they may occur bilaterally in 4% of the cases.[3] Often the choroidal pattern becomes more visible in the area of the dialysis due to the loss of overlying retinal tissue. If the edge of the dialysis remains close to the underlying choroid, the break may not be discovered until scleral depression is performed. The condition is often asymptomatic. In a true dialysis, the posterior border of the vitreous base coincides with the ora serrata. If the posterior border lies slightly posterior to the ora serrata, a skirt of retinal tissue remains attached to the ora (Figures 5-19 and 5-20). Both

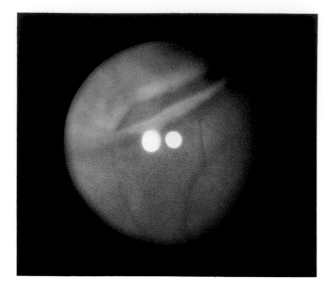

FIGURE 5-19
Superior edge of post-traumatic retinal dialysis in the superior nasal fundus seen through the indirect condensing lens during scleral depression. There is a small rim of detached retinal tissue just posterior to the ora serrata, followed by the dialysis, which allows a view of the choroid. There is another small rim of detached retina on the posterior aspect of the dialysis.

types are usually regarded as retinal ora dialyses,[4] but some consider the latter a retinal tear instead of a true dialysis. Also, because a true retinal dialysis is thought to be caused by separation of the retina from the ora serrata, dentate processes may pull away and remain attached to the torn edge of the retina.[5] As the vitreous contracts, the tears become more elevated in conjunction with increasing retinal detachment. The edge of the dialysis is more scalloped in appearance nasally and smoother temporally due to the anatomic structure of these regions of the ora serrata. Retinal dialyses are usually asymptomatic, unless a clinically significant retinal detachment develops.[6]

The nontraumatic spontaneous dialysis of the young is usually located inferotemporal and is characteristically asymptomatic. The location of the nontraumatic forms suggest a developmental abnormality of the inferotemporal retina and vitreous base region.[7-11] A traumatic retinal dialysis is formed by a contusion blow producing an anterior-posterior compression of the globe, which results in a sudden equatorial expansion; thus, marked traction of the vitreous base area may result in a dialysis.[12] Traumatic retinal dialyses are more commonly found superonasal and are unilateral[3, 13-16]; however, a blow to the eye from an angle to the temporal limbus can result in an inferior, temporal dialysis.[17] Males are more frequently affected than females, probably because males have a higher inci-

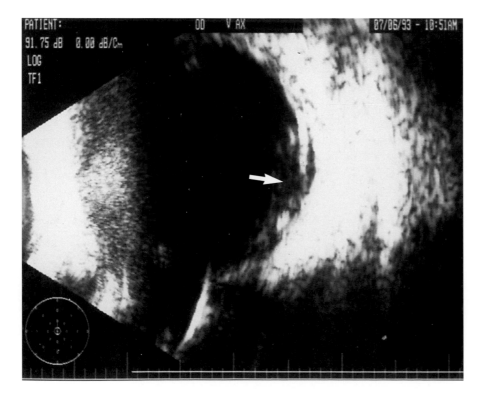

FIGURE 5-20
B-scan ultrasonogram of a recent retinal dialysis with associated vitreous hemorrhage from a torn retinal blood vessel. Arrow indicates the retinal dialysis. Note retinal detachment posterior to the break.

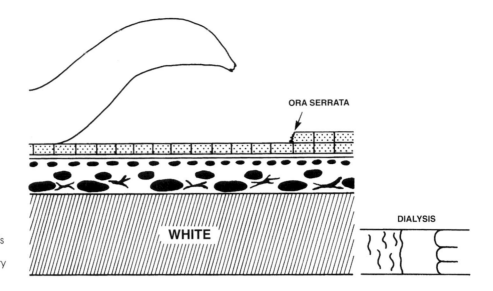

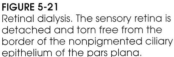

FIGURE 5-21
Retinal dialysis. The sensory retina is detached and torn free from the border of the nonpigmented ciliary epithelium of the pars plana.

dence of ocular trauma. Traumatic retinal dialyses probably occur at the time of the trauma and are most likely the result of equatorial scleral stretching. In patients with a traumatic hyphema, 4–18% of the eyes had either a tear along the posterior vitreous base or a dialysis as soon as the blood absorbed, but no additional breaks were found on follow-up examinations.[18, 19]

Risk factors for a retinal dialysis are family history (especially for the idiopathic form), recent or past trauma, and a more minor association with refractive error, pseudophakia, and various retinal degenerations. A retinal dialysis may be associated with proliferative vitreoretinopathy, proliferative retinal vasculopathies, or chorioretinal inflammatory disease (especially pars planitis).[20]

Histopathology

The retina is separated at or just posterior to the ora serrata (Figure 5-21).[2, 9] The retina itself may appear normal or dysplastic. The overlying vitreous is usually normal in appearance, without liquefaction.

Clinical Significance

A retinal dialysis often progresses to a retinal detachment, and generally the patient is asymptomatic until the macular area becomes involved. The retinal detachment caused by the nontraumatic form is usually slowly progressive and is often associated with multiple demarcation lines.[21, 22] Males are affected more than females, and the bilaterality of this condition stands in marked contrast to traumatic retinal dialyses.

Post-traumatic dialysis may be associated with vitreous hemorrhage (see Figure 5-20) and other stigmata of eye trauma. A traumatic dialysis may not be visible initially due to the presence of retinal or vitreal hemorrhage or retinal edema. Sometimes the trauma induces a chorioretinal inflammation at the site of the dialysis. The inflammation produces a scar and prevents formation of a retinal detachment. The retinal detachment associated with a traumatic dialysis is deceptive in that it often occurs weeks to months after the trauma (> 8 months in at least half of cases).[23] It is often asymptomatic and may be associated with a disinsertion of the vitreous base (vitreous base avulsion). The vitreous usually remains attached to the torn retina and thus, the posterior edge of a dialysis does not tend to form a roll, as is commonly seen in giant retinal tears.[22] The continued vitreous traction can cause the edge of the torn retina to become very elevated. One should suspect a retinal dialysis if the retinal detachment extends onto the pars plana.

The risk of a retinal detachment from a dialysis is reported to be approximately 20%.[24, 25] Retinal dialyses are found in 75–84% of traumatic retinal detachments.[26] Because vitreous detachment is not commonly associated with a dialysis or resultant detachment, photopsia is usually not a symptom in these patients. However, given that these types of detachment are often chronic, it is not unusual to have an anterior chamber reaction or to find cellular debris in the anterior vitreous, which may be inflammatory products, blood, or pigment cells (tobacco dust).[3] The detachment is slowly progressive and is often characterized by successive demarcation lines, which are found in 50% of the cases.[3, 27] Due to the chronicity of these detachments, intra-retinal cysts (macrocysts) are present in 20% of the involved eyes.[3] Shallow macular detachments may be associated with dialysis or detachment; these may be misdiagnosed as idiopathic central choroidopathy. Intraocular pressure may be elevated in eyes with a retinal dialysis, likely secondary to anterior chamber angle recession.[14] Other retinal breaks, chorioretinal atrophy, or chorioretinal scars may appear in these eyes.[28]

A post-traumatic retinal dialysis that is greater than 15 degrees in length, located above the horizontal, or is found in an aphakic eye should be evaluated for treatment.[29] Some authorities say that they should always be treated.[5] Treatment of a retinal dialysis is scleral buckling with cryopexy.[30] The treatment should extend all the way to the ora serrata to completely seal each end of the break.[5] The prognosis is generally favorable for surgical reattachment[3] unless a giant tear develops.

References

1. Leber. Über die Entstehung der Netzhautablosung. Berl Vers Ophthal 1882;14:18.
2. Anderson JR. Anterior dialysis of the retina: Disinsertion or avulsion at the ora serrata. Br J Ophthalmol 1932;16:641–670, 705–727.
3. Hagler HS, North AW. Retinal dialyses and retinal detachment. Arch Ophthalmol 1968;79:376–388.
4. Schepens CL. Retinal Detachment and Allied Diseases. Philadelphia: Saunders, 1983;90–91, 188.
5. Lean JS. Diagnosis and Treatment of Peripheral Retinal Lesions. In WR Freeman (ed), Practical Atlas of Retinal Disease and Therapy. New York: Raven, 1993;211–220.
6. Davis MD. Natural history of retinal breaks without detachment. Arch Ophthalmol 1974;92:183–194.
7. Brown GC, Tasman WS. Familial retinal dialysis. Can J Ophthalmol 1980;15:193–195.
8. Kinyoun JL, Knobloch WH. Idiopathic retinal dialysis. Retina 1984;4:9–14.
9. Smiddy WE, Green WR. Retinal dialysis: Pathology and pathogenesis. Retina 1982;94–116.
10. Verdaguer TJ. Juvenile retinal detachment. Am J Ophthalmol 1982;93:145–156.
11. Verdaguer TJ, Rojas B, et al. Genetical studies in nontraumatic retinal dialyses. Mod Probl Ophthalmol 1975;15:34–39.
12. Schepens CL. Traumatic Retinal Detachment. Clinical and Experimental Study. In New Orleans Academy of Ophthalmology: Symposium on Retina and Retinal Surgery. St. Louis: Mosby, 1969;302–318.
13. Syrdalen R. Trauma and retinal detachment. Acta Ophthalmol Scand Suppl 1970;48:1006–1022.
14. Zion VM, Burton TC. Retinal dialysis. Arch Ophthalmol 1974;98:1971–1974.
15. Straatsma BR, Foos RY, et al. Degenerative Diseases of the Peripheral Retina. In TD Duane, EA Jaeger (eds), Clinical Ophthalmology. Philadelphia: Harper & Row, 1980;26:1–30.
16. Freeman HM, Cox MS, et al. Traumatic retinal detachments. Int Ophthalmol Clin 1974;14:151–170.
17. Weidenthal DT, Schepens CL. Peripheral fundus changes associated with ocular contusion. Am J Ophthalmol 1966;62:465–477.
18. Sellors PJ, Mooney D. Fundus changes after traumatic hyphaema. Br J Ophthalmol 1973;57:600–607.
19. Tasman W. Peripheral retinal changes following blunt trauma. Trans Am Ophthalmol Soc 1972;70:190–198.
20. Cavallerano AA. Retinal dialysis. Photoabstracts. Clin Eye Vision Care 1994;6:88–91.
21. Dobbie JG, Phillips CI. Detachment of ora serrata and pars ciliaris retinae in "idiopathic" retinal detachment. Arch Ophthalmol 1973;68:610–614.
22. Hagler WS. Retinal dialysis: A statistical and genetic study to determine pathogenic factors. Trans Am Ophthalmol Soc 1980;78:886–907.
23. Cox MS, Schepens CL, et al. Retinal detachment due to ocular contusion. Arch Ophthalmol 1966;76:678–685.
24. Straatsma BR, Allen RA. Lattice degeneration of the retina. Trans Am Acad Ophthalmol Otolaryngol 1962;66:600–613.
25. Byer NE. The natural history of the retinopathies of retinal detachment and preventive treatment. Isr J Med Sci 1972;8:1417–1420.
26. Ross WH. Traumatic retinal dialyses. Arch Ophthalmol 1981;99:1371–1374.
27. Benson, WE, Pornsawat N, et al. Characteristics and prognosis of retinal detachments with demarcation lines. Am J Ophthalmol 1978;84:641–644.
28. Schepens CL. Pathogenesis of Traumatic Rhegmatogenous Retinal Detachment. In H Freeman (ed), Ocular Trauma. New York: Appleton-Century-Crofts, 1979;273–284.
29. Lewis H, Kreiger AE. Rhegmatogenous Retinal Detachment. In TD Duane, EA Jaeger (eds), Clinical Ophthalmology. Vol. 3. Philadelphia: Harper & Row, 1980;1–27.
30. Cooling RJ. Traumatic retinal detachment—Mechanisms and management. Trans Ophthalmol Soc UK 1986;105:575–581.

Giant Retinal Tear

Giant retinal tears are an extreme form of retinal dialysis involving more than 90 degrees in circumferential length. They are thought to favor the posterior margin of the vitreous base (Figure 5-22). An important feature of a giant tear is the mobility of the posterior flap, which makes surgical repair such a challenge.[1] One report states that 70% are idiopathic, 20% traumatic, and 10% occur in an area of chorioretinal degeneration.[2] Other reports estimate that ocular trauma is responsible for 25% of cases.[3–5] It occurs four times as often in males as females and most often in young males.[6] Giant retinal tears occur more often in younger patients on average than does the spontaneous form.[7] Myopia, especially over 8 diopters, is a major associated finding. The risk of bilaterality of giant retinal tears is reported to be as high as 75%, and sometimes the fellow eye has extensive lattice degeneration but often appears normal in the periphery.[8] Even giant retinal tears have been the result of PVD.[9] The tears are usually inferotemporal or superonasal, probably because of the greater exposure of the inferotemporal region to trauma and the effect of equatorial expansion from blunt trauma.[7, 10] Tears from penetrating trauma generally tend to be superior in location. There is often a latent period from the time of the trauma to the diagnosis of the tear.[7] This latent period is greater with penetrating trauma, which may result from secondary or delayed vitreous detachment associated with vitreous basal gel incarceration.[11] Giant tears tend to be rapidly symptomatic. The anterior edge of the detaching retina is folded over by vitreous traction. There is extensive liquefaction and collapse of the vitreous, except for anterior adherence to the rolled edge of the torn retina. The retinal detachment frequently progresses, folding over on itself like a taco shell (Figure 5-23). A giant tear may involve 360 degrees.

Idiopathic giant tears often occur along the posterior edge of white-with-pressure. Giant tears may occur along the edge of extensive areas of lattice degeneration or along areas of the retina that have been overtreated with cryotherapy or photocoagulation. They may also occur from a PVD and can be associated with congenital colobomas of the lens and zonules.[12]

Histopathology

The histopathology is similar to that found in retinal dialyses but more extensive (see section on Retinal Dialysis).

Clinical Significance

Giant retinal tears have a poor prognosis due to their tendency to increase in size from both ends. Immediate surgical intervention is indicated to limit their progression. Surgical correction involves vitrectomy, which is required to separate the vitreous traction from the rolled edge of the tear. Scleral buckling in conjunction with vitrectomy, internal fluid gas exchange, expanding gases, low-viscosity liquid fluorochemicals, silicone injection, sodium hyaluronate injection, trans-scleral suturing, retinal incarceration, and retinal tacks has improved the overall prognosis.[3, 4, 13–28] Silicone oil is best removed after reattachment for optical reasons and long-term complications.[29] Heavier-than-water vitreous substitutes can be used to unroll and flatten the retina, even in cases where PVR is present.[26, 30, 31] Placing the patient in a prone posi-

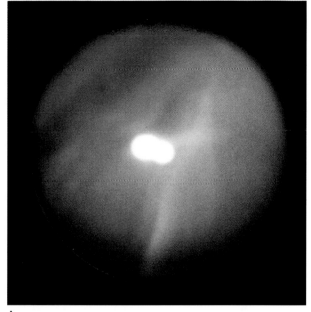

A

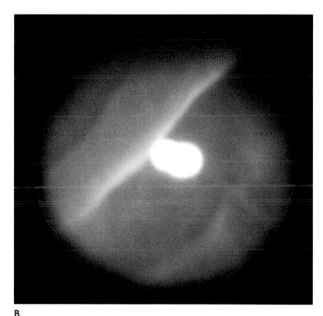

B

FIGURE 5-22
Giant retinal tear extending from 7:00 o'clock to 10:30 in the temporal retina in an aphakic right eye. A. Superior end. B. Midpoint of the break.

tion both operatively and postoperatively is required to unfold and maintain the retina in apposition to the pigment epithelium.[32–34] Sometimes a posterior retinotomy is necessary to aspirate the subretinal fluid to enhance reattachment.[3, 20] Most

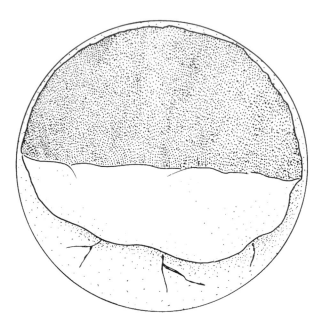

FIGURE 5-23
Diagram of a giant retinal tear of the superior half of the peripheral retina. Note that the flap has folded over on itself to form a "taco shell" appearance.

giant retinal tears without PVR can be managed without scleral buckling.[4, 26, 35] Proliferative vitreoretinopathy is a common postoperative complication.[4] Another common postoperative complication is glaucoma (at least 32% of cases).[3, 7, 36] Glaucoma may be due to the damage to the drainage angle or to the frequent occurrence of aphakia, with its known risk of glaucoma.[29, 37]

Previous successful reattachment of giant tears varied from 5% to 50%, and in cases where the tear was greater than 180 degrees, the success rate ranged from 11% to 25%.[4, 5, 33] Newer surgical techniques are achieving higher repair rates (43–97%).[3, 7, 17, 18, 21, 26, 30, 38–40] The inability to unfold the detached retina accounts for half of the failures in surgical treatments.[4] The success rate for reattachment and visual acuity outcome for giant tears due to penetrating trauma is less than that for blunt trauma or those of a spontaneous origin.[7] One study found that 42% of patients with a giant retinal tear in one eye developed a subsequent retinal detachment in the fellow eye.[5] Therefore, circumferential retinopexy to the follow eye may be considered,[41] although such intensive treatment may lead to chronic iritis, cataract, fixed and dilated pupil, and macular pucker.[42]

References

1. Scott JD. Giant tear of the retina. Trans Ophthalmol Soc UK 1975;95:142–144.
2. Schepens CL. Retinal Detachment and Allied Diseases. Philadelphia: Saunders, 1983;520–549.
3. Leaver PK, Cooling RJ, et al. Vitrectomy and fluid/silicone oil exchange for giant retinal tears: Results at six months. Br J Ophthalmol 1984;64:432–438.
4. Norton EWB, Aaberg TA, et al. Giant retinal tears. I. Clinical management with intravitreal air. Am J Ophthalmol 1969;68:1011–1021.
5. Kanski JJ. Giant retinal tears. Am J Ophthalmol 1975; 79:846–852.
6. Goffstein R, Burton TC. Differentiating traumatic from nontraumatic retinal detachment. Ophthalmology 1982; 89:361–368.
7. Aylward GW, Cooling RJ, et al. Trauma-induced retinal detachment associated with giant retinal tears. Retina 1993;13:136–141.
8. Lean JS. Diagnosis and Treatment of Peripheral Retinal Lesions. In WR Freeman (ed), Practical Atlas of Retinal Disease and Therapy. New York: Raven, 1993;12:211–220.
9. Jaffe NS. Vitreous Detachments. In The Vitreous in Clinical Ophthalmology. Vol. 3. St. Louis: Mosby, 1969;83–98.
10. Weidenthal DT, Schepens CL. Peripheral fundus changes associated with ocular contusion. Am J Ophthalmol 1966;62:465–477.
11. McLeod D. Giant retinal tears after central vitrectomy. Br J Ophthalmol 1985;69:96–98.
12. Hovland KR, Schepens CL, et al. Developmental giant tears associated with lens coloboma. Arch Ophthalmol 1968;80:325–331.
13. Freeman HM, Schepens CL, et al. Current management of giant retinal breaks. II. Trans Am Acad Ophthalmol Otolaryngol 1970;74:59–74.
14. Michels RG, Rice TA, et al. Surgical techniques for selected giant retinal tears. Retina 1983;3:139–153.
15. Darmakusuma IE, Glaser BM, et al. The use of perfluorooctane in the management of giant retinal tears without proliferative vitreoretinopathy. Retina 1994;14:323–328.
16. Brown GC, Benson WE. Use of sodium hyaluronate for the repair of giant retina tears. Arch Ophthalmol 1989;107: 1246–1249.
17. Machemer R, Allen AW. Retinal tears 180 degrees and greater: Management with vitrectomy and intravitreal gas. Arch Ophthalmol 1976;94:1340–1346.
18. Vidaurri-Leal J, Debustros S, et al. Surgical treatment of giant retinal tears with inverted posterior retinal flaps. Am J Ophthalmol 1984;98:464–466.
19. Billington BM, Leaver PK. Vitrectomy and fluid/silicone-oil exchange for giant retinal tears: Results at 18 months. Graefes Arch Clin Exp Ophthalmol 1986;224:7–10.
20. Glaser BM. Treatment of giant retinal tears combined with proliferative vitreoretinopathy. Ophthalmology 1986;93: 1193–1197.
21. Chang S. Low viscosity liquid fluorochemicals in vitreous surgery. Am J Ophthalmol 1987;103:38–43.
22. Federman JL, Shakin JL, et al. The microsurgical management of giant retinal tears with transscleral retinal sutures. Ophthalmology 1982;89:832–839.
23. Peyman GA, Redman KRV, et al. Retinal microincarceration with penetrating diathermy in the management of giant retinal tears. Arch Ophthalmol 1984;102:562–565.
24. Ando F, Kondo J, et al. Surgical techniques for giant reti-

nal tears with retinal tacks. Ophthalmic Surg 1986;17: 408–411.

25. The Retina Society Terminology Committee. The classification of retinal detachment with proliferative vitreoretinopathy. Ophthalmology 1983;90:121–125.

26. Chang S, Lincoff H, et al. Giant retinal tears: Surgical techniques and results using perfluorocarbon liquids. Arch Ophthalmol 1989;107:761–766.

27. Mester U, Rothe R, et al. Use of high-density silicone oil for giant retinal tears. Ophthalmic Res 1986;18:81–86.

28. Chung H, Acosta J, et al. Use of high-density fluorosilicone oil in open-sky vitrectomy. Retina 1987;7:180–182.

29. Franks WA, Leaver PK. Removal of silicone oil: Rewards and penalties. Eye 1991;5:333–337.

30. Lewis JS, McQuen BW II, et al. Current views on giant retinal tears. Pakistan J Ophthalmol 1985;1:215–221.

31. Glaser BM, Carter JB, et al. Perfluorooctane in the treatment of giant retinal tears with proliferative vitreoretinopathy. Ophthalmology 1991;98:1613–1621.

32. Schepens CL, Dobbie JG, et al. Retinal detachments with giant breaks. Preliminary report. Trans Am Acad Ophthalmol Otolaryngol 1962;66:471–479.

33. Schepens, CL, Freeman HM. Current management of giant retinal breaks. Trans Am Acad Ophthalmol Otolaryngol 1967;71:474–487.

34. Michels RG. Vitreous Surgery. St. Louis: Mosby, 1981;250–255.

35. Hoffman ME, Sorr EM. Management of giant retinal tears without scleral buckling. Retina 1986;6:197–204.

36. Lucke K, Laqua H. Silicone Oil in the Treatment of Complicated Retinal Detachment: Techniques, Results and Complications. Heidelberg: Springer-Verlag, 1990.

37. Leaver PK, Billington BM. Vitrectomy and fluid/silicone-oil exchange for giant retinal tears: 5 years follow-up. Graefes Arch Clin Exp Ophthalmol 1989;227:323–327.

38. Freeman HM, Castillejos ME. Current management of giant retinal breaks: Results with vitrectomy and total air fluid exchange in 95 cases. Trans Am Ophthalmol Soc 1981;79:89–102.

39. Charles S. Giant Breaks: Vitreous Microsurgery. Baltimore: Williams & Wilkins, 1987;172–181.

40. Zivojnovic R, Mertens DAE, et al. Das flussige silicon in der amotiochirurge. II. Berich uber 280 falle: Weitere entwichlung der technik. Klin Monatsbl Augenheilkd 1982;181:444–452.

41. Govan JAA. Prophylactic circumferential cryopexy: a retrospective study of 106 eyes. Br J Ophthalmol 1981;65: 364–370.

42. Benson WE. Retinal Detachment. Diagnosis and Management (2nd ed). Philadelphia: Lippincott, 1988.

Chapter 6

Retinal Detachment

A retinal detachment is characterized by a separation of the sensory retina from the retinal pigment epithelium (RPE) (Figure 6-1). Many factors keep the retina in place, and they must be overcome before a retinal detachment can develop. Because the majority of people with a retinal break do not develop a subsequent detachment, the factors keeping the retina on are significant. Between the photoreceptors and the RPE is a material that stains with the properties of an acid mucopolysaccharide. This material serves as a medium for metabolic exchange and acts as a weak-bond "biological glue" between the photoreceptors and the RPE.[1] This bond may be broken by liquefied vitreous (a fluid that is not very viscous and contains hyaluronic acid) percolating through a retinal break or by tractional forces from the vitreous. This bond may be solely or partially responsible for the occurrence of retinal breaks without a significant retinal detachment or a localized detachment (see Figures 3-38, 5-2, 5-9, and 5-14A).

The physical interaction between the apical RPE microvilli and the outer segments of the photoreceptors is important in retinal adhesion.[2] Experimental studies found that RPE cell sheaths play a role in maintaining the retina in position. A cone matrix sheath has been discovered, having a cylinder shape and surrounding the apical ends of the pigment epithelial microvilli and the outer segment of the cones. This matrix serves as a physical bridge between the two structures and therefore helps to keep the two from separating.[3] Electron micrographs have shown that these sheaths are composed of actin-containing material and that they are in close apposition to the outer segments.[4–6] The molecular bridge that exists between the cone matrix and the RPE and cone photoreceptors is composed of insoluble glycoconjugates. The glycoconjugates that comprise the interphotoreceptor matrix are composed mainly of a group of chondroitin sulfate-rich proteoglycans that are distributed heterogeneously into the rod- and cone-associated domains, called the cone and rod matrix sheaths.[7–13] It is believed that these glycoconjugates may mediate the attachment between the retina and the RPE.[14–20]

Chondroitin sulfate proteoglycans have adhesive properties in other tissues.[21–24] In rabbits it was found that mechanical peeling of the retina from the underlying pigment epithelium was reduced after death, which would indicate that there is some active force that keeps the retina in place.[25, 26] The adhesive properties seem to be located between the outer layer segments and the RPE sheaths because when there is mechanical peeling of retina, there is stretching of the RPE sheaths in vivo but not in vitro.[26] It has been found that if mechanical peeling of the retina is done within 2 minutes after death, the cone matrix sheath glycoconjugates become very elongated during retinal peeling.[14, 27] This would indicate that the cone matrix is important in maintaining a tight but flexible adhesion between the RPE and the photoreceptors that allows some degree of mechanical stress capability. During retinal separation the distal tips of the cone matrix may be found still embedded in the microvilli of the RPE, which attests to the strong binding ability of this material.[27] It may be that a change in oxygen tension or other changes in the environment of the space between the RPE and photoreceptors results in a weakening of the cone matrix bonds, which may facilitate a retinal detachment.

Hydrostatic pressure from the vitreous may be helpful in maintaining the retina in position. The highly rich protein content of the choroid produces an osmotic pressure gradient that draws fluid from the subretinal space toward the choroid.[28–30] Because the retina is the barrier that prohibits fluid in the vitreous from diffusing to the choroid,[31] the vitreous pressure holds the retina against the choroid and therefore keeps it in place.[28, 32] The adhesive force also seems dependent on the ionic environ-

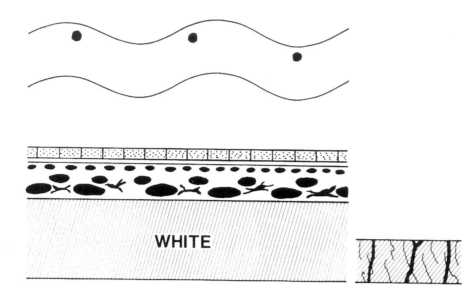

FIGURE 6-1
Retinal detachment shows the sensory retina detached from the pigment epithelium and retinal folds. The separation of the sensory retina from the choriocapillaris, which is the blood supply for the outer retinal layers, will lead to marked degeneration of the outer retinal layers with time.

ment of the space between the RPE and the photoreceptors, and a greatly lowered pH or the loss of extracellular calcium and magnesium markedly reduce the adhesive forces.[33, 34] Thus, it would appear that ionic transport across the RPE is important in maintaining the ionic environment and removal of water in the subretinal space.[29, 35, 36] There is also some question of the effects of the oxygen supply to this anatomic area and that the lack of it may play a role in retinal adhesion.[35] All these mechanisms have some degree (more or less individually) to maintain the physical attachment of the RPE to the photoreceptors and ultimately the attachment of the retina.[8, 16] A breakdown of these mechanisms may be involved in the production of a retinal detachment.

Intraocular pressure (IOP) is believed to be partially responsible for keeping the retina in position.[37] When the vitreous cortex is over a retinal break it may prevent a detachment by not allowing the liquefied vitreous into the break.[38] Also, as the vitreous degenerates with age, it loses its shock-absorbing qualities, and so retinal detachments are more likely to occur. For a retinal detachment to form, all the forces that are used to keep the retina in place have to be overcome by developmental and acquired forces trying to separate the retina. It would appear that vitreous traction is probably the most important force in causing the sensory retina to separate from the pigment epithelium. To maintain the detachment, however, it is also necessary for fluid from the vitreous cavity to gain access through a retinal break to the subretinal space made by separating sensory retina.

Retinal detachments may be detected in the office with the use of many ophthalmic devices, including ophthalmoscopes, biomicroscope with special lenses, ultrasonography, and visual fields. The ophthalmoscopes include the binocular indirect ophthalmoscope, the monocular indirect ophthalmoscope, and the direct ophthalmoscope. The binocular indirect ophthalmoscope with applied scleral depression is the most commonly used instrument for the detection of detachments. The biomicroscope with special fundus lenses can also be used to detect retinal detachments; these lenses are the ultra–wide field contact lenses and precorneal condensing lenses (the 90-diopter being the most popular). The ultra–wide field lenses are almost as useful in detecting a detachment as the binocular indirect ophthalmoscope. If a view of the fundus is not possible due to corneal or vitreous hazy, lens opacification, or other reasons, ultrasonography may enable the clinician to determine if a detachment is present. On occasion, a screening visual field (either confrontation or formal) may discover a visual field loss caused by a detachment.

Symptoms

The signs of a retinal detachment are initially related to vitreous traction on the retina. Light flashes (photopsia) are the result of mechanical traction on the retinal tissue that physically stimulates the photoreceptors. Because the retina has no pain receptors, the only sensory response in the peripheral retina to vitreous traction is photopsia. Vitreous floaters may suddenly appear, possibly the result of blood in the vitreous from a tear of a retinal vessel during the formation of the break (see Figures 4-15, 4-16, and 4-18), or they may appear secondary to a posterior vitreous detachment (PVD) alone (see Posterior Vitreous Detachment and Vitreous Hemorrhage, Chapter 4).

As the retina detaches, the patient experiences a veil or curtain gradually migrating into the visual field from the periphery. As the detachment progresses, more and more vision is lost. A macular detachment results in the loss of central vision. With a total retinal detachment, all useful vision is lost and the patient is usually left with light perception or blindness. The total absence of pain with a progressive retinal detachment is the most insidious aspect of this condition. With normal vision in the fellow eye, it is understandable why many patients are unappreciative of their profound visual loss until they occlude their normal eye.

Clinical Signs

The clinical appearance of a retinal detachment is that of a bullous elevation of whitish, diaphanous (transparent) retina into the vitreous cavity (see Figures 3-79, 3-80, 6-2, 6-13, 6-15, and 6-16). The elevation is most apparent when viewed with the binocular indirect ophthalmoscope, precorneal con-

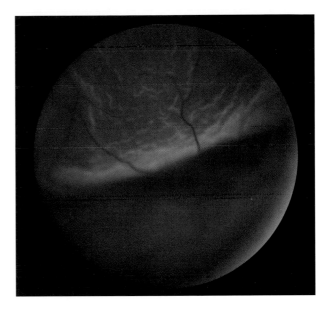

FIGURE 6-2
Large bullous rhegmatogenous retinal detachment in the superior fundus. The detachment looks whitish and displays numerous folds. The detachment hangs down like a curtain in front of the visual axis and thus results in poor vision. After the patient lay down for an hour, the acuity improved to 20/20. The detachment undulated on eye movements.

densing lenses with the biomicroscope, ultra–wide field lenses, and other contact lenses used with the biomicroscope. Elevation of a retinal detachment can be easily seen on ultrasonography (Figures 6-3,

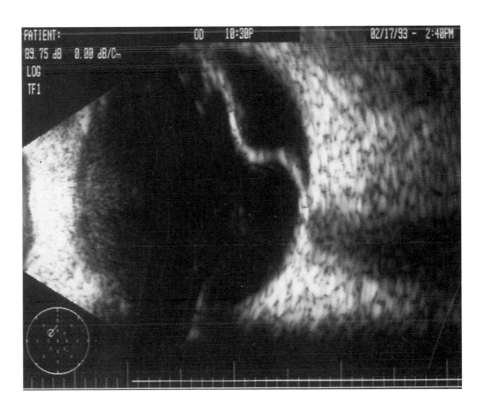

FIGURE 6-3
B-scan ultrasonography of a superior bullous rhegmatogenous retinal detachment. The retinal tear is barely discernible just posterior to the attachment of the retina at the ora serrata, and the posterior detachment is attached to the edge of the optic nerve.

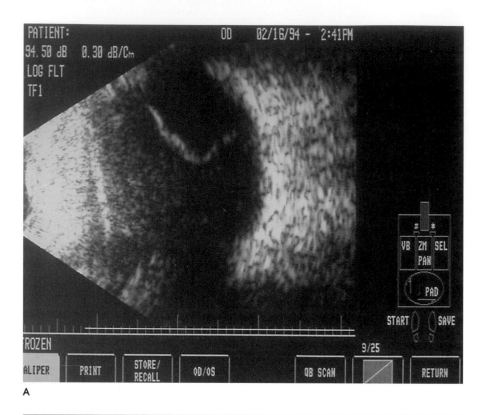

A

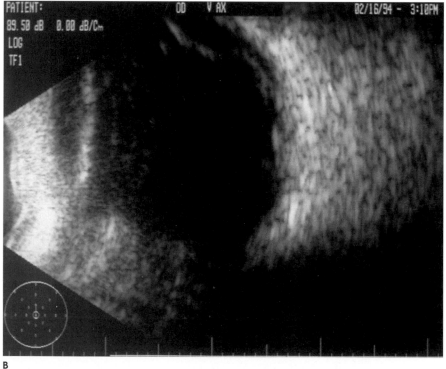

B

FIGURE 6-4
A. B-scan ultrasonogram of a bullous retinal detachment. B. Same detachment after the patient lay down for 15 minutes.

6-4, and 6-6B). Detection of the detached retina is made easier by noting the retinal vessels, which are sometimes more obvious than the semitransparent retina. A fresh retinal detachment appears whitish due to the oblique angle of illumination produced by the bullous detachment and due to ischemic edema of the outer sensory retinal layers after loss of nutritional supply from the choriocapillaris. The retinal blood vessels appear dark and tortuous on the whitish detached retina.

Another hint that the retina is detached is the loss of detail in the underlying choroid pattern (see Figures 3-78, 3-79, 3-80, 5-14C, 6-5 and 6-14). Choroidal detail is lost when fluid accumulates between the retina and the underlying choroid, and the higher the fluid level the greater the loss of underlying detail. The detached retina forms folds, either small (indicating a shallow detachment) or large (bullous detachment) (Table 6-1). The folds are due to the fact the detached retina is longer than the chord distance across the vitreous cavity, causing the folds to develop in the free-floating retina.

In some cases, detached retina in the far periphery is markedly thinner than the posterior retina, which can be seen in some patients as a zone of 360 degrees of peripheral, lighter-appearing fundus. When these patients have a retinal detachment, this very thin peripheral retina can just barely be seen (even with the fundus mirror or precorneal fundus lens) (see Figure 6-6A) and so resembles a retinal dialysis. The transparency of the peripheral retina in a detachment is also due to the finding that it is not white and edematous, as is the posterior retina. But if there is a retinal break in the thin retina, it is more easily identified. The thinner peripheral retina can be demonstrated on ultrasonography (see Figure 6-6B).

A shallow retinal detachment is more difficult to detect because it is low in elevation, it has less obvious folds, the detachment more closely approximates the curvature of the inner eye wall, and the detached retina has far less movement during eye movements (see Figures 5-11, 5-14C, 6-4B, 6-7, 6-12, and 6-14). However, even a shallow detachment results in a loss of underlying choroidal detail, a phenomenon that is often responsible for its detection. Ultrasonography can easily detect shallow detachments. Scleral depression allows a view that enhances a slight retinal elevation, and depression of a shallow detachment places the detachment on a cross-sectional view during the dynamic rolling process, which may allow the area above the roll to take on a "fogbank" appearance. The fogbank phenomenon is very suggestive of a shallow retinal detachment or shallow retinoschisis (see Figure 3-64). Scleral depression also causes the shallow detachment to become more opaque when seen from an oblique angle, and indentation may cause small parallel folds in the detached retina. In addition, the retinal vessels may cast a shadow on the underlying choroid,

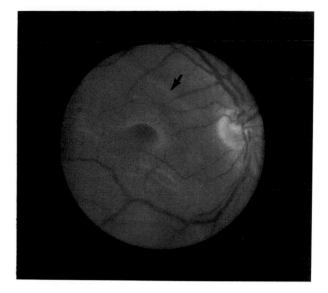

FIGURE 6-5
Shallow rhegmatogenous retinal detachment extending from the inferior ora serrata to a line just superior to the macula (*arrow*). The macula is detached and has a distinctive hazy, dimpled appearance. Note the folds in the retina, whitish appearance, and loss of choroidal detail.

which gives the appearance of a double vessel traveling through the involved area (see Figures 6-7 and 6-8 and Table 6-1). Small retinal breaks in shallow detachments are more difficult to see, but their detection can be enhanced by applying scleral depression.

With a large amount of subretinal fluid, the bullous detachment may appear as an undulating (wavelike) membrane on eye movement. If there is no such undulation, one should suspect that the lesion may be a retinoschisis rather than a retinal detachment. However, a long-standing detachment mimics a retinoschisis, and there is little if any movement of such a detachment (see Long-Standing Retinal Detachment in this chapter).

A careful evaluation should be made of the retinal detachment with binocular indirect ophthalmoscopy with or without scleral depression, or with contact fundus lenses or precorneal lenses with the biomicroscope, to locate and identify all the retinal breaks associated with the detachment. These breaks are usually found in the far periphery of the retina. They frequently occur in areas of lattice degeneration (see Figures 3-78 through 3-80) or in hyperpigmented areas (pigment clumps) that are the locus of firm vitreoretinal adhesions. Old chorioretinal scars should also be carefully examined for

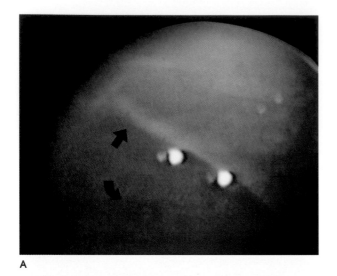

A

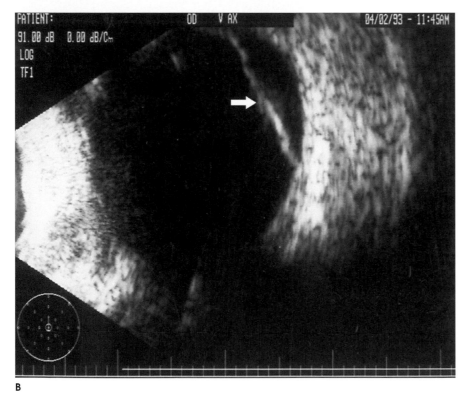

B

FIGURE 6-6
A. A retinal detachment with a very thin peripheral retina that fails to become edematous like the posterior thicker retina (arrow indicates transition zone). This gives the peripheral fundus a transparent appearance, as if a retinal dialysis had occurred. The small round lesion in the thin peripheral retina is an operculated tear (*curved arrow*), which caused the detachment. B. B-scan of retina showing the marked thinner peripheral retina (arrow indicates transition area).

retinal breaks that occur at the edges of the scar. If no retinal break is found, a nonrhegmatogenous retinal detachment must be suspected. Because the detached retina is elevated above the choroid, light reflected from the choroid may retroilluminate a retinal tear. During the retinal examination, therefore, the clinician may detect the fleeting glimpse of a small orange glow indicating the location of the break. The transillumination glow is seen only when the reflected light from the choroid or sclera is just right, so it may be very difficult to make it

reappear. The discovery of small breaks can be a very laborious task, sometimes taking an hour or two of ophthalmoscopy with and without scleral depression, three-mirror contact lens, 90-diopter precorneal condensing lens, or ultra–wide field contact lens. Small breaks may be located in folds in the detachment, and this may make their discovery very difficult. The finding of pigment in the detached retina indicates previous areas of pigment clumping due to isolated vitreous traction. Such pigmented areas are likely to be the location of retinal breaks. All areas of pigment clumping should be located on the retinal drawing. The discovery of small retinal breaks may be complicated by the clarity of the intraocular view. Peripheral cataracts may haze the view of the peripheral retina and make it hard to see small peripheral breaks. Pseudophakic eyes may have obscuration of the peripheral retina due to posterior capsular fibrosis, cortical remnants, optical distortions caused by the edge of the intraocular lens, and a small pupil.[39] Another difficulty in observing the retina is vitreous haze, either from vitreous hemorrhaging, vitreous degeneration, and opacification. Even after finding a retinal break, the clinician must be careful to proceed with the retinal examination to determine if other breaks are present. It must be kept in mind that the major reason for the production of a rhegmatogenous detachment is vitreous traction and that scleral depression reduces transvitreal vitreous traction by foreshortening the diameter of the globe; therefore, scleral depression does not exacerbate the tear or detachment.

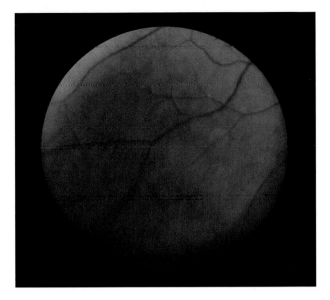

FIGURE 6-7
Shallow retinal detachment in periphery demonstrating the double vessel effect, which is caused by a retinal vessel on the detachment casting a shadow on the underlying pigment epithelium and choroid.

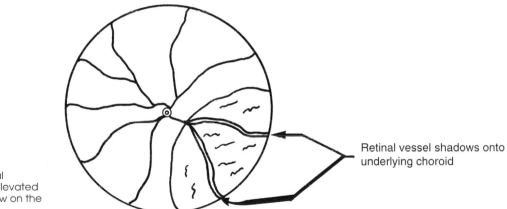

FIGURE 6-8
Diagram of a shallow retinal detachment in which the elevated retinal vessels cast a shadow on the underlying choroid.

Retinal vessel shadows onto underlying choroid

Table 6-1. Shallow vs. Bullous Retinal Detachment

Shallow retinal detachment	Bullous retinal detachment
Not elevated very much	Very elevated
Whitish in color if recent	White in color if recent
May have a few small retinal folds if recent	Usually has many large retinal folds of varying size if recent
Mild to moderate loss of underlying choroidal detail	Marked loss of choroidal detail
Retinal vessels may cast shadow onto underlying choroid	No shadow of retinal vessels
Slight to moderate undulations seen on eye movements if recent	Usually marked undulations on eye movements if recent
May demonstrate only a moderate visual acuity loss in involved area if recent	Marked visual acuity loss in involved area
Scleral depression may demonstrate "fog banking" on the scleral roll as the shallow detachment is seen on cross section	No "fog banking" on scleral depression

In case of a vitreous bleed, the fresh blood is usually found spread out close to the location of the tear that caused the hemorrhage, but in time the blood gravitates inferiorly in the retro-hyaloidal space and allows a good view of the retina, except for the inferior region. To facilitate the inferior gravitation of the blood, the patient is instructed to go home and maintain an upright body posture as much as possible (such as sitting to watch television, which has the added benefit of requiring less eye movement), sleep with the head elevated approximately 45 degrees (two pillows), limit activities that may jar the head, and not bend over to a low head position. In severe cases, the patient may be hospitalized and have bilateral ocular patching to obtain greater gravitational effects on the blood in a shorter time span. Generally, within only a few days to a week most of the blood will be located in the inferior fundus, but if a rebleed occurs, then persistent obscuration of the fundus will occur. The patient is examined every 1–2 days to determine the quality of the fundus view and to find a reason for the bleed. When the vitreous hemorrhage markedly decreases visualization of the fundus, ultrasonography may be used in an attempt to find a retinal detachment or a large retinal tear.

Pathologic Mechanisms

The pathologic mechanisms for the production of a retinal detachment vary from developmental factors found in myopia and Marfan's syndrome that change the overall size of the globe; vitreoretinal maldevelopments, such as coloboma; retinal vascular disease, such as sickle cell disease and forms of vasculitis; metabolic diseases, such as diabetes; inflammation, such as acute retinal necrosis; neoplasms, such as metastatic choroidal tumors; degenerations, such as lattice degeneration; and trauma, both blunt and perforating. There has also been a report of a retinal detachment secondary to an anterior staphyloma.[40–43]

In general, retinal detachments assume three basic shapes: lateral detachments that extend into the superotemporal or nasal quadrants, superior detachments that cross the vertical meridian and progress down both sides, and inferior detachments.[44] Location is thought to be somewhat important in the progression of a detachment. A superiorly located detachment is more likely to progress because gravity helps facilitate downward movement of the subretinal fluid; the opposite is true of a detachment

located in the inferior region of the fundus. A retinal detachment found in the superotemporal quadrant of the fundus is more hazardous to the visual status of the patient because its downward movement can easily result in macular involvement. A superonasal detachment is not as visually threatening, however, because the optic disc acts as an obstruction to macular involvement. The speed at which a retinal detachment progresses toward the posterior pole depends on the amount of vitreous traction, the number and size of the breaks, their distance from the posterior pole, and the degree of preretinal organization. A detachment from equatorial breaks usually involves the posterior pole sooner than one from oral breaks.

The first report of retinal detachment associated with atopic dermatitis was made by Balyeat[45] in 1937, and numerous other reports have followed.[46–53] Retinal detachments have been found in patients with atopic dermatitis, the disease is found in about 3–10% of the population.[54–56] Retinal detachment has been considered fairly rare, and retinal tears have been found to cause the detachment in up to 97% of cases.[57–59] The retinal tears are usually located near the vitreous base (up to 82.5%)[49–53] and rarely in the pars plicata,[53, 60–62] with one report of 16.3%.[52] Recently, however, crescent-shaped tears in the equatorial region[63–65] and retinal dialysis have been reported.[63, 66] The etiology of retinal detachment has been thought to be associated with retinal edema secondary to allergy or vascular abnormalities.[59, 67] Some think that inflammation of the peripheral retina is the cause,[48, 68] which is consistent with the clinical finding of cells and flare found in the anterior chamber of patients with this condition. Cells in the anterior chamber of patients with a retinal detachment are photoreceptors outer segments.[69] Some believe that the detachment may be caused by chronic eye rubbing due to the severe itching associated with this dermatitis.[51, 63, 70]

Incidence

The incidence of phakic nontraumatic retinal detachment in the general population is reported to be about 1 to 5 in 10,000 per year or 0.005% to 0.05%.[71–78] The inclusion of traumatic retinal detachment only slightly increases this percentage. The incidence of retinal breaks in the general population is reported to be about 3.3%.[79] Therefore, the difference in incidence between retinal breaks and detachment indicates that the chances of developing a phakic nontraumatic retinal detachment from most breaks is fairly low at 1:330. Rhegmatogenous retinal detachments are found bilaterally in about 10–15% of cases and occur in 16% of aphakic cases.[80–83] The time from the first detachment to the fellow eye detachment was 5 years in 71% of the cases, and it was simultaneous 18% of the time. In bilateral cases there was at least one predisposing factor in 85% and two or more factors in 53% of cases.[82]

Retinal detachments can occur at any age, but as age increases, so does the frequency of detachments.[71, 76, 84] They are most likely to occur between the ages of 40 and 70,[85] with an average age of about 55.[86] The average age for males is 53–57 and for females is 51–62.[76, 83] The prevalence of detachment in patients older than 40 years is 0.14%.[87] Only 3–4% of retinal detachments occur in people under age 16.[88] Retinal detachments in general are more commonly found in males than females (61% vs. 39%)[85, 89–91]; however, some have reported that nontraumatic retinal detachments are more common in females (65.1%) than males (55.7%),[92] and some report no difference.[83] Retinal detachments are less frequent in blacks, even though they have the same incidence of PVD.[85, 93–95]

Associated Conditions

The most common conditions associated with retinal detachments are myopia (40–55%), aphakia (23–40%), and ocular trauma (10–20%).[83, 85, 89, 96] In one 4-year study, other conditions that predispose to retinal detachments included lattice degeneration (21%), granular tufts (7%), retinal tears (5%), and retinoschisis (6%).[97]

Myopia

High myopia (>8 diopters or >24 mm in axial length) is another risk factor,[80, 92, 98] with a reported incidence of 0.7–6.0%.[96, 98–101] One study found that people with myopia over 5 diopters who live to be 60 years of age had a lifetime risk of developing retinal detachment of 2.4% as compared to the emmetropes who reached age 60 with a risk of 0.06%.[71, 102] Also, patients with over 8 diopters of myopia have about 10% of all retinal detachments but are only 1% of the general population.[71, 103] Myopes account for about 42% of all retinal detachments[103] but represent only about 10% of the population.[71] All myopic patients who undergo cataract surgery are at risk. However, two separate studies showed that even myopes with asymptomatic breaks were unlikely to progress to a retinal detachment,[104, 105] and therefore most do not

need to be treated.[106] It has been determined that the equatorial dimension and the axial length are important risk factors in myopes developing detachments. Biometric studies have found an increase in the occurrence of retinal detachments in eyes with a greater equatorial diameter as compared to eyes without retinal detachment, and this was true for emmetropic and myopic eyes.[107] Patients with high myopia develop retinal detachments due to premature vitreous syneresis,[108–110] greater incidence of PVD,[111–115] lattice degeneration, and thinning of the anterior region of retina. Incidence of retinal detachment is increased in high-myopic patients undergoing clear lens extraction to correct the axial refractive error[116–118] and has been reported to be in 7.3% of patients.[119] The detachments in one study occurred on average 2 years and 3 months after surgery.[120] It is fairly common to treat these patients with prophylactic photocoagulation or cryotherapy to prevent subsequent detachments,[121–124] but this prophylactic treatment does not prevent the future development of retinal detachment.[125, 126] Often, retinal breaks occur along the posterior border of the circumferential band of photocoagulation.[120] It has been postulated that with large posterior lacunae, an unusually rigid thin layer of vitreous cortex that forms the wall of the lacuna is a factor in the development of holes and breaks in highly myopic eyes.[127, 128]

Aphakia and Pseudophakia

Aphakia also leads to a greater risk of a nontraumatic rhegmatogenous detachment. The incidence of phakic and aphakic nontraumatic retinal detachment has been reported to be about 11.0 per 100,000 per year, 6.1 for nontraumatic phakic, 4.9 for nontraumatic aphakic, 1.0 for traumatic phakic, and 0.4 for traumatic aphakic.[14] Patients with aphakia have an incidence of 1–5% (half of which occur in the first year after surgery),[89, 129–131] and presumably this is secondary to PVD, which frequently occurs during this period of time.[88, 89, 105, 130, 132–134] Whereas only about 2.9% of the older population have had cataract surgery, approximately 40% of patients with a retinal detachment have had prior cataract extraction.[135, 136] The rate of retinal detachment after the surgical loss of vitreous is reported to increase significantly, to around 7%.[137, 138] Compared to the general population, aphakes are 15.7 times more likely to develop a detachment.[113] Aphakes who are high myopes have a 6–8% chance of developing a detachment,[139–141] and in one study of myopes over 10 diopters, the chance increases to about 40%.[142] Studies have found that patients with pathologic myopia who have cataract surgery develop retinal detachments at an earlier age.[140, 143, 144] Aphakic as compared to phakic detachments are more often total (38% vs. 20%), the macula is more often detached (83% vs. 65%), and fixed retinal folds (a possible early sign of proliferative vitreoretinopathy) are present.[103] No retinal breaks are found in 7–16% of aphakic detachments, as compared to phakic detachments, where no breaks are found in 2–11.6% of cases.[83, 103, 129, 145] In patients with a previous history of retinal detachment, an increased risk of redetaching after cataract removal has been reported.[146] Aphakic detachments progress rapidly, and the time of detachment is rather close to the time of the break.[89] Over half of the detachments in aphakia occur in the first year after cataract surgery, with an additional 10–20% occurring over 2 years.[131, 147]

Often, in aphakes the retinal breaks are small and located close to the ora serrata.[129] The increased prevalence of detachments in aphakes is caused by the removal of the crystalline lens, which allows the vitreous to have a greater degree of mobility and a greater incidence of PVD.[148–153] One study found that more than 75% of aphakic eyes over 1 year after cataract extraction had a PVD.[148] Because these eyes usually have a complete PVD, the tractional forces are on the posterior margin of the vitreous base (this is the anterior limit in the anterior progression of a PVD) during eye movements. Thus, it is not uncommon to find small tears at the posterior margin of the vitreous base responsible for the detachment. And because a PVD is more common after cataract surgery, retinal tears long after surgery are more likely to occur at the posterior margin of the vitreous base. These small tears found at the posterior margin of the vitreous base are more common in older patients.[154] Such retinal tears have been reported to occur in one eye in more than 60% of people over 70 years of age, and this is in a population that has a detachment rate of around 0.2–0.032%.[76, 84] Retinal detachments occurring late after a PVD are relatively unusual.[155] Therefore, a complete PVD is a good prognostic sign because there are most likely no areas of vitreoretinal adhesions remaining to induce a retinal tear. As a matter of fact, it has been reported that very few retinal detachments occur after the acute stage of a PVD, and one report claims that the chance of a detachment occurring in the fellow aphakic eye of a patient with an aphakic detachment is ten times higher if no PVD is present as compared to the same type of patient with a PVD in the fellow eye.[156, 157] Many of the same type of findings have been seen in

pseudophakic eyes,[154] but the incidence of PVD is lower if the posterior capsule remains intact.[149, 154] If the posterior capsule is broken, the incidence of PVD after extracapsular cataract extraction is comparable to aphakia.[149] The higher incidence of retinal detachment may also be due to the loss of hyaluronic acid after cataract removal, which leads to a more liquefied state of the vitreous body that produces greater tractional forces on the retina.[105, 148–151] Some have hypothesized that the loss of hyaluronic acid following a capsulotomy may play a part in pseudophakic detachments.[158]

Cataract patients with extracapsular cataract extraction (ECCE) have an incidence of only 0–2% of pseudophakic retinal detachment in the first postoperative year.[71, 72, 132, 159–165] A posterior capsulotomy, however, essentially negated the advantage of an ECCE, and the incidence of detachment increased to 1–3%.[166–172] Other studies found that the incidence of retinal detachment was 0.8% for patients with an intact posterior capsule compared to 2.3% for those who had a primary nonlaser discission and 3.2% for secondary nonlaser discission.[173] The most important factor in developing a retinal detachment in patients with ECCE is the loss of integrity of the posterior lens capsule, which allows for anterior vitreous mobility and thus, retinal traction.[140, 142, 144, 174] More than half the retinal detachments in pseudophakia occur in the first year, with an additional 10–20% occurring over 2 years.[131, 147] The rate of detachment after a neodymium-yttrium-aluminum-garnet (Nd-YAG) laser capsulotomy is reported to be 1.0–3.6%,[160, 161, 171, 172, 175–178] which is about the same for mechanical capsulotomies; thus, it would seem apparent that opening the capsule is mostly responsible for an increase in the incidence of detachment. The risk for a detachment after Nd-YAG capsulotomy is four times greater than without a capsulotomy.[132, 168] Most detachments occur within the first year,[172] and the median time span from Nd-YAG capsulotomy to detachment in one report was 6 months,[179] whereas another study found that 47–59% occurred within 3 months.[147] Risk factors for developing a detachment after Nd-YAG capsulotomy are lattice degeneration, high axial myopia, and a history of detachment in the fellow eye.[172, 179] It has been suggested that Nd-YAG capsulotomies that preserve the anterior vitreous structure may be useful in lowering postlaser complications such as retinal detachment.[158] Reports have linked retinal detachment formation with photorefractive keratectomy; this is believed to be related to the PVD formation secondary to the shock wave produced by the procedure.[180] However, many other authorities do not believe that this is possible and that because most of the patients are moderate to high myopes, PVDs occurred as a natural course of the myopic condition.

In patients with pathologic myopia, the incidence of retinal detachment after cataract surgery ranged from 5.5% to 8%,[142, 144, 159, 161, 181] after intracapsular cataract extraction (ICCE) from 5.74% to 11.11%, and with ECCE it was 0.66–2.17%.[144, 161, 174] The overall risk of a retinal detachment in ICCE is 8 times greater than with ECCE.[144, 159, 174] Therefore, ECCE significantly lowers the incidence of detachment in high myopes. Peripheral retinal degenerations can increase the risk of retinal detachment after ECCE, and myopic eyes have an incidence of such retinal lesions in up to 11% of eyes.[119] With clear-lens extraction for the treatment of myopia, the incidence of retinal detachment is reported to be 7.3%, which is significant compared to the same procedure by ECCE (0.66–2.17%). The incidence of retinal detachment in this group increased to numbers twice as high with posterior capsulotomy or surgical discission compared to those having no procedures performed on the posterior capsule and those who were pseudophakic had no detachments.[119] Patients considering clear-lens extraction should be well educated on the risks of retinal detachment.

The breaks found in pseudophakic detachments, as in aphakic detachments, are typically small flap tears located along the posterior vitreous base and are more frequently seen within 2 years of surgery.[129, 154, 182, 183] However, a significant number of equatorial tears are found in pseudophakic and aphakic detachment, and they occur more frequently within the first 6 months of surgery.[89, 129, 184–186] Not only is the incidence of detachment less with pseudophakia, there is less likelihood of a total detachment or macular involvement and fewer signs of proliferative vitreoretinopathy. It is interesting that the rate of pseudophakic detachments are the same as phakic detachments and that they share most of the same characteristics.[89, 129, 183–186] The time from cataract surgery to detachment in one study was 18% in 0–3 months, 10% in 3–6 months, 24% in 6–12 months, 20% in 12–24 months, and 28% after 24 months[154]: More than 50% of detachments occur in the first year.[89, 129] Because well over 90% of cataract surgery involves intraocular lenses,[187] pseudophakic detachments are now more common than aphakic detachments.[154]

With congenital cataract extraction, the incidence of retinal detachment in one study was 1.5% over 5.5 years.[188] However, the rate is likely to be higher than that because the average time span between surgery and detachment is around 22.8 years.[189]

Patients with congenital cataracts and a retinal detachment in one eye must be followed carefully because 70% may develop a detachment in the contralateral eye.[190]

Trauma

Trauma significantly increases the risk of retinal detachment because it may produce a retinal tear or dialysis. Severe ocular trauma has a 90% prevalence in males, and patients are on average 25 years younger than those with nontraumatic unilateral retinal detachments,[92, 191, 192] with boxers being especially at risk.[193] Most tears occur at the time of the traumatic event, but the time interval between the trauma and the appearance of the detachment can vary. In one study of 160 patients, this interval was 1 month (30%), 8 months (50%), and 2 years (80%).[191, 194] Thus, a long interval after the trauma does not eliminate the injury as the cause of the detachment. Blunt trauma is the leading cause of retinal detachment in adolescents and children.[182, 191]

Retinal tears are likely due to the fact that blunt trauma produces an anterior-posterior compression of the globe that results in an equatorial expansion. During the equatorial expansion, the vitreous is not able to stretch enough, and therefore marked vitreous traction in the region of the vitreous base may produce a tear along the posterior margin.[191] Such tears along the posterior margin are usually linear and may form a retinal dialysis. Two studies found that such tears occurred in 4–18% of traumatic eyes and that only 4% of the breaks were located in the posterior fundus.[195, 196] Retinal detachments due to a dialysis characteristically progress very slowly and display such associated clinical findings as demarcation lines, tobacco dust, and macrocyst (intraretinal cysts).[197] The tears of the posterior margin of the vitreous base and dialyses have been most frequently found in the superonasal location[191]; another report found them more commonly in the inferotemporal region.[197] Most often the tear occurs at the time of the traumatic event. If the vitreous traction is severe enough, the nonpigmented epithelium may tear along the anterior margin of the vitreous base on the pars plana.[198] The success of retinal reattachment caused by a dialysis is excellent unless the tear enlarges into a giant retinal tear.[191] Another theory for the production of tears is the traction caused by the sudden acceleration of the vitreous during the traumatic event. Retinal tears may be flap tears if the resultant traction is severe on an isolated small area of firm vitreoretinal adhesion. The trauma may also cause an area of posttraumatic necrosis, which may cause a retinal tear with ragged edges.[199] The trauma necessary to produce a retinal tear in most cases probably directly compresses the globe; therefore, head trauma itself most likely will not result in a tear or detachment. A study of 247 cases of severe head trauma failed to find any retinal breaks.[200] There have even been reported cases of retinal detachment in golf-related injuries.[201]

Penetrating injuries of the posterior segment are much more likely to produce a retinal detachment (20% of cases), and detachments are 4.5 times more frequent if a vitreous hemorrhage is present.[202] Late-occurring retinal tears are usually caused by episcleral fibrovascular tissue that proliferates through the break in the wall of the globe into the vitreal cavity. The tears usually occur at the opposite side of the retina from the entry wound site of the foreign body.[173, 202, 203] The prognosis for such cases is very poor.[173, 204]

Glaucoma

Glaucoma has also been reported to be a risk factor for detachment. Some clinical studies have reported that 4–7% of patients with chronic open-angle glaucoma developed a retinal detachment.[205–207] This is especially evident in patients with pigmentary dispersion syndrome, where it has been reported to occur in 6.4% of the cases.[208] Miotic therapy for glaucoma (both parasympathomimetics and anticholinesterases) may be associated with retinal detachment formation, and greater risk seems to accompany the initiation of therapy and the use of stronger miotics.[209–215] However, there are thousands of patients on such miotic therapy and a very small number of cases have been reported. In one study of 34 eyes the miotic treatment resulted in a detachment in detachment-prone eyes: myopia (62%), aphakia (24%), ipsilateral lattice degeneration (38%), and retinal disease in fellow eye (50%); virtually all detachments were rhegmatogenous.[215] All glaucoma patients on miotic therapy should have a periodic dilated fundus examination; if there is a sudden decrease in IOP or dramatic change in the visual field despite good pressure control, a dilated fundus examination is necessary.[216] Congenital glaucoma is associated with retinal detachment and is likely due to the progressive enlargement of the globe, but visualization to detect peripheral lesions may be difficult because of opacification of the cornea or cataracts.[217, 218]

Lattice Degeneration

Lattice degeneration is also frequently associated with retinal detachment formation (see Lattice Degeneration in Chapter 3). Less often associated with retinal detachment formation is retinoschisis (see Retinoschisis in Chapter 3).

Fellow Eye

Patients with a history of a retinal detachment in one eye are at increased risk of retinal detachment formation in the fellow eye. The incidence in the fellow eye with no predisposing lesions is about 5%, and in eyes with predisposing factors it is 10% or more.[73, 74, 156, 219–227] Several studies have shown that if the fellow eye of patients with a history of retinal detachment develops retinal tears, it will progress to a retinal detachment in 25–30% of cases.[221, 225, 228] Another study found that phakic fellow eyes of patients with a history of retinal detachment and lattice degeneration who did not receive prophylactic treatment have a 2.5 times greater chance of developing a retinal detachment compared to those who do not receive treatment.[229] Many studies have shown a benefit of prophylactic treatment of fellow eyes,[75, 97, 222, 230–233] but there is a lack of consensus about which eyes should be treated.[229] A family history of a rhegmatogenous retinal detachment places the patient at an increased risk for developing a detachment.[129, 220–223, 234] The type of retinal tear or peripheral lesion in the fellow eye also affects the risk of detachment in that eye. In one study, seven of 42 eyes with flap tears developed a detachment, but none of 26 fellow eyes with operculated tears developed a detachment. The study also found detachments in nine of 38 fellow eyes with lattice degeneration, 11 of 68 eyes with pigment clumping, and four of 51 eyes with vitreoretinal tags with traction.[155]

Bilaterality

The world incidence of bilateral retinal detachments is reported to be 15.52%.[97] The incidence in fellow eyes is greater in aphakic than in phakic eyes. In patients where the fellow eye is aphakic, the incidence of retinal detachment is reported to be two to four times higher, or 21–41% compared to 7–10% if the eye was phakic.[155, 159, 235, 236] Myopes were more at risk of developing bilateral detachments.[237] One study reported that of 100 patients with bilateral surgical aphakia and a rhegmatogenous retinal detachment in one eye, the fellow eye went on to develop a detachment in 26% of cases.[157] Therefore, it is highly beneficial to use prophylactic treatment of flap tears in aphakic fellow eyes; however, the treatment of round retinal holes in lattice degeneration or other peripheral lesions in aphakic fellow eyes is far less clear, with some reports advising treatment and others questioning the need.[235, 238, 239] But if treatment is performed on these lesions, care must be taken to not overtreat, which may result in a detachment.[199] Pseudophakia reduces the incidence of detachment to 6% in the fellow eye.[173]

Subclinical Detachment

A subclinical detachment is a peripheral retinal detachment that is at least 1 disc diameter from the break but no more than 2 disc diameters posterior to the equator. These detachments are more likely to lead to a clinically significant retinal detachment as compared to eyes with breaks but without detachment.[219, 222] Treatment is usually required because 30% will advance.[222] Such a detachment does not necessarily require a scleral buckling procedure, especially if minor or no vitreous traction is present. Walling off the detachment with at least 3–4 mm of laserpexy[232] or cryopexy that extends to the ora serrata usually stabilizes the detachment and often results in a flattening or reattachment over months. This type of treatment has a 95% success rate,[240] but failure is often the result of not extending the treatment all the way anterior to the ora serrata.

Rhegmatogenous, Nonrhegmatogenous, and Total Retinal Detachments

Rhegmatogenous Retinal Detachment

Retinal detachment secondary to a retinal break is known as a rhegmatogenous detachment (*rhegma* means "to rend or tear") (see Figures 3-78 through 3-80, 5-11, 5-13, 5-14C, 6-6 and 6-9). The development of a rhegmatogenous detachment requires (1) a full-thickness retinal break, (2) vitreous traction, and (3) the ingress of fluid through the break. One that is not produced by a retinal break is called a nonrhegmatogenous detachment. It is usually caused by the accumulation of an exudate or transudate in the subretinal space. A tractional retinal detachment without retinal breaks is also a nonrhegmatogenous detachment.

It is not uncommon to find a whitish rim of retina around a retinal break in an area of retinal detachment (Figure 6-9). The most likely explanation for this phenomenon is that a localized retinal detachment around the break for months to years has caused whitish degeneration of the localized detachment. When a large detachment involves the area, the old localized detachment appears more white than a recent larger detachment.

In recent rhegmatogenous detachments, the protein content of the subretinal fluid is much lower than that of the plasma, but with time the composition of the fluid slowly becomes more like plasma. As a matter of fact, the total protein concentration increases, and so does the amount of enzymes normally found in the plasma.[241] Even though the subretinal fluid becomes more like the plasma, experimental studies have not found a breakdown in the blood-retinal barrier, even in long-standing detachments.[242, 243] As the protein content of the subretinal fluid increases, so does the viscosity, and therefore fluid drained from a recent detachment is watery, whereas that from a long-standing detachment is quite viscous.[199] One component of the subretinal fluid is hyaluronic acid, which is found in the vitreous and not in plasma.[244] The routes of passage of plasma constituents into the subretinal fluid are most likely via retinal blood vessels (this has been documented as leaky vessels on fluorescein angiography)[245] or degenerated pigment epithelium. The subretinal fluid can be absorbed due to osmotic pressure from the choroid and from metabolic transport across the pigment epithelium.[246, 247]

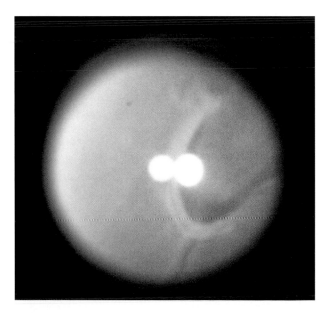

FIGURE 6-9
Large flap tear can be seen in whitish retinal detachment that undulated with eye movements. The white border to retinal break denotes localized retinal detachment for months to years before the bullous detachment.

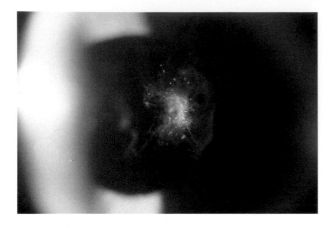

FIGURE 6-10
"Tobacco dust" (pigment cells) in the anterior vitreous seen during biomicroscopy of a patient with a rhegmatogenous detachment.

Vitreous and retinal hemorrhages are common in rhegmatogenous detachments and are the result of either vitreous traction on a superficial retinal blood vessel or the shearing of a retinal vessel during the formation of a tear. The blood in the vitreous often appears as a plume of reddish smoke that moves with the vitreous on eye movements. The release of red blood corpuscles in the posterior vitreous cavity that float close to the retinal surface cast shadows that the patient appreciates as numerous tiny black specks that slowly move across the peripheral visual field toward the central field of view. These disappear as they degenerate and finally rupture. It is not uncommon to find retinal hemorrhages adjacent to the tear caused by a ruptured blood vessel crossing the area of the torn retina,which often indicates a newly formed break. This type of juxtapositional retinal hemorrhage slowly disappears over a few weeks to months.

The finding of numerous brown specks in the anterior vitreous during biomicroscopy strongly suggests a retinal break with associated rhegmatogenous retinal detachment (Figure 6-10).[248–250] These specks represent free-floating RPE cells[251] ("tobacco dust" or Shaffer's sign of the vitreous). The cells float off the RPE into the subretinal fluid beneath the detachment, then migrate through the retinal break into the vitreous cavity. Those that float in the anterior vitreal cavity can be seen with the biomicroscope. These pigmented cells have a light brown appearance and tend to remain stationary in the anterior vitreous (except if there is a PVD). This condition is usually associated with a clinically significant rhegmatogenous detachment, which allows

for a large area of pigment epithelium to be exposed to the overlying fluid environment. The pigment epithelial cells in this abnormal fluid environment degenerate and migrate off the basal lamina. There has been a report that this condition occurs with retinal tears without an associated detachment.[252] Mild anterior uveitis is often associated with a clinically significant retinal detachment; therefore, biomicroscopy can be useful in the diagnosis. Some misdiagnosed uveitis has occurred due to mistaking the pigment cells for inflammatory cells; thus it is important to look carefully at the cells floating in the anterior vitreous with the biomicroscope for a slight brown color. When clumps of pigment cell macrophages form on the outer surface of the detached retina, they have the appearance of white dots and are called subretinal precipitates. The appearance of subretinal precipitates indicates chronicity.[253–255]

The region of the retina involved in a rhegmatogenous detachment can aid in localizing the retinal break. A detachment that is superior and travels approximately the same distance inferior in the nasal and temporal halves of the fundus probably indicates a break close to the 12-o'clock position. A retinal break at the 6-o'clock position would produce a detachment that is approximately a mirror image of the one produced by the 12-o'clock break. A retinal detachment that ranged from the superonasal to the inferonasal region to partly into the inferotemporal region would be most indicative of a break in the superonasal region of the fundus. The billowing movement of a retinal detachment studied with an understanding of gravitational forces can facilitate the discovery of retinal breaks, for often the breaks are found in the most bullous area or areas of the detachment. Most retinal breaks that cause a nontraumatic retinal detachment have been located in the superior temporal quadrant of the retina.[81, 89, 90]

A retinal detachment may extend past the ora serrata, causing the nonpigmented epithelium of the pars plana to separate from the pigmented epithelium. This is frequently observed in cases of traumatic retinal dialysis or giant retinal tear (see Retinal Dialysis and Giant Retinal Tear in Chapter 5). It can also occur whenever there is marked vitreous traction on the vitreous base, and it is frequently seen in proliferative vitreoretinopathy (PVR) (see Proliferative Vitreoretinopathy in Chapter 7). Detached ciliary epithelium is invisible when viewed straight on but appears as a translucent membrane when seen in profile during scleral depression or on a scleral buckle. Detachment of the ciliary epithelium occurs more often above the horizontal meridian and nasally than below and temporally. The detachment can extend as far anterior as the ciliary processes. The detached ora serrata is seen as a narrow lightly pigmented scalloped zone that separates the transparent ciliary epithelium from the thicker detached retina. A faint pigment line in the underlying choroid denotes where the ora serrata was attached and has the contour of the ora bays and teeth.[92, 256] The finding of signs of PVR, such as fixed retinal folds and equatorial traction bands, strongly suggests the possibility of a rhegmatogenous detachment.

Usually the IOP in an eye with a rhegmatogenous detachment decreases in proportion to the extent and duration of the detachment.[257–259] Studies have determined that the reason for the reduction in IOP is due to misdirection of the aqueous flow posteriorly through the retinal break and absorbed by the RPE and choroid.[241, 260–264] Rhegmatogenous detachments can lead to an increase in IOP, however, and if the detachment is not discovered, the patient may be inadvertently treated for glaucoma or uveitis.[199]

Incidence

The median age for idiopathic rhegmatogenous retinal detachment was 57 for males and 62 for females.[76] Frequency in children is small: Only 3–4% of rhegmatogenous retinal detachments occur in people under age 16.[88] Another study found that the age-adjusted annual incidence of nontraumatic phakic retinal detachments was 3.4 per 100,000 in patients less than 50 years of age, 28.9 per 100,000 in patients aged 50–64, and 31.3 in patients over 65.[76] One study reported 12.9 per 100,000 per year for idiopathic rhegmatogenous retinal detachment and 13.0 per 100,000 when aphakic detachment was added.[76] Another study reported a combined incidence of 8.9 per 100,000 per year for phakic and aphakic retinal detachment.[78] Also, patients with a pre-existing retinal hole have an increase in retinal detachment formation following cataract extraction.[219] The most common type of retinal break in pseudophakic detachments is a flap tear, and the incidence varies from 46 to 90%.[154, 155, 183, 185] These flap tears are usually small and located at the posterior margin of the vitreous base.[265] Patients with aphakia have retinal tears of similar type and location and retinal detachments with similar morphologic characteristics and time of onset as those found in pseudophakic patients.[89, 129, 183–185, 265, 266] Round or oval holes in one study were found in 57% of 4,000 cases of nontraumatic phakic retinal detachments.[89] Single retinal breaks causing retinal detachments were found in 41–54%,[89, 155] and multiple breaks were found in 46% of patients.[155] One study found that a single break that developed a nontraumatic retinal detachment is more frequent in patients over age 40 compared to younger patients (28% vs. 19%).[81] The incidence of anterior breaks and the relatively extensive detachments increases in eyes that have undergone cataract surgery.[81, 89, 129, 154] Retinal breaks located at the posterior vitreous base that result in a retinal detachment range from 12% to 30%.[81, 89, 129, 155] Also, anterior breaks are more likely to be the cause of a detachment if it occurs more than 2 years after surgery compared to less than 6 months.[154] This may be explained by the fact that after a total PVD, all the remaining vitreous traction is at the posterior margin of the vitreous base.

Retinal breaks are far more common than retinal detachments. One study suggested that the risk of any break leading to detachment may be only one in 70.[87] A retinal detachment is bilateral in a range from 6.7–40.0% in all patients, which is much greater than the incidence of retinal detachment in the general population.[76, 80, 81, 225, 267, 268] Therefore, a retinal detachment in one eye greatly enhances the risk for the fellow eye. Family history is very important, as persons with hereditary diseases, such as Wagner's disease (see Hereditary Hyaloideoretinopathies in Chapter 3) and high myopia, are more likely to develop a retinal detachment. Patients with vitreal and retinal diseases are at substantial risk. It is helpful to note that approximately 50% of rhegmatogenous retinal detachments are caused by retinal tears demonstrating vitreous traction, about 30% are associated with lattice degeneration, and approximately 20% are the result of retinal dialyses or holes.[269, 270] Another study reported that symptomatic retinal tears account for 30–50% of rhegmatogenous retinal detachments, and asymptomatic breaks only account for 10%.[219] Therefore, it is not very common for an asymptomatic retinal break to progress to a retinal detachment, and many authorities suggest following such breaks. The risk of a retinal tear present prior to cataract surgery progressing to a retinal detachment increases substantially after extraction, perhaps to 50%.[219]

Macular Hole

A macular hole can result in a rhegmatogenous retinal detachment, but this does not occur very often. It is usually accompanied by a very flat perimacular detachment, although a large bullous detachment can occur (Figures 6-11 and 6-12). If a retinal detachment does not involve the peripheral fundus but is

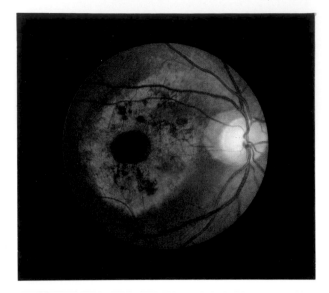

FIGURE 6-11
A large posttraumatic macular hole with a white collar that presents a previous small surrounding retinal detachment. Note the surrounding chorioretinal atrophy with pigment proliferation and migration.

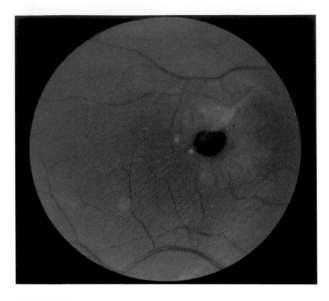

FIGURE 6-12
A posttraumatic macular hole within a long-standing retinal detachment. Note many retinal folds, giant drusen beneath the detachment, whitish-looking thin retina, attenuated retinal vessels, and loss of underlying choroidal detail.

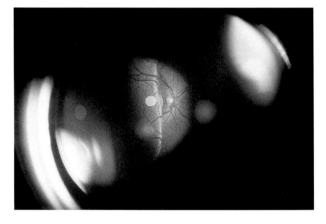

FIGURE 6-13
A rhegmatogenous retinal detachment of the temporal half of the retina with the macula seen on the rolled posterior edge of the detachment as a small yellow area. The view is through the ultra–wide field fundus lens.

limited to the posterior pole, a macular break should be suspected if no other obvious etiology is present. Differentiating between macular cyst, partial macular break, and full-thickness hole may be difficult. High magnification with a biomicroscope and precorneal condensing lenses, contact lenses, or Hruby lens is usually required to detect a macular cyst. Rupture of the inner wall of a cyst will not result in a retinal detachment if the outer wall is intact. Only a full-thickness break results in a retinal

detachment. True full-thickness macular holes were present in only 0.62% of 5,442 cases of retinal detachment in one study.[256]

A detached macula appears edematous, and its yellow color is more obvious, and it appears to cover a larger area than the normal attached macula (Figure 6-13). Sometimes the thin macular area seems to have a dimpled appearance, which may be due to the fovea being only half the retinal thickness (see Figure 6-4). A shallow macular detachment may be detected by looking for loss of underlying choroidal detail, very small retinal folds, and little to no movement on eye movements. Visual acuity drops when the macula is off, although it is better in a fresh shallow retinal detachment than in a high detachment. The closer the detached macula is to the underlying choroid and RPE, the better the photoreceptor functioning. Even if the macula is only slightly detached, however, there is a great deal of uncertainty in recovering pre-existing acuity.[271] The obscuration of choroidal detail along with the loss of visual acuity is often the best way to tell when the macula is detached.

Lattice Degeneration

Patients with lattice degeneration are at risk for retinal detachment formation; the incidence is 0.3–0.5%.[272, 273] Lattice degeneration has, however, been reported to be responsible for approximately

20–30% of all retinal detachments.[21, 274] Several studies found that 30–45% of retinal detachments were caused by atrophic holes in lattice degeneration,[273, 274] with 70% of such detachments occurring in myopic eyes and 70% in patients younger than 40 years of age.[275] Detachments caused by atrophic holes in lattice tend to progress slowly, and demarcation lines are fairly common. Some 55–70% of detachments caused by lattice result from a tear along the posterior margin of the lattice lesion,[273, 274] with 90% of such detachments occurring in patients older than age 50; only 43% of the eyes were myopic.[274] These detachments caused by retinal tears progress more rapidly and usually do not have demarcation lines.

Diabetes

Diabetics with proliferative retinopathy rarely develop a peripheral flap tear induced detachment; rather, the breaks are usually oval and located next to areas of fibrovascular proliferation.[199, 276] Due to the vitreous traction, these types of detachments spread very quickly.[199, 276] Branch retinal vein occlusions rarely result in a detachment.[277–280] The cause is probably the anoxic retina producing areas of neovascular proliferation that adhere to the overlying vitreous cortex; during PVD formation, traction on these areas may result in a tear and subsequent detachment.[199]

Intraocular Infections

Patients with intraocular infections may develop a rhegmatogenous retinal detachment. Eyes with endophthalmitis after cataract surgery have an incidence of retinal detachment of close to 90% if they are treated with antibiotics alone and 21% if vitrectomy is added to the treatment plan.[281] A detachment may develop in 50% of cases of acute retinal necrosis syndrome.[282–285] The resultant detachments often develop multiple large tears or giant tears that frequently result in PVR. Only about 60% of these cases are successfully surgically repaired.[199] Virus retinal infections can lead to retinal destruction and retinal breaks. Cytomegalovirus (CMV) retinitis causes rhegmatogenous detachments in about 15–24% of the patients with AIDS.[286, 287] Bilateral CMV retinitis is more common in patients with retinal detachment (60–80%)[288, 289] compared to the 42% rate of bilaterality in CMV retinitis.[290] Due to the destruction of the retina in CMV cases, visual loss in such detachments is substantial.[291] A small percentage of patients with AIDS develop retinal detachments due to the necrotizing retinitis associated with herpes simplex or zoster and the rate of retinal detachment is much higher, at approximately 70–80%.[292, 293] Other infections associated with retinal detachments are toxoplasmosis, toxocariasis, and pars planitis.

Hereditary Hyaloideoretinopathies

Patients with hereditary hyaloideoretinopathies, such as Wagner's disease, Stickler's syndrome, and Goldmann-Favre syndrome, are at risk for retinal detachments due to the vitreous degeneration with associated whitish bands and membranes that adhere to the retina (see Hereditary Hyaloideoretinopathies in Chapter 3). Patients with congenital and acquired retinoschisis are at a low risk for developing a retinal detachment (see Retinoschisis in Chapter 3). Entities and procedures that are associated with retinal detachment are Ehlers-Danlos syndrome,[216] Marfan's syndrome, retinopathy of prematurity and homocystinuria.[199] Procedures associated with retinal detachment are penetrating keratoplasty, pars plana vitrectomy, retinal laserpexy and cryopexy, and scleral perforation from strabismus surgery and retrobulbar injection. Miotic medications for glaucoma can induce a rhegmatogenous detachment.

Trauma

Traumatic retinal detachments are usually rhegmatogenous, with retinal breaks most often found in the far retinal periphery and the posterior pole.[92] The trauma is usually direct to the globe. Indirect trauma can also result in a retinal detachment, but it seems to occur at sites of pre-existing retinal degeneration such as lattice degeneration. Severe ocular trauma has nearly a 90% prevalence in males, and patients are on average 25 years younger than those with nontraumatic unilateral retinal detachment.[92] The time interval between the trauma and the appearance of the detachment in a series of 160 cases was 1 month (30%), 8 months (50%), and 2 years (80%).[191, 194] Thus a long interval after ocular trauma does not eliminate the injury as the etiology of the detachment. A rhegmatogenous detachment has been reported to be associated with noncontact pneumatic tonometry.[294] Retinal detachment after noncontact pneumatic tonometry.

Far less common is an asymptomatic rhegmatogenous detachment found on a routine dilated fundus examination. Often, in these cases there is a demarcation line, macrocyst, underlying pigment epithelial alterations, and other signs of chronicity.[295] The lack of symptoms probably indicates that

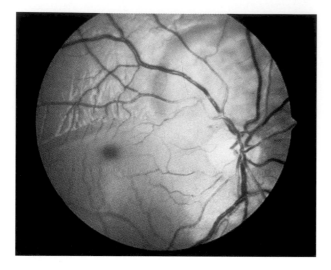

FIGURE 6-14
A serous retinal detachment temporal to the optic disc involves the macula; a detachment of the pigment epithelium can be seen above the optic disc. The subject is a young female with eclampsia.

strong vitreous traction may not have been totally responsible for the tear and subsequent detachment. There is debate on whether to treat such detachments, with some in favor[296–298] and others favoring follow-up only.[295, 299] With follow-up, educating the patient to the symptoms of a progressive retinal detachment and self-testing of the peripheral visual field is of paramount importance.

Nonrhegmatogenous Retinal Detachment

A nonrhegmatogenous retinal detachment frequently occurs in association with retinal angiomata (such as Coats' disease) in the presence of a choroidal inflammatory process (chorioretinitis) or other choroidal pathology (such as intrinsic or metastatic malignant tumors). Other causes include uveal effusion, pars planitis, sympathetic ophthalmia, eclampsia, Harada's disease, and trauma.

A nonrhegmatogenous detachment may appear essentially similar to a rhegmatogenous detachment, except there are no retinal breaks and the bullous appearance rarely shows retinal folds. The subretinal fluid in a nonrhegmatogenous detachment is rich in blood proteins and is more viscous than the liquefied vitreous and aqueous under a rhegmatogenous detachment. It tends to migrate or move easily with changes in head position; therefore, the detachment shifts toward the dependent part of the fundus due to gravity. A nonrhegmatogenous detachment generally does not extend to the ora serrata, but a rhegmatogenous detach-

ment commonly extends to the ora. The reasons for this may be that in a nonrhegmatogenous detachment the subretinal fluid is more viscous and there is the absence of vitreous traction; both of which generally do not enhance far anterior separation of the sensory retina. Sometimes such a detachment can become so bullous that it may be seen immediately behind the lens.[199]

The presence of a nonrhegmatogenous retinal detachment without obvious etiology should be suspected of harboring a choroidal tumor; therefore, it is important to examine the detachment carefully to determine if a retinal tear is present. Metastases from lung and breast carcinomas are the most frequent origins of choroidal tumors in adults.[299] Tumors may be small and flesh-colored and are often initially overlooked on routine examinations. Intrinsic choroid melanomas also can produce a nonrhegmatogenous shifting detachment, but their pigmented appearance usually allows for early detection and diagnosis (see Figures 3-19 and 3-21); the retinal detachment associated with a choroidal tumor may conceal the tumor beneath it. About 75% of choroidal melanomas have a secondary retinal detachment[96] (see Choroidal Nevus and Malignant Melanoma in Chapter 3).

Also, a tumor in the superior fundus may produce a shifting retinal detachment that migrates to the inferior fundus. Thus, two retinal detachments may be seen during ophthalmoscopy, one superior over the tumor and the other in the dependent region of the fundus. Experimental studies have found that the IOP in nonrhegmatogenous detachments is reduced, and this ocular hypotony seems to be related to the retinal detachment itself.[300] The detection of a subretinal mass may be found on indirect ophthalmoscopy, ultrasonography, fluorescein angiography, and magnetic resonance imaging (MRI). Sometimes a tumor may look like a nonexistent retinal detachment by elevating the pigment epithelium along with the sensory retina, which, in the past, has been known as a solid retinal detachment.

A rather rare type of nonrhegmatogenous detachment results from eclampsia and preeclampsia in pregnant women.[301–303] It seems to occur around the thirty-second week of gestation, and it has in one case occurred in a woman with a normal pregnancy.[304] There is an incidence rate of 1 in 18,524 pregnancies.[302] It usually appears as bilateral exudative detachments in the posterior poles (Figure 6-14) and generally resolves shortly after delivery. The incidence of this complication seems to be decreasing in recent years, most likely due to better antenatal care.

Other causes of nonrhegmatogenous detachments are Vogt-Koyanagi-Harada syndrome, idiopathic central serous chorioretinopathy,[305–308] posterior scleritis,[309] optic pit,[310] choroidal coloboma,[311] morning glory syndrome,[312, 313] nanophthalmos,[314, 315] and uveal effusion syndrome.[316, 317] Choroidal detachments are sometimes mistaken for a nonrhegmatogenous detachment.

Tractional Retinal Detachment

A tractional nonrhegmatogenous retinal detachment results from the physical separation of the sensory retina from the RPE and is caused by vitreous membrane traction. Usually advanced vitreous degeneration is present with accompanying scarring and band formation. The contraction of these bands is the primary cause of a tractional detachment. Several disease conditions can produce a tractional retinal detachment—for example, diabetic retinopathy, sickle cell retinopathy, pars planitis, Wagner's vitreoretinal degeneration, retrolental fibroplasia, proliferative vitreoretinopathy (see Proliferative Vitreoretinopathy in Chapter 7), vitreous hemorrhage, long-standing intraocular inflammation, and trauma (especially perforating trauma). About 8% of retinal detachments secondary to perforating injury are nonrhegmatogenous.[96] The retinal detachment commonly has a smooth taut surface, is immobile, is usually concave to the anterior segment, and rarely extends to the ora serrata. This appearance can be confused with a retinoschisis.

Tractional rhegmatogenous detachments are caused by a vitreous traction producing a tear in the retina that results in a typical-appearing rhegmatogenous detachment (white bullous retina that has folds and undulates on eye movements). Diabetics may have strong vitreoretinal adhesions that can produce a retinal tear during PVD formation, and it may even produce a tear in the posterior pole. However, the most common type of retinal detachment in diabetics is that of a nonrhegmatogenous tractional detachment. These detachments have a smooth appearance, do not move on eye movements, are usually concave to the anterior segment of the eye, and rarely extend to the ora serrata.[199] Often the tractional detachment remains stationary for years, whereas in others it may progress to the macula, and only in severe cases does the detachment extend from equator to equator.[199] The treatment for tractional detachments that involve the macula requires a vitrectomy to release the tension on the retina.

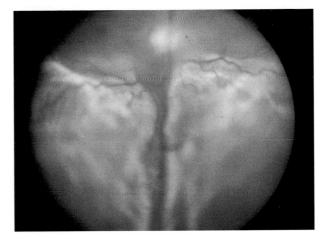

FIGURE 6-15
Total retinal detachment with two large whitish triangular-shaped bullae pointing to the optic disc. Just temporal to the optic disc is the reddish, dimpled appearance of the detached macula.

Total Retinal Detachment

A total retinal detachment results from the separation of the entire sensory retina from the pigment epithelium. This most often occurs in eyes with large retinal breaks (especially giant retinal tears or with numerous breaks); however, sometimes a single, small break can produce a total detachment if a large amount of liquefied vitreous is available and continued significant vitreous tractional forces on the retina (Figure 6-15). Total detachments are more likely to be found in aphakic than phakic eyes.

If the detached retina remains fixed to the ora serrata and the optic disc, it produces a funnel-shaped structure (funnel detachment) with the wide end anterior and the optic disc at the narrow end (Figures 6-16 and 6-17). Total retinal detachments can be imaged with ultrasonography (Figure 6-18) and CT scan (Figure 6-19). Usually, the optic disc can be seen at the apex of the funnel; however, if the detached retina is pulled together near the apex of the funnel, the optic nerve head is hidden beneath the retina (Figures 6-20 and 6-21). This whitish funnel-shaped structure is also known as a "morning glory detachment" due to its resemblance to the horn-shaped flower. If the detached retina separates from the ora serrata, it will collapse toward the center of the vitreous cavity and form a chord of detached retina emanating from the optic disc (Figure 6-22). Both the anatomic and visual prognoses for reattachment of a totally detached retina are rather poor. When a detachment becomes total, the electroretinogram becomes unrecordable and the electro-oculogram is markedly reduced.[318, 319]

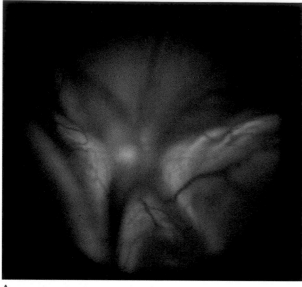

A

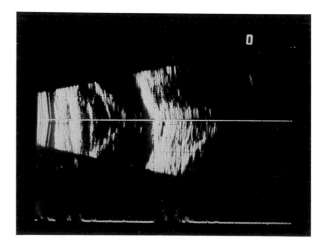

FIGURE 6-17
An anterior-posterior cut through an enucleated eye showing a total retinal detachment. The retina is still attached at the optic disc (*straight arrow*) and the ora serrata (*small curved arrow*). There is a superior chorioretinal scar from cryopexy (*large straight arrow*) and below at the encircling band (*large curved arrow*). Note the encircling band above and below and the scleral sponge above with a groove in it for the band.

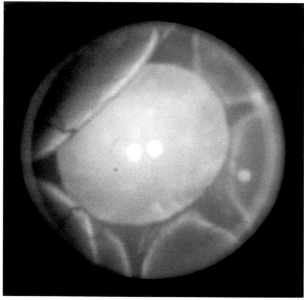

B

FIGURE 6-16
A. Total retinal detachment "morning glory detachment," which has whitish detached triangular retinal folds pointing toward the optic disc. This occurred in an eye with a long-standing luxated lens in the vitreous secondary to past ocular trauma. B. With time, while the patient was in a supine position in the examination chair, the dislocated cataractous lens came to rest at the bottom of the funnel detachment, obscuring the optic disc.

FIGURE 6-18
B-scan ultrasonogram of a total retinal detachment seen as a funnel-shaped structure in the vitreous cavity.

Histopathology

Sections of detached retinas show fluid accumulation in the subretinal space, degeneration of the photoreceptor layer, reduced protein synthesis, and an edematous retina, which is mostly seen in the inner retinal layers. Some of the earliest damage (as soon as 1 hour in animal studies)[320] is the loss of the

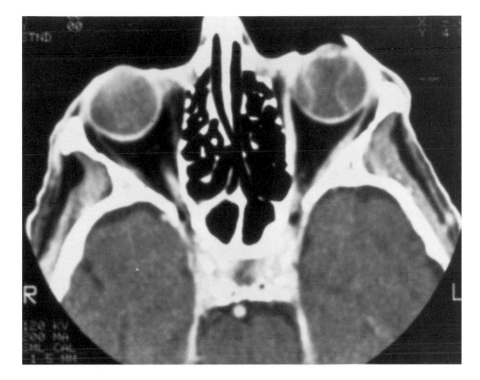

FIGURE 6-19
Computerized tomography scan of a globe with a total retinal detachment in the left eye. Because the 2-mm cut was off center it produced a baseball-like configuration inside the globe.

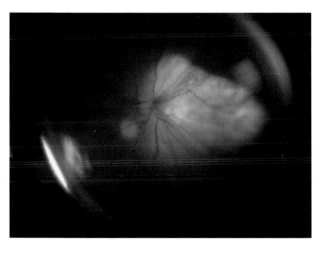

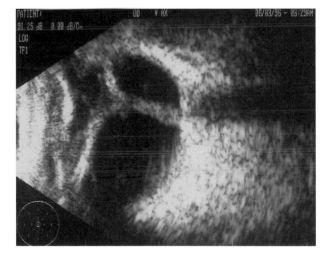

FIGURE 6-20
This patient was a boxer 40 years ago and now shows a total long-standing retinal detachment in one eye that has collapsed at the posterior region of the funnel and prohibits a view of the optic disc. View is through the ultra–wide field fundus lens.

FIGURE 6-21
B-scan of total retinal detachment that has collapsed anteriorly, and therefore there is no view of the optic disc.

photoreceptors. The blue-sensitive cones seem to be the most fragile, showing rapid irreversibility (totally irreversible in only 2.5 days).[321–325] The earliest change is that of the outer segments losing their horizontal orientation of the discs and showing swelling, along with ruptured plasma membranes and pyknotic and displaced nuclei.[321, 326, 327] The red and green cones seem to be more resistant to degeneration and are even functional in acutely detached retinas.[328] The red and green cones are primarily responsible for spatial resolution,[324] so their preservation is likely to be the reason for attaining good visual acuity after quick reattachment of the macula. Rods also show some of the same degenerative

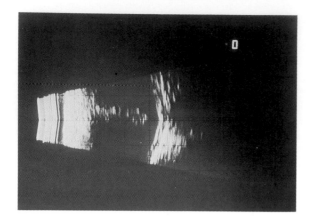

FIGURE 6-22
B-scan ultrasonogram of a total retinal detachment that has suffered so much traction and degeneration that it has collapsed on itself into the center of the vitreous cavity and therefore formed a chord of degenerated retinal tissue.

changes but usually at a later time. The retinal edema produces folds in the outer layers, which are seen ophthalmoscopically as decreased transparency and irregular corrugations.[253, 254] Given that the retinal circulation remains intact and that the degree of retinal degeneration is proportional to the height of the detachment; it is believed that most of these changes are due to the separation of the retina from the pigment epithelium and choroid.[254] At first, the pigment epithelial cells become larger, but with time they tend to separate from the basal lamina and float under the detachment and through the break into the vitreous cavity.[254, 327, 329] Under ophthalmoscopy, these cells are called tobacco dust or Shaffer's sign. In traumatic detachments the proposed mechanisms for photoreceptor death include toxic blood products, neovascular membranes, and apoptosis (programmed cell death).[330, 331]

After 2–3 months of detachment, there is degenerative atrophy of the outer layers, which causes the remaining sensory retina to look thin and transparent. Microcystoid degeneration is initially seen, followed by coalescence of the cystoid spaces into a larger cyst with time. This microcystoid degeneration causes the honeycomb appearance to the detached retina on clinical examination.[329] Some proliferation of glial and connective tissue occurs and increases with time.

The fluid under a retinal detachment can be seen on histology sections as a pink area beneath the detachment (see Figure 3-18B); if no fluid is seen, the retinal separation is artifactual in origin. The char-

acteristics of this fluid can indicate the etiology of the detachment; for example, eosinophils are found in a nematode endophthalmitis, foamy macrophages and periodic acid-Schiff (PAS)–positive fluid in Coats' disease, and serous proteinaceous fluid in choroidal tumors.

Clinical Significance

The clinical significance of a retinal detachment is that it may lead to a peripheral or central loss of vision. A peripheral loss of vision may or may not noticeably affect the visual performance of the patient because the visual field of the eyes overlaps to some degree. However, a loss of central vision can markedly affect the daily performance of the patient, especially if depth perception and stereoacuity are demands on the visual world. The significance of asymptomatic rhegmatogenous retinal detachment is that it usually leads to total blindness if not accurately diagnosed and surgically corrected. The significance of a nonrhegmatogenous retinal detachment depends on the underlying pathology; the most worrisome causes are malignant intraocular tumors.

A subclinical retinal detachment is one that is more than 1 disc diameter from the break but less than 2 disc diameter posterior to the equator. Another definition is a peripheral retinal detachment that has not yet produced symptoms. One report states that 30% of such detachments progress, and therefore treatment is usually indicated.[332] Often just delimiting such a detachment with photocoagulation is adequate treatment, but it is likely to fail if the treatment is not placed to the ora serrata at each end of the detachment.[261, 333] The anterior treatment to the ora should prevent fluid leakage into the subretinal space from an anterior route.

Once the macula is detached, the patient rarely retains full pre-existing visual acuity, and the final visual acuity is often disappointing.[334, 335] The longer the macula is off, the less the visual recovery.[336] If the macula is off less than 1 week, the retinal recovery is rapid and within hours of reattachment, protein synthesis increases and regeneration of the outer segments begins.[332, 337–339] Also, the higher the detached macula, the worse the vision, and when the macula is on a bullous detachment, visual recovery is less.[340, 341] In experimental studies, the further the photoreceptors are away from the pigment epithelium, the greater the permanent photoreceptor damage.[39] This is probably due to the photoreceptors being further away from their nutritional supply of the pigment epithelium and the choriocapillaris. Rod outer segments recover faster than cone outer segments.[342] In reattachment of a total detachment, the electroretinogram may be recordable within 5 hours.[318] Intraretinal edema starts to resolve within hours and is usually nearly completely gone within 9 hours. The electroretinogram will continue to improve for about 12 weeks,[318] which is about the time that the outer segments return to normal histologically.[342, 343] Even if the macula is only off for a day, 20/20 acuity is seldom retained.[336, 344] In humans the visual acuity may continue to improve for 6 months or longer.[199, 345] If the detachment remains for over a month, the morphologic recovery is poor.[337] After 1 month, the best visual acuity that could be recovered is 20/70, and after 3 months 20/200 would be the best that could be anticipated. A retina that is totally detached for over 2 years is not likely to demonstrate visual improvement after reattachment, but some remarkable exceptions have occurred.[149]

The preoperative visual acuity can be a prognosis for postoperative acuity. Vision limited to hand motion may still show vast improvement after reattachment; however, in the absence of light perception, no functional recovery is possible. Exceptions are patients with high ocular tension of fairly recent origin associated with retinal detachment and no light perception vision; measurable vision may return after reattachment and lowering of intraocular tension.[149] As compared to visual acuity, color vision loss occurs early and may be permanent.[346, 347]

Metamorphopsia may occur after successful surgical reattachment of the macula and can have a profound affect on the visual performance of the patient. If an encircling band is used to surgically repair a retinal detachment, this may induce axial myopia. If the induced myopia is great enough, symptomatic anisometropia and aniseikonia may occur, which can have a significant affect on the patient's visual performance.

Glaucoma is another complication of retinal detachment, which may be due to the release of degenerating rods' and cones' outer segments into the vitreous cavity and then into the anterior chamber, where they become lodged in the trabecular meshwork. There is also an accompanying uveitis without keratic precipitates or ciliary injection, which is unresponsive to corticosteroids. This has been called the Schwartz syndrome.[348] The IOP comes back down to normal ranges in most instances within a few days of successful surgical reattachment of the retina.[349]

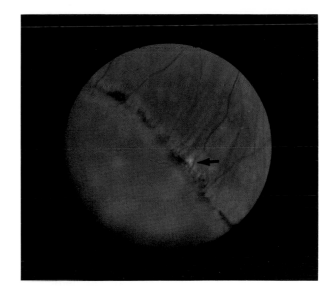

FIGURE 6-23
Long-standing bullous retinal detachment shows typical pigmented demarcation line at posterior edge and a small area of chorioretinal atrophy (*arrow*). The detached retina looks whitish and hides the underlying choroidal pattern. This detachment has a taut appearance, without any folds.

Demarcation Lines

Clinical Description

A pigmented demarcation line is sometimes found with a retinal detachment, past or present. If an edge of a retinal detachment remains stationary for at least 3–6 months, hyperplasia of the pigment epithelium at the detachment margin may occur, producing a pigmented demarcation line (Figures 6-23 and 6-24).[350] This tractional force may be the result of vitreous traction on the detached retina or the undulating action of the detached retina on eye movements pulling on the margin of the detachment. It is probably the result of tractional stimulation to the border caused by the detached retina pulling on the attached retina. Pigmented demarcation lines may be continuous along the entire extent of the margin of the detachment or may appear as a broken line. It is likely that strong tractional forces result in a continuous line and mild traction in a broken line. White or gray-white demarcation lines (sometimes called a friction line or high water mark) are likely secondary to the same tractional forces causing irritative inflammation, with resultant fibrosis along the edge of a detachment (Figures 6-25 and 6-26).

The pigmented demarcation line is usually found along the posterior edge of a detachment, just posterior to the border (Figure 6-27). Sometimes the pigmentation is seen as a narrow band on the

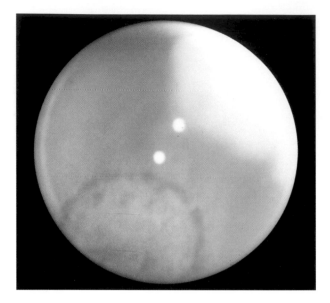

FIGURE 6-24
Long-standing localized retinal detachment shows typical pigmented demarcation line surrounding the detachment. The pigmented area in the center of the detachment, which denotes an area of previous vitreous traction, is where the retinal break was located. This detachment has a taut appearance, without any folds. The view is through the indirect condensing lens (the white spot is an artifact).

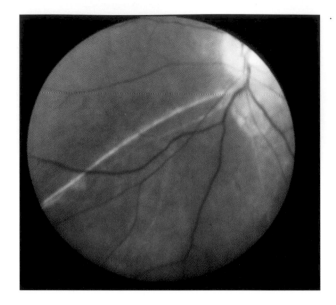

FIGURE 6-25
A whitish demarcation line remains after the reattachment of the inferonasal retina; it extends from the optic disc to the periphery.

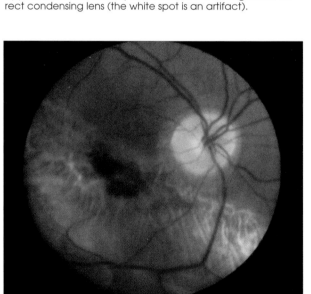

FIGURE 6-26
A demarcation line, between the normal retina above and previously detached atrophic retina below. This line of demarcation is known as a high water mark. Choroidal vessels can be seen through the atrophic retina, and pigment proliferation can be seen close to the demarcation line in the macular area.

detachment side of the border. A retinal hole or operculated retinal tear may develop a small surrounding detachment that may have a surrounding

pigmented demarcation line (see Figures 5-6 and 6-24). An inferiorly located detachment is most likely to produce a pigmented demarcation line because, without the aid of gravity, it advances slowly. One of the most common causes of slowly advancing retinal detachment is a retinal dialysis, and demarcation lines are found in about 50% of patients with such a break.[351, 352] Demarcation lines commonly occur in the inferior half of the retina and are frequently associated with a retinal dialysis that often produces a slowly advancing retinal detachment.

If a detachment progresses intermittently, each stationary period may result in a demarcation line; multiple demarcation lines may be associated with a detachment. They can occur so close together that they seem to coalesce into one large pigmented band. After spontaneous or surgical reattachment of a detached retina, single or multiple pigmented demarcation lines can be a residual finding (Figure 6-28). Degeneration of a detached retina may occur, so that even after reattachment there can be a line separating the normal retina from the previously detached retina. This demarcation line forming an inferior detachment is known as a high water or high tide mark. On rare occasions, instead of a pigmented demarcation line at the leading edge of a detachment, a band of chorioretinal atrophy may occur in front of the detachment.

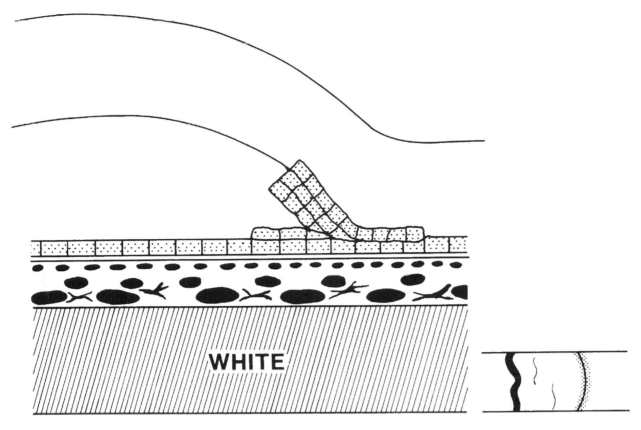
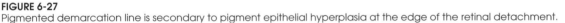

FIGURE 6-27
Pigmented demarcation line is secondary to pigment epithelial hyperplasia at the edge of the retinal detachment.

Cryotherapy can cause the release of pigment epithelial cells and pigment into the subretinal space ("pigment fallout"); these can migrate inferiorly due to gravity[353] and deposit along the lower margin of the detachment (a pseudo-demarcation line).[354] In the case of a total retinal detachment, the pigment may settle in the posterior pole. It has been shown that this pigment does not affect vision.[355]

Histopathology

Pigmented demarcation lines show proliferation of the pigmented epithelial cells from the pigmented epithelium across the angle made by the detached retina with the attached retina. The white demarcation lines are composed of fibrocytic proliferation with fibrin deposition.

Clinical Significance

A demarcation line indicates that the detachment has been stationary for at least 3–6 months.[356, 357] Therefore, demarcation lines are an indication of

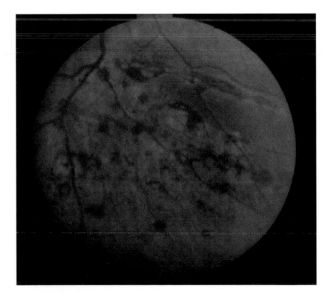

FIGURE 6-28
Multiple pigmented demarcation lines were produced by the halting progression of a retinal detachment, which has since been reattached.

chronicity of a detachment. Pigmented demarcation lines are believed to increase retinochoroidal adherence because the pigment epithelial cells that proliferated across the angle made by the detached retina meeting the attached retina possess intercellular bonding. This intercellular bonding is believed to hinder further progression of the detachment. In 23% of cases, demarcation lines are strong enough to prevent progression of a detachment.[358] Therefore, it is a positive prognostic sign, but it may also be said that if there is enough traction on a detachment to produce a pigmented line, enough traction may remain to produce further advancement of the detachment. Therefore, this demarcation barrier can be broken with progression of the detachment.[358] Thus, the existence of demarcation lines do not carry the assurance of complete stability of the detachment. Vision can be permanently decreased if a demarcation line passes through the macula. Occasionally, retinal tears occur at the margin of a demarcation line.

References

1. Zimmerman LE, Eastham AB. Acid mucopolysaccharide in the retinal pigment epithelial and visual cell layer of the developing mouse eye. Am J Ophthalmol 1959;47:488–500.
2. Yao X-Y, Marmor MF, et al. Interphotoreceptor matrix plays an important role in retinal adhesiveness. Invest Ophthalmol Vis Sci 1989;30(Suppl):240.
3. Sebag J. Vitreous Pathology. In W Tasman, EA Jaeger (eds), Clinical Ophthalmology. Vol. 3. Philadelphia: Harper & Row, 1992;39:1–26.
4. Burnside B, Laties A. Actin filaments in apical projections of the primate pigmented epithelial cell. Invest Ophthalmol Vis Sci 1976;15:570–575.
5. Hogan MJ, Alvarado JA, et al. Histology of the Human Eye. Philadelphia: Saunders, 1971:405–421.
6. Spitznas M, Hogan MJ. Outer segments of photoreceptors and the retinal pigment epithelium. Inter-relationships in the human eye. Arch Ophthalmol 1970;84:810–619.
7. Johnson LV, Hageman GS, et al. Restricted Extracellular Matrix Domains Ensheath Cone Photoreceptors in Vertebrate Retina. In CDB Bridges, AJ Adler (eds), The Interphotoreceptor Matrix in Health and Disease. New York: Liss, 1985.
8. Johnson LV, Hageman GS, et al. Domains of photoreceptors matrix ensheath cone photoreceptors in vertebrate retina. Invest Ophthalmol Vis Sci 1986;27:129–135.
9. Hageman GS, Johnson LV. Biochemical characterization of the major peanut agglutinin-binding glycoproteins in vertebrate retinae: a species comparison. J Comp Neurol 1986;249:499–510.
10. Hollyfield JG, Rayborn ME, et al. Insoluble interphotoreceptor matrix domain surround rod photoreceptors in the human retina. Exp Res 1990;51:107–110.
11. Tien L, Rayborn ME, et al. Characterization of the interphotoreceptor matrix surrounding rod photoreceptors in the human retina. Exp Eye Res 1992;55:297–306.
12. Fariss RN, Anderson DH, et al. Comparison of photoreceptor-specific matrix domains in cat and monkey retinas. Exp Eye Res 1990;51:473–485.
13. Mieziewska KM, van Veen T, et al. Red and cone-specific domains in the interphotoreceptor matrix. J Comp Neurol 1991;308:371–380.
14. Hageman GS, Johnson LV. The cone matrix sheath: structural composition and functional analyses [abstract]. Invest Ophthalmol Vis Sci 1988;29(Suppl):108.
15. Hollyfield JG, Varner HH, et al. Retinal detachment to the pigment epithelium. Retina 1989;9:59–68.
16. Yao X-Y, Hageman GS, et al. Retinal adhesiveness is weakened by enzymatic modification of the interphotoreceptor matrix in vivo. Invest Ophthalmol Vis Sci 1990;31:2051–2058.
17. Yao X-Y, Hageman GS, et al. Recovery of retinal adhesion after enzymatic perturbation of the interphotoreceptor matrix. Invest Ophthalmol Vis Sci 1992;33:498–503
18. Hageman GS, Johnson LV. Structure, Composition and Function of the Retinal Interphotoreceptor Matrix. In N Osborne, G Chader (eds), Progress in Retinal Research. Oxford, England: Pergamon, 1991:207–249.
19. Hageman GS, Johnson LV. Molecular and structural organization of the extracellular matrix associated with primate cone photoreceptors [abstract]. J Cell Biol 1987;105:1656a.
20. Rayborn ME, Varner HH, et al. Analysis of the cone matrix sheath in the human retina using cupromeronic blue as a stain for proteoglycans [abstract]. Invest Ophthalmol Vis Sci 1988;29(Suppl):108.
21. Alpin JD, Hughs RC. Complex carbohydrates of the extracellular matrix: structures, interactions and biological roles. Biochem Biophys Acta 1982;694:375–418.
22. Hassell JR, Kimura JH, et al. Proteoglycan core protein families. Annu Rev Biochem 1986;55:539–567.
23. Fransson LA. Structure and function of cell-associated proteoglycans. Trends Biochem Sci 1987;12:406–411.
24. Ruoslahti E. Structure and biology of proteoglycans. Annu Rev Cell Biol 1988;4:229–255.
25. Kain HL. New model for examining choroidal adhesion experimentally. Arch Ophthalmol 1984;102:608–611.
26. Zauberman H, de Guillebon H. Retinal traction in vivo and post mortem. Arch Ophthalmol 1972;87:549–554.
27. Hageman GS, Marmor MF, et al. The interphotoreceptor matrix mediates primate retinal adhesion. Arch Ophthalmol 1995;113:655–660.
28. Bill A. Blood circulation and fluid dynamics in the eye. Physiol Rev 1975;55:383–417.
29. Frambach DA, Marmor MF. The rate and route of fluid from the subretinal space of the rabbit. Invest Ophthalmol Vis Sci 1982;22:292–302.
30. Hughes BA, Miller SS, et al. Effects of cyclic AMP on fluid absorption and ion transport across frog retinal pigment epithelium: Measurements in the open-circuit state. J Gen Physiol 1984;83:875–899.
31. Orr G, Goodnight R, et al. Relative permeability of retina and retinal pigment epithelium to diffusion of tritiated water from vitreous to choroid. Arch Ophthalmol 1986;104:1678–1680.
32. Fatt I, Shantinath K. Flow conductivity of retina and its role in retinal adhesion. Exp Eye Res 1971;12:218–226.
33. Marmor MF, Maack T. Local environment factors and retinal adhesion in the rabbit. Exp Eye Res 1982;34:727–733.
34. Marmor MF, Yao X-Y. The enhancement of retinal adhesiveness by quabain appears to involve cellular edema. Invest Ophthalmol Vis Sci 1989;30:1511–1514.

35. Marmor MF, Yao X-Y. The metabolic dependency of retinal adhesion in rabbit and primate. Arch Ophthalmol 1995;113:232–238.

36. Marmor MF, Abdul-Rahim AS, et al. The effect of metabolic inhibitors on retinal adhesion and subretinal fluid resorption. Invest Ophthalmol Vis Sci 1980;19:893–903.

37. Nigi A, Kawano SI, et al. Effects of intraocular pressure and other factors on subretinal fluid resorption. Invest Ophthalmol Vis Sci 1987;28:2099–2102.

38. Pederson JE, Cantrill HI, et al. Experimental retinal detachment. II. The role of the vitreous. Arch Ophthalmol 1982;100:1155–1159.

39. Williams GA, Aaberg TM Sr. Techniques of Scleral Buckling. In W Tasman, EA Jaeger (eds), Clinical Ophthalmology. Vol. 6. Philadelphia: Harper & Row, 1994;39:1–40.

40. Robertson DM. Retinal detachment with equatorial staphyloma. Arch Ophthalmol 1996;114:496–497.

41. Watzke RC. Scleral staphyloma and retinal detachment. Arch Ophthalmol 1963;70:796–804.

42. Faris B, Freeman HM, et al. Scleral dehiscence, anterior staphyloma, and retinal detachment. I. Incidence and pathogenesis. Trans Am Acad Ophthalmol Otolaryngol 1975;79:851–853.

43. Freeman HM, Schepens CL, et al. Scleral dehiscence, anterior staphyloma, and retinal detachment. II. Surgical management. Trans Am Acad Ophthalmol Otolaryngol 1975;79:854–857.

44. Lincoff H, Kreissig I. Management of Rhegmatogenous Retinal Detachment. In WR Freeman (ed), Practical Atlas of Retinal Diseases and Therapy. New York: Raven, 1993:221–235.

45. Balyeat RM. Complete retinal detachment (both eyes), with special reference to allergy as a possible primary etiologic factor. Am J Ophthalmol 1937;20:580–582.

46. Coles RS, Laval J. Retinal detachment occurring in cataract associated with neurodermatitis. Arch Ophthalmol 1952;48:30–39.

47. Garrity JA, Kuesegang TJ. Ocular complications of atopic dermatitis. Can J Ophthalmol 1984;19:21–24.

48. Katsura H, Hida T. Atopic dermatitis: Retinal detachment associated with atopic dermatitis. Retina 1984;4:148–151.

49. Danjo S, Morimoto K, et al. Ocular complications of atopic dermatitis. Jpn J Clin Ophthalmol 1989;43:715–718.

50. Nagansaki H, Ideta H, et al. Trauma-induced retinal detachment with atopic dermatitis. Jpn J Clin Ophthalmol 1989;43:725–728.

51. Oka C, Ideta H, et al. Retinal detachment with atopic dermatitis similar to traumatic retinal detachment. Ophthalmology 1994;101:1050–1054.

52. Katura H, Nomura M, et al. Clinical features of retinal detachment associated with atopic dermatitis. Floria Ophthalmol Jpn 1994;45:380–385.

53. Nakatsu A, Wada Y, et al. Retinal detachment in patients with atopic dermatitis. Ophthalmologica 1995;209:160–164.

54. Toshihito M, Fumio S, et al. Intraocular observation of the vitreous base in patients with atopic dermatitis and retinal detachment. Retina 1995;15:286–290.

55. Taylor B, Wadsworth M. Changes in the reported prevalence of childhood eczema since 1939–45 war. Lancet 1984;2:1255–1258.

56. Larsen FS, Holm NV, et al. Atopic dermatitis: A genetic-epidemiologic study in a population-based twin sample. J Am Acad Dermatol 1986;15:487–497.

57. Azuma N, Hida T, et al. Retrospective survey of surgical outcomes in rhegmatogenous retinal detachments associated with atopic dermatitis. Arch Ophthalmol 1996; 114:281–285.

58. Klemens F. Dermatose, kararact und ablatio retinae. Klin Monastbl Augenheilkd 1962;140:657–663.

59. Ingham RM. Retinal detachment associated with atopic dermatitis and cataract. Br J Ophthalmol 1965;49:96–97.

60. Lijima Y, Wagai K, et al. Retinal detachment with breaks in the pars plicata of the ciliary body. Am J Ophthalmol 1989;108:349–355.

61. Nishihara M, Kusaka S, et al. Retinal detachment due to a break of the ciliary body of an atopic dermatitis patient. Jpn J Clin Ophthalmol 1994;48:116–117.

62. Katsura H, Oda H, et al. Breaks in the pars plicata following surgery for atopic cataract. Ophthalmic Surg 1994; 25:514–515.

63. Kusaka S, Ohashi Y. Retinal detachments with crescent-shaped retinal breaks in patients with atopic dermatitis. Retina 1996;16:312–316.

64. Honda M, Kojima N, et al. A case of atopic dermatitis with retinal detachment and giant falciform tear. Jpn J Clin Ophthalmol 1985;39:1344–1345.

65. Nakai Y, Kitaooji H, et al. A case of atopic dermatitis with retinal detachment and deep retinal break. Jpn J Clin Ophthalmol 1993;47:748–749.

66. Kawahima S, Yano K, et al. A case of retinal detachment with an irregular retinal break. Nihon No Ganka 1987;58:823–827.

67. Mylius K. Doppelseitige spontane Netzhautabloesung bei 2 jungendichen, seit jahren an Neurodermatitis dissemiata leidnden Patienten. Klin Monastbl Augenheilkd 1949;115:247–250.

68. Matsuo T, Shiraga F, et al. Intraoperative observation of the vitreous base in patients with atopic dermatitis and retinal detachment. Retina 1995;15:286–290.

69. Matsuo N, Matsuo T, et al. Photoreceptor outer segments in the aqueous humor of patients with atopic dermatitis and retinal detachment. Am J Ophthalmol 1993;115:21–25.

70. Cordes FC, Cordero-Moreno R. Atopic cataracts: Report of four cases. Am J Ophthalmol 1946;29:402–407.

71. Bohringer Von HR. Staistisches zu haufigkeit und risiko der netzhautablosung. Ophthalmol 1951;131:331–334.

72. Haimann MH, Burton TC, Brown CK, Epidemiology of retinal detachment. Arch Ophthalmol 1982 100;282–292.

73. Haut J, Massin M. Frequency of incidence of retina detachment in the French population: Percentage of bilateral detachment. Arch Ophtalmol 1975;35:533–536.

74. Paufique L. The present status of the treatment of retinal detachment. Trans Ophthalmol Soc UK 1959;69:221–248.

75. Stein R, Feller-Ofry V, Romano A. The Effect of Treatment in the Prevention of Retinal Detachment. In IC Michaelson, ER Berman (eds), Causes and Prevention of Blindness. New York: Academy, 1972:409–410.

76. Wilkes SR, Beard CM, Kurland LT, et al. The incidence of retinal detachment in Rochester, Minnesota, 1970–1978. Am J Ophthalmol 1982;94:670–673.

77. Phelps CD, Burton TC. Glaucoma and retinal detachment. Arch Ophthalmol 1977;95:418–422.

78. Michaelson IC, Stein R. A study in the prevention of retinal detachment. Ann Ophthalmol 1963;1:49–55.

79. Straatsma BR, Foos RY, Feman SS. Degenerative Diseases of the Peripheral Retina. In TD Duane, EA Jaeger (eds), Clinical Ophthalmology. Vol. 3. Philadelphia: Harper & Row, 1980:1–29.

80. Schepens CL, Marden D. Data on the natural history of retinal detachment. I. Age and sex relationship. Arch Ophthalmol 1961;66:631–644.

81. Schepens CL, Marden D. Data on the natural history of retinal detachment. Further characterization of certain unilateral nontraumatic cases. Am J Ophthalmol 1966; 61:213–226.

82. Laatikainen L, Harju H. Bilateral rhegmatogenous retinal detachment. Acta Ophthalmologica 1985;63:541–545.

83. Laatikainen L, Tolppanen EM. Characteristics of rhegmatogenous retinal detachment. Acta Ophthalmologica 1985;63:146–154.

84. Haimann NH, Burton TC, et al. Epidemiology of retinal detachment. Arch Ophthalmol 1982;100:289–292.

85. Lewis H, Kreiger AE. Rhegmatogenous Retinal Detachment. In TD Duane, EA Jaeger (eds), Clinical Ophthalmology. Vol. 3. Philadelphia: Harper & Row, 1993:1–12.

86. Laatikainen L, Tolppanen EM, et al. Epidemiology of rhegmatogenous retinal detachment in a Finnish population. Acta Ophthalmologica 1985;63:59–64.

87. Okun E. Gross and microscopic pathology in autopsy eyes. Part III. Retinal breaks without detachment. Am J Ophthalmol 1961;51:369–391.

88. Tasman W. Retinal detachment in children. Trans Am Acad Ophthalmol Otolaryngol 1967;71:455–460.

89. Ashrafzadeh MT, Schepens CL, et al. Aphakic and phakic retinal detachment. Arch Ophthalmol 1973;89:476–483.

90. Everett WG, Katzin D. Meridional distribution of retinal breaks in aphakic detachments. Am J Ophthalmol 1968;66:928–932.

91. Schepens CL, Marden D. Data on the natural history of retinal detachment: Further characterization of certain unilateral cases. Am J Ophthalmol 1966;61:213–226.

92. Schepens CL. Retinal Detachment and Allied Diseases. Philadelphia: Saunders, 1983.

93. Foos RY, Wheeler NC. Vitreoretinal juncture: Synchysis senilis and posterior vitreous detachment. Ophthalmology 1982;89:1502–1512.

94. Brown PR, Thomas RD. The incidence of primary retinal detachment in the Negro. Am J Ophthalmol 1965;60:109–110.

95. Weiss H, Tasman WS. Rhegmatogenous retinal detachment in blacks. Ann Ophthalmol 1978;10:799–806.

96. Yanoff M, Fine SF. Ocular Pathology (2nd ed). Philadelphia: Harper & Row, 1982:461,563.

97. Laatikaimen L. The fellow eye in patients with unilateral retinal detachment: Findings and prophylactic treatment. Acta Ophthalmologica 1985;63:546–551.

98. Curtin BJ. The Myopias: Basic Science and Clinical Management. Philadelphia: Harper & Row, 1985:337.

99. Morita H, Funata M, et al. A clinical study of the development of posterior vitreous detachment in myopia. Retina 1995;15:117–124.

100. Pierro I, Camesasa FI, et al. Peripheral retinal changes and axial myopia. Retina 1992;12:12–17.

101. Hogan MJ, Alvarado JA, Weddell JE. Histology of the Human Eye: An Atlas and Textbook. Philadelphia: Saunders, 1971:607–637.

102. Ruben M, Rajpurohit P. Distribution of myopia in aphakic retinal detachments. Br J Ophthalmol 1976;60:517–521.

103. Constable IJ, Tolentino FI, et al. Clinico-Pathologic Correlations of Vitreous Membranes. In RC Pruett, CDJ Regan (eds), Retina Congress. New York: Appleton-Century-Croft, 1974:245–257.

104. Neumann E, Hyams S. Conservative management of retinal breaks: A follow–up study of subsequent retinal detachment. Br J Ophthalmol 1972;56:482–486.

105. Hyams SW, Neumann E, Friedman Z. Myopia-aphakia. II. Vitreous and peripheral retina. Br J Ophthalmol 1975; 59:483–485.

106. Neumann E. The Natural History of Retinal Holes with Specific Reference to the Development of Retinal Detachment and the Time Factor Involved. In IC Michaelson, ER Berman (eds), Causes and Prevention of Blindness. New York: Academic, 1972:404–408.

107. Meyer-Schwickerath G, Gerke E. Biometric studies of the eyeball and retinal detachment. Br J Ophthalmol 1984; 68:29–31.

108. Akiba J. Prevalence of posterior vitreous detachment in high myopia. 1993;100:1384–1388.

109. Rieger H. Uber die bedeutug der aderhautveranderungen fur die entstehung der glaskorperabhebung. Graefes Arch Clin Exp Ophthalmol 1937;136:118–165.

110. Singh A, Paul SD, et al. A clinical study of vitreous body (emmetropia and refractive errors). Orient Arch Ophthalmol 1970;8:11–17.

111. Lindner B. Acute posterior vitreous detachment and its retinal complications: a clinical biomicroscopic study. Acta Ophthalmol Scand Suppl 1966;87:1–108.

112. Jaffe NS. Complications of acute posterior vitreous detachment. Arch Ophthalmol 1968;79:368–371.

113. Byer NE. Natural history of posterior vitreous detachment with early management as the premier line of defense against retinal detachment. Ophthalmology 1994;101: 1503–1514.

114. Tasman WE. Posterior vitreous detachment and peripheral retinal breaks. Trans Am Acad Ophthalmol Otolaryngol 1968;72:217–224.

115. Novak MA, Welch RB. Complications of acute symptomatic posterior vitreous detachment. Am J Ophthalmol 1984;97:308–314.

116. Rodrigues A, Gutierrez E, et al. Complications of clear lens extraction in axial myopia. Arch Ophthalmol 1987;105: 1522–1523.

117. Rodrigues A, Rodriquez FM, et al. Retinal Detachment, Giant Tears and PVR in Clear Lens Extraction for Axial Myopia. In K Heimann, P Wiedelmann (eds), Proliferative Vitreoretinopathy. Heidelberg, Germany: Kaden, 1989: 29–31.

118. Stirpe M, Michels R. Retinal Detachment After Removal of the Clear Crystalline Lens to Treat Axial Myopia. In AE Maumenee, WJ Stark, I Esente (eds), Cataract and Refractive Microsurgery. Milan: Fogliazza, 1989:321–323.

119. Barraquer C, Cavelier C, et al. Incidence of retinal detachment following clear-lens extraction in myopic patients. Arch Ophthalmol 1994;112:3336–3339.

120. Ripandelli G, Billi B, et al. Retinal detachment after clear lens extraction in 41 eyes with high axial myopia. Retina 1996;16:3–6.

121. Colin J, Robinet A. Clear lensectomy and implantation of low powered posterior chamber intraocular lenses for the correction of high myopia. Ophthalmology 1994;101: 107–112.

122. Buratto L. Considerations on clear lens extraction in high myopia. Eur J Implant Refract Surg 1991;3:221–226.

123. Verzella F. Microsurgery of the lens in high myopia for optical purposes. Cataract 1984;1:8–12.

124. Verzella F. High myopia in the bag refractive implantation. Ophthalmic Forum 1985;3:174–175.

125. Bonnet M, Aracil P, et al. Rhegmatogenous retinal detachment after prophylactic argon laser photocoagulation. Graefes Arch Clin Exp Ophthalmol 1987;225:5–8.

126. Byer NE. Rethinking Prophylactic Treatment of Retinal Detachment. In M Stirpe (ed), Advances in Vitreoretinal Surgery. New York: Ophthalmic Communications Society, 1992:399–411.

127. Stirpe M, Michaels M, et al. Retinal detachment in highly myopic eyes due to macular holes and epiretinal traction. Retina 1990;10:113–114.

128. Stripe M, Varano M, et al. Firm Adhesions Between Cortical Vitreous and Posterior Retina in Highly Myopic Eyes. In M Stirpe (ed), Advances in Vitreoretinal Surgery. New York: Ophthalmic Communications Society, 1992: 129–133.

129. Norton EWD. Retinal detachment in aphakia. Am J Ophthalmol 1964;58:111–124.

130. Scheie HG, Morse PH, Aminlari A. Incidence of retinal detachment following cataract extraction. Arch Ophthalmol 1973;89:293–295.

131. Smith PW, Stark WJ, et al. Retinal detachment after extracapsular cataract extraction with posterior chamber intraocular lens. Ophthalmology 1987;94:495–503.

132. Javitt JC, Vitale S, Canner JK, et al. National outcomes of cataract extraction. I. Retinal detachment after inpatient surgery. Ophthalmology 1991;98:895–902.

133. Ober RR, Wilkinson CR, Fiore JV, et al. Rhegmatogenous retinal detachment after neodymium-YAG laser capsulotomy in aphakic and pseudophakic eyes. Am J Ophthalmol 1986;101:1396–1402.

134. Koch DD, Liu JF, Gill EP, et al. Axial myopia increases the risk of retinal complications after neodymium–YAG posterior capsulotomy. Arch Ophthalmol 1989;107:986–990.

135. Haimann MH, Burton TC, Brown CK. Epidemiology of retinal detachment. Arch Ophthalmol 1982;100:289–292.

136. Hager WS. Pseudophakic retinal detachment. Trans Am Ophthalmol Soc 1982;80:45–59.

137. Schachat A, Beauchamp G, et al. Retinal Detachment: Preferred Practice Pattern. San Francisco: American Academy of Ophthalmology, 1990.

138. Vail D. After-results of vitreous loss. Am J Ophthalmol 1965;59:573–586.

139. Barraquer K. Surgery of the Anterior Segment of the Eye. Vol. 1. New York: McGraw-Hill, 1964:289.

140. Lusky M, Weinberger D, et al. The prevalence of retinal detachment in aphakic high myopic patients. Ophthalmic Surgery 1987;18.444–445.

141. Stein R, Pinchas A, et al. Prevention of retinal detachment by circumferential barrage prior to lens extraction in highly myopic eyes. Ophthalmologica 1972;165:125–136.

142. Ruben M, Rajpurohit P. Distribution of myopia in aphakic retinal detachment. Br J Ophthalmol 1976;60:517–521.

143. Hyams SW, Bialik M, et al. Myopia-aphakia. I. Prevalence of retinal detachment. Br J Ophthalmol 1975;59:480–482.

144. Jaffe N. Retinal Detachment in Aphakia. In EA Klein (ed), Cataract Surgery and Its Complications (5th ed). St. Louis: Mosby, 1990:653–665.

145. Griffith RD, Ryan EA, et al. Primary retinal detachments without apparent breaks. Am J Ophthalmol 1976;81: 420–427.

146. Ackerman AL, Seelenfreund MH, et al. Cataract extraction following retinal detachment surgery. Arch Ophthalmol 1970;84:41–44.

147. Greven CM, Sanders RJ, et al. Pseudophakic retinal detachment: Anatomic and visual results. Ophthalmology 1992;99:257–262.

148. Heller MD, Straatsma BR, et al. Detachment of the posterior vitreous in phakic and aphakic eyes. Mod Probl Ophthalmol 1972;10:23–26.

149. McDonald PJ, Green WR. Comparison of intracapsular and extracapsular cataract surgery: Histopathologic studies of eyes obtained post mortem. Ophthalmology 1985; 92:1208–1223.

150. Osterlin S. Vitreous Changes after Cataract Extraction. In HM Freeman, T Hirose, CL Schepens (eds), Vitreous Surgery and Advances in Fundus Diagnosis and Treatment. Boston: Appleton-Century-Croft, 1975:15–21.

151. Kangro M, Osterlin S. Hyaluronic concentration in the pseudophakic eye. ARVO abstracts, 1985:28.

152. Friedman Z, Newman E. Posterior vitreous detachment after cataract extraction in non-myopic eyes and the resultant retinal lesions. Br J Ophthalmol 1975;59:451–454.

153. Jaffe NS, Light DS. Vitreous changes produced by cataract surgery. A study of 1058 aphakic eyes. Arch Ophthalmol 1966;76:541–553.

154. Bradford JD, Wilkinson CP. Pseudophakic retinal detachment. The relationships between retinal tears and the time following cataract surgery at which they occur. Retina 1989;9:181–186.

155. Wilkinson CP. Phakic retinal detachments in the elderly. Retina 1995;15:220–223.

156. Davis MD, Segal PP, et al. A Natural Course Followed by the Fellow Eye in Patients with Rhegmatogenous Retinal Detachment. In RC Pruett, CDJ Regan (eds), Retina Congress. New York: Appleton-Century-Croft, 1972: 643–600.

157. Hovland KR. Vitreous findings in the fellow eyes of aphakic retinal detachment. Am J Ophthalmol 1978;86:350–353.

158. Smith RT, Moscoso WE, et al. The barrier function in neodymium–YAG laser capsulotomy. Arch Ophthalmol 1995;113:645–652.

159. Clayman HM, Jaffe NS, et al. Intraocular lenses, axial length, and retinal detachment. Am J Ophthalmol 1981; 92:778–780.

160. Coonan P, Fung WE, et al. The incidence of retinal detachment following extracapsular cataract extraction: A ten-year study. Ophthalmology 1985;92:1096–1101.

161. Percival SPB, Anand V, Das DK. Prevalence of aphakic retinal detachment. Br J Ophthalmol 1983;67:43–45.

162. Seward HC, Doran RML. Posterior capsulotomy and retinal detachment following extracapsular lens surgery. Br J Ophthalmol 1984;68:379–382.

163. Smith PW, Stark WJ, et al. Retinal detachment after extracapsular cataract extraction with posterior chamber intraocular lens. Ophthalmology 1987;94:495–504.

164. Little J. Discussion: Aphakia and retinal detachment. In J Emery (ed), Current Concepts in Cataract Surgery: Selected Proceedings of the Fourth Biennial Cataract Congress. St. Louis: Mosby, 1976:345.

165. Shafer DN. Symposium: Phacoemulsification. Retinal detachment after phacoemulsification. Trans Am Acad Ophthalmol Otolaryngol 1974;78:28.

166. McPherson AR, O'Malley RE, Bravo J. Retinal detachment following late posterior capsulotomy. Am J Ophthalmol 1983;95:593–597.

167. Troutman RC. Cataract survey of the cataract phacoemulsification committee. Trans Am Acad Ophthalmol Otolaryngol 1975;79:178–185.

168. Ninn-Pedersen K, Bauer B. Cataract patients in defined Swedish population, 1985 to 1990. Arch Ophthalmol 1996;114:382.

169. Watzke RC. Retinal detachment following phacoemulsification [letter]. Ophthalmology 1978;85:546–547.

170. Wilkinson CP, Anderson LS, Little JH. Retinal detachment following phacoemulsification. Ophthalmology 1978;85: 151–156.

171. Goldberg MF. Clear lens extraction for axial myopia. Ophthalmology 1987;94:571–582.

172. Rickman-Barger L, Florine C, et al. Retinal detachment

after neodymium-YAG laser posterior capsulotomy. Am J Ophthalmol 1989;101:531–543.

173. Cox MS, Freeman HM. Retinal detachment due to ocular penetration. I. Clinical characteristics and surgical results. Arch Ophthalmol 1978;96:1354–1361.

174. Jaffe N, Clayman H, et al. Retinal detachment in myopic eyes after intracapsular and extracapsular cataract extraction. Am J Ophthalmol 1984;97:48–52.

175. Liesegang TJ, Bourne WM, et al. Secondary surgical and neodymium-YAG laser discussions. Am J Ophthalmol 1985;100:510–519.

176. Winslow RL, Taylor BC. Retinal complications following YAG laser capsulotomy. Ophthalmology 1985;92:785–789.

177. Lindstrom L, Lindquist TD, et al. Retinal Detachment in Axial Myopia Following Extracapsular Cataract Surgery. In DR Caldwell (ed), Cataracts: Transactions of the New Orleans Academy of Ophthalmology. New York: Raven, 1988:146–148.

178. Chambless WS. Incidence of anterior and posterior segment complications in over 3000 cases of extracapsular cataract extractions: Intact and open capsules. J Am Intraocular Implant Soc J 1985;11:146–148.

179. Leff SR, Welch JC, et al. Rhegmatogenous retinal detachment after YAG laser posterior capsulotomy. Ophthalmology 1987;94:1222–1225.

180. O'Donald FE. Alleged link between PRK and retinal detachment dismissed by ophthalmologist. Ocular Surgical News 1996;14:46–47.

181. Irvine A. The pathogenesis of aphakic retinal detachment. Ophthalmic Surg 1985;16:101–107.

182. Wilkinson CP. Pseudophakic retinal detachment. Retina 1985;5:1–4.

183. Hawkins WR. Aphakic retinal detachment. Ophthalmic Surg 1975;6:66–74.

184. Wilkinson CP. Retinal detachments following intraocular lens implantation. Ophthalmology 1981;88:410–413.

185. Cousins S, Boniuk I, et al. Pseudophakic retinal detachments in the presence of various IOL types. Ophthalmology 1986;93:1198–1207.

186. Ramsey RC, Cantrill HI, et al. Pseudophakic retinal detachment. Can J Ophthalmol 1983;18:262–265.

187. Stark WJ, Terry AC, et al. Intraocular Lenses: Changing Indications. In WJ Stark, WJ Terry, AE Maumenee (eds), Anterior Segment Surgery. Baltimore: Williams & Wilkins, 1987:69–76.

188. Chrousos GA, Parks MM, et al. Incidence of chronic retinal detachment and secondary membrane surgery in pediatric aphakic patients. Ophthalmology 1984;91:1238–1241.

189. Toyofuku H, Hirose T, et al. Retinal detachment following congenital cataract surgery. Arch Ophthalmol 1980;98:669–675.

190. Jagger JD, Cooling RJ, et al. Management of retinal detachment following congenital cataract surgery. Trans Ophthalmol Soc UK 1983;103:103–107.

191. Cox MS, Schepens CL, et al. Retinal detachment due to ocular contusion. Arch Ophthalmol 1966;76:678–685.

192. Ross WH. Traumatic retinal dialyses. Arch Ophthalmol 1981;99:1371–1374.

193. Maguire JL, Benson WE. Retinal injury and detachment in boxers. JAMA 1986;255:2451–2453.

194. Freeman HM, Cox MS, Schepens CL. Traumatic retinal detachments. Int Ophthalmol Clin 1974;14:151–170.

195. Sellors PJ, Mooney D. Fundus changes after traumatic hyphemas. Fr J Ophthalmol 1973;57:600–607.

196. Tasman W. Peripheral retinal changes following blunt trauma. Trans Am Ophthalmol Soc 1972;70:190–198.

197. Hagler WS, North AW. Retinal dialyses and retinal detachment. Arch Ophthalmol 1968;79:376–388.

198. Wilhelm JL, Zakov ZN, et al. Erythropheresis in treating retinal detachments secondary to sickle-cell retinopathy. Am J Ophthalmol 1981;92:582–583.

199. Benson WE (ed). Retinal Detachment: Diagnosis and Management. New York: Lippincott, 1987.

200. Doden W, Stark N. Retina and vitreous findings after serious indirect eye trauma. Klin Monatsbl Augenheilkd 1974;32:32–40.

201. Mieler WF, Sumit K, et al. Golf-related ocular injuries. Arch Ophthalmol 1995;113:1410–1413.

202. Percival SPB. Late complications from posterior segment intraocular foreign bodies. Br J Ophthalmol 1972;56:462–468.

203. Labelle P, Brunet M, et al. Retinal detachment following intraocular foreign body. Can J Ophthalmol 1974;9:2–8.

204. Benson WE, Machemer R. Severe perforating injuries treated with pars plana vitrectomy. Am J Ophthalmol 1976;81:728–732.

205. Becker B. In discussion: Smith JL. Retinal detachment and glaucoma. Trans Am Acad Ophthalmol Otolaryngol 1963;67:731–732.

206. Kolker AE, Hetherington J Jr. Becker-Shaffer's Diagnosis and Therapy of the Glaucomas (3rd ed). St. Louis: Mosby, 1970:246–248.

207. Phelps CD, Burton TC. Glaucoma and retinal detachment. Arch Ophthalmol 1977;95:418–422.

208. Phelps CD. Glaucoma Associated with Retinal Disorders. In R Ritch, MB Shields (eds), The Secondary Glaucomas. St. Louis: Mosby, 1982:150–161.

209. Ackerman AL. Retinal Detachments and Miotic Therapy. In RC Pruett, CDJ Regan (eds), Retina Congress. New York: Appleton-Century-Croft, 1972:533–539.

210. Alpar JJ. Miotics and retinal detachment: A survey and case report. Ann Ophthalmol 1979;35:395–401.

211. Beasley H, Fraunfelder FT. Retinal detachments and ocular miotics. 1979;86:95–98.

212. Freilich DB, Seelenfreund MH. Miotic drugs, glaucoma and retinal detachment. Mod Probl Ophthalmol 1975;15:318–322.

213. Heimann K, Kyrieleis E. Retinal detachment during therapy with miotics. Klin Monatsbl Augenheilkd 1970;156:98–104.

214. Kraushar MF, Podell DL. "Miotic-Induced" Retinal Detachment. In RC Pruett, CDJ Regan (eds), Retina Congress. New York: Appleton-Century-Croft, 1972:541–545.

215. Pape LG, Forbes M. Retinal detachment and miotic therapy. Am J Ophthalmol 1978;85:558–566.

216. Pemberton JW, Freeman HM, et al. Familial retinal detachment and the Ehlers-Danlos Syndrome. Arch Ophthalmol 1966;76:817–824.

217. Cooling RJ, Rice NSC, et al. Retinal detachment in congenital glaucoma. Br J Ophthalmol 1980;64:417–421.

218. Winslow R, Tasman W. Juvenile retinal detachment. Int Ophthalmol Clin 1976;16:97–105.

219. Davis MD. Natural history of retinal breaks without detachment. Arch Ophthalmol 1974;92:183–194.

220. Delaney WV Jr, Oates RP. Retinal detachment in the second eye. Arch Ophthalmol 1978;96:629–634.

221. Folk JC, Burton TC. Bilateral phakic retinal detachment. Ophthalmology 1981;89:815–820.

222. Merin S, Feiler V, et al. The fate of the fellow eye in retinal detachment. Am J Ophthalmol 1971;71:477–481.

223. Tornquist R. Bilateral retinal detachment. Acta Ophthalmol Scand Suppl 1963;41:126–133

224. Sigelman H. Vitreous base classification of retinal tears: Clinical application. Surv Ophthalmol 1980;25:59–70.

225. Robertson DM, Priluck IA. 360-degree prophylactic cryoretinopexy: A clinical and experimental study. Arch Ophthalmol 1979;97:2130–2134.

226. Dollfus M. Le traitement preventif du decollement de la retine. XVIII Concilium Ophthalmologicum. Bruxelles: Imprimerie Medicale et Scientifique 1958:988–989.

227. Meyer-Schwickerath G, Fried M. Prophylaxis of retinal detachment. Trans Ophthalmol Soc UK 1980;100:56–65.

228. Hyams SW, Meir E, et al. Chorioretinal lesions predisposing to retinal detachment. Am J Ophthalmol 1974, 78:429–437.

229. Folk JC, Arrindell EL, Klugman MR. The fellow eye of patients with phakic lattice retinal detachment. Ophthalmology 1989;96:72–79.

230. Morse PH, Sheie HG. Prophylactic cryoretinopexy of retinal breaks. Arch Ophthalmol 1974;77:619–649.

231. Colyear BHJ, Pischell DK. Preventative treatment of retinal detachment by means of light coagulation. Trans Pacific Coast Otolaryngol Ophthalmol Soc 1960;41:193–217.

232. Pollak A, Oliver M. Argon laser photocoagulation of symptomatic flap tears and retinal breaks of fellow eyes. Br J Ophthalmol 1981;65:469–472.

233. Okun E, Cibis PA. Photocoagulation in "Limited" Retinal Detachments and Breaks Without Detachment. In A McPherson (ed), New and Controversial Aspects of Retinal Detachment. International Symposium, Proceedings. New York: Harper & Row; 1968:164–171.

234. Michels RG, Wilkinson CP, Rice TA. Retinal Detachment: Diagnosis and Management. St. Louis: Mosby, 1990.

235. Benson WE, Grand MG, Okun E. Aphakic retinal detachment. Arch Ophthalmol 1975;93:245–249.

236. Campbell CJ, Rittler MC. Cataract extraction in the retinal detachment-prone patient. Am J Ophthalmol 1972;73:17–24.

237. Tournquist R, Stenkula S, et al. Retinal detachment: A study of a population-based patient material in Sweden. Acta Ophthalmologica 1987;65:213–222.

238. McPherson A, O'Malley R, Beltangady SS. Management of the fellow eyes of patients with rhegmatogenous retinal detachment. Ophthalmology 1981;88:922–934.

239. Govan JAA. Prophylactic circumferential cryopexy: A retrospective study of 106 eyes. Br J Ophthalmol 1981;65:364–370.

240. Roseman RL, Olk RJ, et al. Limited retinal detachment: A retrospective analysis of treatment with transconjunctival retinocryopexy. Ophthalmology 1986;93:216–223.

241. Kaufman PL, Podos SM. The subretinal fluid in primary rhegmatogenous retinal detachments. Surv Ophthalmol 1973;18:100–116.

242. Toris CB, Pederson JE. Experimental retinal detachment. VII. Intravitreous horseradish peroxidase diffusion across the blood–retinal barrier. Arch Ophthalmol 1985;102:752–756.

243. Toris CB, Pederson JE. Experimental retinal detachment. VIII. Retinochoroidal horseradish peroxidase diffusion across the blood–retinal barrier. Arch Ophthalmol 1985;103:266–269.

244. Godtfredsen E. Investigations into hyaluronic acid and hyaluronidase in the subretinal fluid in retinal detachment, partly due to ruptures and partly secondary to malignant choroidal melanoma. Br J Ophthalmol 1949;33:721–732.

245. Rosen E. A photographic investigation of simple retinal detachment. Trans Ophthalmol Soc UK 1968;88:331–342.

246. Negi A, Marmor MF. Effects of subretinal and systemic osmolarity on the rate of subretinal fluid absorption. Invest Ophthalmol Vis Sci 1984;25:616–620.

247. Negi A, Marmor MF. Mechanisms of subretinal fluid resorption in the cat eye. Invest Ophthalmol Vis Sci 1986;27:1560–1568.

248. Hamilton AM, Taylor W. Significance of pigment granules in the vitreous. Br J Ophthalmol 1972;56:700–702.

249. Shafer DM. Comment. In CL Schepens, CDJ Regan (eds), Controversial Aspects of the Management of Retinal Detachment. Boston: Little, Brown, 1965:51.

250. Stratford T. Comment. In CL Schepens, CDJ Regan (eds), Controversial Aspects of the Management of Retinal Detachment. Boston: Little, Brown, 1965:51.

251. Machemer R. Massive periretinal proliferation: A logical approach to therapy. Trans Am Ophthalmol Soc 1977;75:556–586.

252. Dana MR, Werner MS, et al. Spontaneous and traumatic vitreous hemorrhage. Ophthalmology 1993;100:1377–1383.

253. Lagua H, Machemer R. Clinical-pathological correlation in massive periretinal proliferation. Am J Ophthalmol 1975;80:913–929.

254. Machemer R, Norton EWD. Experimental retinal detachment in the owl monkey. I. Methods of production and clinical picture. Am J Ophthalmol 1968;66:388–396.

255. Machemer R. Experimental retinal detachment in the owl monkey. II. Histology of the retina and pigment epithelium. Am J Ophthalmol 1968;66:396–410.

256. von Pirquet SR, Jaugschaffer O. Treatment of Macular Holes by Photocoagulation. In CL Schepens, CDJ Regan (eds), Controversial Aspects of the Management of Retinal Detachment. Boston: Little, Brown, 1966:181.

257. Dobbie JG. A study of intraocular fluid dynamics in retinal detachment. Arch Ophthalmol 1963;69:159–164.

258. Langham ME, Regan CDJ. Circulation changes associated with the onset of primary retinal detachment. Arch Ophthalmol 1969;81:820–829.

259. Steinert RF, Puliafito, et al. Cystoid macular edema, retinal detachment, and glaucoma after Nd-YAG laser posterior capsulotomy. Arch Ophthalmol 1991;112:373–380.

260. Pederson JE, Cantrill HL. Experimental retinal detachment. V. Fluid movement through the retinal hole. Arch Ophthalmol 1984;102:136–139.

261. Pederson JE. Experimental retinal detachment. IV. Aqueous humor dynamics in rhegmatogenous detachment. Arch Ophthalmol 1982;100:1814–1816.

262. Tsuboi S, Noie-Taki J, et al. Fluid dynamics in the eye with rhegmatogenous retinal detachment. Am J Ophthalmol 1985;99:673–676.

263. Tsuboi S, Pederson JE. Permeability of the blood-retinal barrier to carboxy fluorescein in eyes with rhegmatogenous retinal detachment. Invest Ophthalmol Vis Sci 1987;28:96–100.

264. van Heuven WAJ, Lam K-W, et al. Source of subretinal fluid on the basis of ascorbate analyses. Arch Ophthalmol 1982;100:976–978.

265. O'Connor PR. External buckling without drainage for selected detachments in aphakic eyes. Am J Ophthalmol 1976;82:358–364.

266. Ramsay RC, Cantrill HL, Knobloch WH. Pseudophakic retinal detachment. Can J Ophthalmol 1983;18:262–265.

267. Siegelman J. Vitreous base classification of retinal tears: Clinical application. Surv Ophthalmol 1980;25:59–70.

268. Amsler M, Schiff-Wertheimer S. In P Bailliart (ed), Le decollement de la retinae in traite de ophthalmologie. Vol. 5. Paris: Masson, 1939:559–576.

269. Byer NE. The natural history of the retinopathies of retinal detachment and preventive treatment. Isr J Med Sci 1972;8:1417–1420.

270. Straatsma BR, Allen RA. Lattice degeneration of the retina. Trans Am Acad Ophthalmol Otolaryngol 1962;66:600–613.

271. Pischel DK. Retinal detachment: A manual. Am Acad Ophthalmol Otolaryngol 1965;1085:197–199.

272. Byer NE. Lattice degeneration of the retina. Surv Ophthalmol 1979;23:213–248.

273. Byer NE. Changes in and prognosis of lattice degeneration of the retina. Trans Am Acad Ophthalmol Otolaryngol 1974;78:114–125.

274. Benson WE, Morse PH. The prognosis of retinal detachment due to lattice degeneration. Ann Ophthalmol 1978;10:1197–1200.

275. Tillery WV, Lucier AC. Round atrophic holes in lattice degeneration—an important cause of aphakic retinal detachment. Trans Am Acad Ophthalmol Otolaryngol 1976;81:509–518.

276. Tasman W. Retinal detachment secondary to proliferative diabetic retinopathy. Arch Ophthalmol 1972;87:286–289.

277. Gutman FA, Ryan EA, et al. The natural course of temporal branch retinal vein occlusion. Trans Am Acad Ophthalmol Otolaryngol 1974;78:178–192.

278. Joondeph HC, Goldberg MF. Rhegmatogenous retinal detachment after tributary vein occlusion. Am J Ophthalmol 1975;80:253–257.

279. Regenbogen L, Godel V, et al. Retinal breaks secondary to vascular accidents. Am J Ophthalmol 1977;84:187–196.

280. Zauberman H. Retinopathy of retinal detachment after major vascular occlusion. Br J Ophthalmol 1968;52:117–121.

281. Nelsen PT, Marcus DA, et al. Retinal detachment following endophthalmitis. Ophthalmology 1985;92:1112–1117.

282. Clarkson JG, Blumenkrans MS, et al. Retinal detachment following the acute retinal necrosis syndrome. Ophthalmology 1984;91:1165–1668.

283. Culbertson WW, Blumenkrans MS, et al. The acute retinal necrosis syndrome. Part 2. Histopathology and etiology. Ophthalmology 1982;89:1317–1325.

284. Fisher JP, Lewis ML, et al. The acute retinal necrosis syndrome. Part 1. Clinical manifestations. Ophthalmology 1982;89:1309–1312.

285. Kreiger AE. Discussion of Clarkson JG, Blumenkrans MS, Culbertson WW, et al. Retinal detachment following the acute retinal necrosis syndrome. Ophthalmology 1984;91:1665–1668.

286. Jabs DA, Enger C, et al. Retinal detachments in patients with cytomegalic retinitis. Arch Ophthalmol 1911;109:794–799.

287. Freeman WR, Qicerno JI, et al. Surgical repair of rhegmatogenous retinal detachment with cytomegalic retinitis. Ophthalmology 1992; 99:466–474.

288. Kupperman BD, Flores-Aguilar M, et al. A masked prospective evaluation of outcome parameters for cytomegalovirus-related retinal detachment surgery in patients with acquired immune deficiency syndrome. Ophthalmology 1994;101:46–55.

289. Lim JI, Enger C, et al. Improved visual results after surgical repair of cytomegalovirus-related retinal detachment. Ophthalmology 1994;101:264–269.

290. Studies of Ocular Complications of AIDS Research Group. Foscarnet-Ganciclovir Retinitis Trial, 4: Visual outcomes. Ophthalmology 1994;101:1250–1261.

291. Matsuo T, Morimoto K, et al. Factors associated with poor visual outcome in acute retinal necrosis. Br J Ophthalmol 1991;75:450–454.

292. Clarkson JG, Blumenkranz MS, et al. Retinal detachment following the acute retinal necrosis syndrome. Ophthalmology 1984;91:1665–1668.

293. Engstrom RE, Holland GN, et al. The progressive outer retinal necrosis syndrome: A variant of necrotizing herpetic retinopathy in patients with AIDS. Am J Ophthalmol 1994;101:1488–1502.

294. Axer-Siegel R, Weinberger D. Retinal detachment after noncontact pneumatic tonometry. Retina 1996;16:80–81.

295. Brod RD, Flynn HW Jr, et al. Asymptomatic rhegmatogenous retinal detachments. Arch Ophthalmol 1995;113:1030–1032.

296. Jarrett WH. Retinal detachment. Trans Am Ophthalmol Soc 1988;86:307–320.

297. Benson WE, Pornsawat N, et al. Characteristics and prognosis of retinal detachments with demarcation line. Am J Ophthalmol 1977;84:641–644.

298. Byer NE. The long-term natural history of lattice degeneration of the retina. Ophthalmology 1989;96:1396–1402

299. Jones WL. Intraocular metastatic disease to the eye. J Am Optom Assoc 1981;52:741–744.

300. Pederson JE. Experimental retinal detachment. I. The effect of subretinal fluid composition on reabsorption rate and intraocular pressure. Arch Ophthalmol 1982;100:1150–1154.

301. Riss B, Skorpik C, et al. Severe changes in the fundus oculi in pregnancy toxemia: 3 cases. Wien Klin Wochenschr 1983;95:692–695.

302. McEvoy M, Runciman J, et al. Bilateral retinal detachment in association with preeclampsia. Aust NZ J Obstet Gynaecol 1981;21:246–247.

303. Gitter KA, Houser BP, et al. Toxemia of pregnancy. An angiographic interpretation of fundus findings. Arch Ophthalmol 1968;80:449–454.

304. Brismar G, Schimmelpfenning W. Bilateral exudative retinal detachments in pregnancy. Acta Ophthalmologica 1989;67:699–702.

305. Benson WE, Shields JA, et al. Idiopathic central serous retinopathy with bullous retinal detachment. Ann Ophthalmol 1980;12:920–924.

306. Gass JDM. Bullous retinal detachment. An unusual manifestation of idiopathic central serous choroidopathy. Am J Ophthalmol 1973;75:810–821.

307. Mazzuca DE, Benson WE. Central serous retinopathy: Variants. Surv Ophthalmol 1986;31:170–174.

308. Tsukahara I, Uyama M. Central serous retinopathy with bullous retinal detachment. Graefes Arch Klin Ophthalmol 1978;206:169–178.

309. Benson WE, Shields JA, et al. Posterior scleritis. A cause of diagnostic confusion. Arch Ophthalmol 1979;97:1482–1486.

310. Gass JDM (ed). Stereoscopic Atlas of Macular Disease (2nd ed). St. Louis: Mosby, 1977:368–371.

311. Wang K, Hilton GF. Retinal detachment associated with coloboma of the choroid. Trans Am Ophthalmol Soc 1985;83:49–62.

312. Haik BG, Greenstein SH, et al. Retinal detachment in the morning glory anomaly. Ophthalmology 1984;91:1638–1647.

313. Irvine AR, Crawford JB, et al. The pathogenesis of retinal detachment with morning glory disc and optic pit. Retina 1986;6:146–150.

314. Brockhurst RJ. Nanophthalmos with uveal effusion: A new clinical entity. Arch Ophthalmol 1975;93:1989–1999.

315. Singh OS, Simmons RJ, et al. Nanophthalmos: A prospective on identification and therapy. Ophthalmology 1982;89:1006–1012.

316. Gass JDM, Jallow S. Idiopathic serous detachment of the choroid, ciliary body, and retina (uveal effusion syndrome). Ophthalmology 1982;89:1018–1032.
317. Schepens CL, Brockhurst RJ. Uveal effusion. I. Clinical picture. Arch Ophthalmol 1963;70:189–201.
318. Hamasaki DI, Machemer R, et al. Experimental retinal detachment in owl monkey. VI. The electroretinogram of the detached and reattached retina. Graefes Arch Klin Ophthalmol 1969;177:212–221.
319. Lobes LA. The electro-oculogram in human retinal detachment. Br J Ophthalmol 1978;62:223–226.
320. Erickson PA, Fisher SK, et al. Retinal detachment in the cat: The outer plexiform and nuclear layers. Invest Ophthalmol Vis Sci 1983;24:927–942.
321. Nork TM, Millecchia LL, et al. Selective loss of blue cones and rods in human retinal detachment. Arch Ophthalmol 1995;113:1066–1073.
322. Hart WMJ, Burde RM. Three-dimensional topography of the visual field: Sparing of foveal sensitivity in macular disease. Ophthalmology 1983;90:1028–1038.
323. Cook B, Lewis GP, et al. Photoreceptor degeneration in experimental retinal detachment: Evidence for an apoptotic mechanism. Invest Ophthalmol Vis Sci 1994;35 (Suppl):1833.
324. Winthrop SR, Clearly PE, et al. Penetrating eye injuries: A histopathological review. Br J Ophthalmol 1980;64:809–817.
325. Blight R, Hart JC. Structural changes in the outer retinal layers following blunt mechanical non-perforating trauma to the globe: An experimental study. Br J Ophthalmol 1977;61:573–587.
326. Kroll AJ, Machemer R. Experimental detachment and reattachment in the rhesus monkey: Electron microscopic comparison of rods and cones. Am J Ophthalmol 1969;68:58–77.
327. Kroll AJ, Machemer R. Experimental retinal detachment in the owl monkey. III. Electron microscopy of the retina and pigment epithelium. Am J Ophthalmol 1968;66:410–427.
328. Frieberg TR, Eller AW. Prediction of visual recovery after scleral buckling of macula–off retinal detachment. Am J Ophthalmol 1992;114:715–722.
329. Hogan MJ, Zimmerman LE. Ophthalmic Pathology: An Atlas and Textbook (2nd ed). Philadelphia: Saunders, 1962:549–569.
330. Chang C-J, Lai WW, et al. Apoptotic photoreceptor cell death after traumatic retinal detachment in humans. Arch Ophthalmol 1995;113:880–886.
331. Ryan SJ, Mitti RN, et al. The disciform response: An historical perspective. Graefes Arch Klin Exp Ophthalmol 1980;215:1–20.
332. Kroll AJ, Machemer R. Experimental retinal detachment in the owl monkey. VIII. Photoreceptor proteins renewal in early retinal detachment. Am J Ophthalmol 1971;72:356–366.
333. Vander JF, Tasman W. Photocoagulation of Posterior Segment Disorders. In W Tasman, EA Jaeger (eds), Clinical Ophthalmology. Vol. 6. Philadelphia: Harper & Row, 1992;76:1–15.
334. Liggett PE, Gauderman WJ, et al. Pars plana vitrectomy for acute retinal detachment in penetrating ocular injuries. Arch Ophthalmol 1990;108:1724–1728.
335. Sjostrand J, Anderson C. Micropsia and metamorphopsia in the re-attached macula following retinal detachment. Acta Ophthalmologica 1986;64:425–432.
336. Burton TC. Recovery of visual acuity after retinal detachment of the macula. Trans Am Ophthalmol Soc 1982;80:475–497.
337. Anderson DH, Guerin CJ, et al. Morphological recovery in the reattached retina. Invest Ophthalmol Vis Sci 1986;27:168–183.
338. Machemer R, Buettner H. Experimental retinal detachment in the owl monkey. IX. Radioautographic study of protein metabolism. Am J Ophthalmol 1973;73:377–389.
339. Machemer R, Kroll AJ. Experimental retinal detachment in the owl monkey. VII. Photoreceptor protein renewal in normal and detached retina. Am J Ophthalmol 1971;71:690–695.
340. Tani P, Robertson DM, et al. Prognosis for central vision and anatomic reattachment of rhegmatogenous retinal detachment with macula detached. Am J Ophthalmol 1981;92:611–620.
341. Davidorf FH, Havener WH, et al. Macular vision following retinal detachment surgery. Ophthalmic Surg 1975;6:74–81.
342. Kroll AJ, Machemer R, et al. Experimental retinal detachment in the owl monkey. V. Electron microscopy of the reattached retina. Am J Ophthalmol 1969;67:117–130.
343. Machemer R. Experimental retinal detachment in the owl monkey. IV. The reattached retina. Am J Ophthalmol 1968;66:1075–1091.
344. Grupposo SS. Visual acuity following surgery for retinal detachment. Arch Ophthalmol 1975;93:327–330.
345. Ueda M, Adachi-Usami E. Assessment of central visual function after successful retinal detachment surgery by pattern visual evoked cortical potentials. Br J Ophthalmol 1992;76:482–485.
346. Kollner H. Untersuchegen uber die farbenstorung bei netzhautablosung. Z Augenheilkd 1907;17:117 121.
347. Marre M. The investigation of acquired colour vision deficiencies. In A Hilger, ed. Colour 73. New York: Wiley, 1973:99–135.
348. Schwartz A. Chronic open-angle glaucoma secondary to rhegmatogenous retinal detachment. Am J Ophthalmol 1973;75:205–211.
349. Lambrou FH, Vela MA, et al. Obstruction of the trabecular meshwork by retinal rod outer segments. Arch Ophthalmol 1989;107:742–745.
350. Hogan MJ, Zimmerman LE. Ophthalmic Pathology. Philadelphia: Saunders, 1962:549–568.
351. Hagler HS, North AW. Retinal dialysis and retinal detachment. Arch Ophthalmol 1969;79:376–388.
352. Benson WE, Pornsawat N, et al. Characteristics and prognosis of retinal detachments with demarcation lines. Am J Ophthalmol 1978;84:641–644.
353. Abraham RK, Shea M. Cryopexy for improved results in the prophylaxis of retinal detachment. Trans Ophthalmol Soc UK 1968;88:297–311.
354. Sudarsky RD, Yanuzzi LA. Cryomarcation line and pigment migration after retinal cryosurgery. Arch Ophthalmol 1970;83:395–401.
355. Hilton GF. Subretinal pigment migration. Arch Ophthalmol 1974;93:445–450.
356. Zion VM, Burton TC. Retinal dialysis. Arch Ophthalmol 1980;98:1971–1974.
357. Kinyoun JL, Knoblach WH. Idiopathic retinal dialysis. Retina 1984;4:9–14.
358. Benson WE, Nantawan P, et al. Characteristics and prognosis of retinal detachments with demarcation lines. Am J Ophthalmol 1977;84:641–644.

Long-Standing Retinal Detachment

In a long-standing retinal detachment (RD), marked degenerative changes demonstrate extensive degeneration and atrophy of the outer retinal layers and, to a lesser degree, the inner retinal layers. There is proliferation of glial and connective tissues (Figure 6-29), which contract with time to shorten the detached retina and tightly stretch it, thus flattening a bullous detachment (Figure 6-30). With a total RD, the retina is pulled into the center region of the vitreous cavity as a funnel-shaped detachment (see Figure 6-18). The result is a detached retina that does not undulate on eye movement but may quiver or remain in a fixed position. This thin and transparent appearance of a long-standing detachment often makes it difficult to detect, and it is sometimes mistaken for a retinoschisis.

Fibrosis of the detached retina can produce radial or circular folds and contraction stars. Numerous white strands may also be seen in the subretinal space, which may bridge the detached sensory retina and produce a napkin ring deformity in the detached retina. The contraction bands must be severed to flatten the retina for surgical reattachment.

Deep folds may form between bullae, and the bullae attach to each other. The site of adherence shows interruptions of the internal limiting membrane.[1] Severe fixed folds may produce sharp bends or kinks in the retinal vessels, which may

embarrass the existing circulation and result in hemorrhages. Hemorrhage on long-standing detachments is not uncommon. The retinal vessels may become white and sclerotic with time on long-standing detachments.

A new detachment seems white due to ischemic edema of the outer layers secondary to separation from the choriocapillaris and RPE, but with time, this ischemic condition of the outer layers is lost due to degenerative atrophy. Therefore, long-standing detachments become transparent and thin with time, making it possible to see underlying structures clearly.[2] Small retinal breaks may be more difficult to detect in long-standing detachments because there is less contrast of the break in clear retina. A long-standing detachment may be seen draping off a scleral buckle, looking like a sheet of taut, transparent membrane elevated off the buckle and anchored some distance posteriorly. Large macrocysts (retinoschisis) may develop in the middle layers of the detached retina (Figures 6-31, 6-32, and 6-33).[3, 4]

A retinal dialysis is a common cause of long-standing detachments, and intraretinal macrocysts are present in about 20% of such detachments.[5] Sometimes, a long-standing detachment from a dialysis can cause a shallow detachment of the macula, which may be misdiagnosed as an idiopathic central serous maculopathy.[6] Other changes seen are reactive pigment proliferation, degeneration of the RPE, thickening of the lamina vitrea (posterior vitreous cortex), and formation of drusen. The choroid often shows marked degenerative changes, and the walls of the vessels of the choriocapillaris become hyalinized.[1] Long-standing detachments have a greater frequency of total detachment. There may be subretinal precipitates on a long-standing detachment. They look like tiny white dots, and it is believed that the dots are composed of clusters of RPE macrophages.[2, 7, 8] Yellowish-white subretinal precipitates have also been found associated with detachments secondary to choroidal melanoma and retinoblastoma.[9]

In long-standing detachments, the IOP can actually increase due to decrease in aqueous outflow, which may be the result of accumulation of pigment cells, "tobacco dust," or outer photoreceptor segments in the trabecular meshwork.[10–12] The IOP may return to normal levels after reattachment of the detachment.[8]

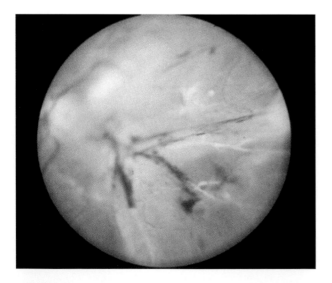

FIGURE 6-29
A long-standing retinal detachment showing a taut, thin, atrophic surface with sclerotic blood vessels and hemorrhages. The optic disc is on the left edge of the photograph. A pigment spot and gliosis are on the detached retina.

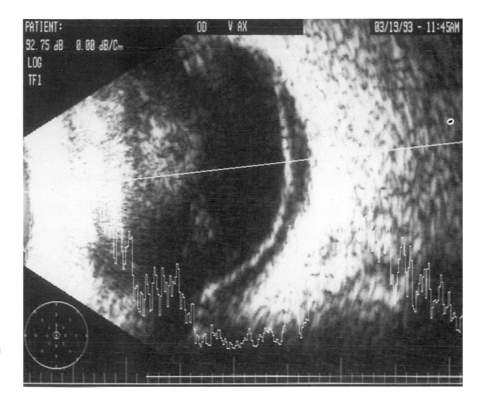

FIGURE 6-30
B-scan ultrasonogram of long-standing retinal detachment. The detachment is thin, and contraction has pulled the detached retina posteriorly; therefore, it now has almost the same curvature as the inner eye wall.

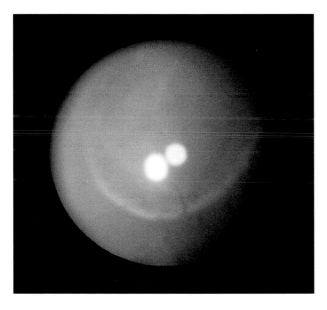

FIGURE 6-31
Macrocyst in long-standing retinal detachment, seen as a bullous area in the center of the indirect condensing lens.

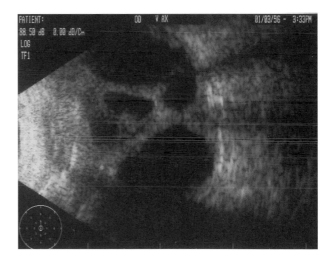

FIGURE 6-32
B-scan ultrasonogram of a posttraumatic phthisical globe with a long-standing total retinal detachment showing multiple macrocysts.

Histopathology

The deterioration of the retina results in a progressive loss of opsin and outer segments of the photoreceptors in the subretinal space and a gradual atrophy and depigmentation of the RPE.[1, 13]

Clinical Significance

Generally, long-standing detachments remain stationary and require no intervening surgical procedures. In recent detachments, the protein content of the subretinal fluid is much lower than that of

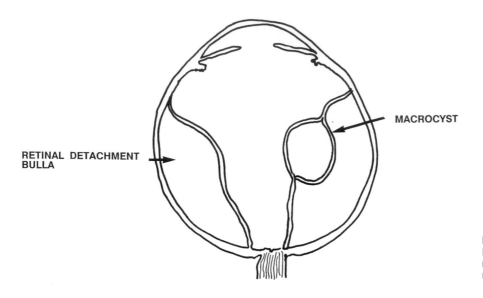

RETINAL DETACHMENT
BULLA

MACROCYST

FIGURE 6-33
Diagram of a long-standing total
retinal detachment with a large
macrocyst.

the plasma, but with time the composition of the fluid slowly becomes more like that of the plasma. As a matter of fact, the total protein concentration increases, and so does the amount of enzymes that are normally found in the plasma.[14] As the protein content of the subretinal fluid increases, so does the viscosity; therefore, fluid drained from a recent detachment is watery, whereas it is quite viscous from a long-standing detachment.[2] It is possible for a long-standing detachment to decrease in elevation or possibly reattach. The subretinal fluid can be absorbed due to osmotic pressure from the choroid and from metabolic transport across the RPE.[15, 16] However, it is much more difficult to reabsorb viscous fluid and therefore, even if the retinal breaks on a long-standing detachment sealed completely, it may take months to absorb the fluid. Other delay mechanisms in delayed reabsorption are degeneration of the RPE and choriocapillaris.[2] Sometimes the folding and proliferation of glial tissue seals the retinal breaks on the detached retina, thus trapping the subretinal fluid. Subsequently, macrophages, proliferating pigment cells, cholesterol crystals from small hemorrhages, and other toxic products accumulate to act as irritants in the trapped subretinal fluid, producing secondary uveitis. The uveitis may cause secondary glaucoma, which can eventually lead to enucleation. Hemorrhaging from degenerating retina and choroid is not uncommon and can result in further intraocular inflammation.[1]

References

1. Hogan MJ, Zimmerman LE. Ophthalmic Pathology: An Atlas and Textbook (2nd ed). Philadelphia: Saunders, 1962;549–569.
2. Benson WE (ed). Retinal Detachment: Diagnosis and Management. New York: Lippincott, 1987.
3. Machemer R. Experimental retinal detachment in the owl monkey. II. Histology of the retina and pigment epithelium. Am J Ophthalmol 1968;66:396–410.
4. Yanoff M, Fine SF. Ocular Pathology (2nd ed). Philadelphia: Harper & Row, 1975;461,563.
5. Hagler HS, North AW. Retinal dialysis and retinal detachment. Arch Ophthalmol 1969;79:376–388.
6. Gutner RK. Retinal dialysis. Clin Eye Vision Care 1994;6:88–91.
7. Lagua H, Machemer R. Clinical-pathological correlation in massive periretinal proliferation. Am J Ophthalmol 1975;80:913–929.
8. Machemer R, Norton EWD. Experimental retinal detachment in owl monkey. I. Methods of production and clinical picture. Am J Ophthalmol 1968;66:388–396.
9. Takagi T, Tsuda N, et al. Subretinal precipitates of retinal detachments associated with intraocular tumors. Ophthalmologica 1988;197:120–126.
10. Linner E. Intraocular pressure in retinal detachment. Arch Ophthalmol 1966;84(suppl):101–106.
11. Schwartz A. Chronic open-angle glaucoma secondary to rhegmatogenous retinal detachment. Am J Ophthalmol 1973;75:205–211.
12. Matsuo N, Takabatake M, et al. Photoreceptor outer segments in the aqueous humor in rhegmatogenous retinal detachment. Am J Ophthalmol 1986;101:673–679.
13. Hara S, Ishiguro S, et al. Immunoreactive opsin content in subretinal fluid from patients with rhegmatogenous retinal detachment. Arch Ophthalmol 1987;105:260–263.
14. Kaufman PL, Podos SM. The subretinal fluid in primary rhegmatogenous retinal detachment. Surv Ophthalmol 1973;18:100–116.

15. Negi A, Marmor MF. Effect of subretinal and systemic osmolarity on the rate of subretinal fluid absorption. Invest Ophthalmol Vis Sci 1984;25:616–620.

16. Negi A, Marmor MF. Mechanisms of subretinal fluid absorption in the cat eye. Invest Ophthalmol Vis Sci 1986;27:1560–1563.

Treatment

Leber, at the end of the nineteenth century, was the first to implicate the importance of vitreous traction and the formation of retinal breaks in the subsequent development of an RD.[1] Later, Gonin was the first ophthalmologist to advance the theory of the importance of closing lesions responsible for causing idiopathic RDs and draining the subretinal fluid.[2,3] Because of the poor reattachment rates during the 1930s to 1950s, there was a strong argument for the prophylactic treatment of retinal breaks with detachment. Not all surgeons of these times believed in the universal treatment of breaks, however; Colyear and Pischel[4] believed that specific groups of patients needed only prophylactic treatment. Treatment of retinal breaks became even more popular when the binocular indirect ophthalmoscope with scleral depression was able to detect many more peripheral retinal lesions and breaks.[5] Also adding to the popularity of treatment was the invention of photocoagulation by Meyer-Schwickerath.[6] Custodis popularized the use of episcleral explants to close retinal breaks.[7–9] Today, with better instruments and surgical techniques demonstrating greater success rates and visual outcomes, prophylactic treatment is increasingly reserved for specific higher-risk cases.

The preoperative examination consists of drawing the location and extent of the RD and finding all the retinal breaks. Drawing of an RD may take as long as an hour or more, but the use of an ultra–wide field contact lens can reduce the time to 15–30 minutes. This time saving occurs because wide views of the detachment are obtained, and relationships to anatomic points inside the eye are more easily visualized. Because the detached retina is elevated above the choroid, light reflected from the choroid may retroilluminate a retinal tear. Consequently, during the retinal examination the clinician may get a fleeting glimpse of a small orange glow, indicating the location of the break. The light must be in just the right position to show the transillumination of the break, so even after detecting the transient glow of the retinal break, it may be very difficult to see again. The discovery of small breaks can be a very laborious task, sometimes taking an hour or two of ophthalmoscopy with and without scleral depression, three-mirror or 90-diopter precorneal condensing lens, or ultra–wide field contact lens. Small breaks may be located in folds in the detachment, which may make their discovery very difficult. The finding of pigmented areas in the detached retina indicates previous areas of pigment clumping due to isolated vitreous traction. Such pigmented areas are likely to be the location of retinal breaks. The discovery of small retinal breaks may be complicated by the clarity of the intraocular view. Peripheral cataracts may haze the view of the peripheral retina and make it hard to see small peripheral breaks. Pseudophakic eyes may produce hazy views of the peripheral retina due to posterior capsular fibrosis, which results in optical distortions caused by the edge of the intraocular lens, cortical remnants, and small pupils. Another difficulty in seeing the retina is caused by vitreous haze, either from vitreous hemorrhaging, vitreous degeneration, or opacification. Even after finding a retinal break, the clinician must be careful to continue to proceed with the retinal examination to determine if other breaks are present. It must be kept in mind that the major reason for the production of a rhegmatogenous detachment is vitreous traction. Because scleral depression reduces transvitreal vitreous traction by foreshortening the diameter of the globe, it does not exacerbate the tear or detachment.

Immobilization of the eyes with bilateral ocular occlusion is attempted in some patients with a bullous rhegmatogenous detachment, especially if it threatens the macula. This often allows for flattening of the bullous detachment, which may make visualization of retinal breaks easier; in a few patients, it may allow for complete reattachment. The earliest sign of settling of the bullous detachment is crinkling of the detached retina next to the posterior border.[10]

The surgical procedure used depends on the clinical findings and the surgeon's personal preference of possible reparative procedures. Surgical repair of a symptomatic rhegmatogenous detachment is almost always recommended.[11] There are always potential complications in RD procedures, but it is well recognized that the benefits outweigh the risks in symptomatic eyes.[12-14] The treatment of asymptomatic RDs found on routine examinations is not as well defined. Often, the reason for proceeding with scleral buckling in patients without symptoms is the progression of the detachment, especially if it threatened the macula. In one study, eight of 16 cases of asymptomatic detachments underwent scleral buckling due to documented progression (one involving the macula), whereas the remaining eight cases were followed for 10 years without any signs of progression.[15]

Treatment of a nonrhegmatogenous RD is directed at the underlying pathology and may require the use of irradiation, chemotherapy, corticosteroids, antimicrobial drugs, photocoagulation, diathermy, cryotherapy, or metal or plastic retinal tacks. Retinal tacks have been able to preserve useful vision in many surgical cases of complicated RD.[16-24] Treatment of a retinal detachment necessitates sealing the retinal break. If the detachment is shallow, this may be done by transconjunctival cryopexy or laser photocoagulation. If the detachment is more elevated, scleral buckling in conjunction with transscleral cryotherapy is required. After successful sealing of the retinal break, the fluid beneath the break is actively removed by the RPE. Because the fluid cannot be replenished, the detached retina reattaches to the inner eye wall. Reattachment generally occurs in 16–24 hours.[10] Cryopexy has the disadvantages of causing cystoid macular edema (CME),[25, 26] dispersion of RPE cells,[27] and breakdown of the blood-retinal barrier, which may enhance the potential for proliferative vitreoretinopathy (PVR).[28]

Scleral Buckling Materials and Procedures

In more complicated cases involving tractional detachment, tenacious vitreous bands, or PVR, a closed pars plana vitrectomy in conjunction with scleral buckling is required for successful reattachment. In difficult cases, internal fluid-gas exchange or intravitreal silicone injection may be necessary. Such vitreous substitutes work as a tamponade to force the detached retina back onto the inner eye wall.

Expandable Gases

Expandable gases, such as sulfurhexafluoride (SF6) and perfluoropropane (C3F8), are used in the management of complicated cases of retinal detachment, such as PVR, giant tears, and advanced vitreoretinal degenerations.[29, 30] The gas bubbles can be seen as shiny spheres in the vitreous cavity, and they can be imaged on ultrasonography (Figure 6-34). Perfluoro-

carbon gases expand from two to five times in nonvitrectomized eyes due to diffusion of blood gases into the gas bubble. The nonvitrectomized eye can accept 0.2–0.3 ml of the gas injected via a needle through the pars plana. In the vitrectomized eye, the amount of injected gas can be greater due to the loss of the vitreous, which results in more space for the gas to expand. Perfluoropropane expands to 2.3 ml, which is enough to fill half the vitreous cavity. One of the major advantages of C3F8 is that its half-life is relatively short (12 days), which is enough time to achieve a secure retinal adhesion.[10] In complicated retinal detachment, where vitrectomy is combined with gas-fluid exchange, nonexpansile concentration of gas, such as 20% SF6 or 14% C3F8, is used. The 20% gas stays in the eye for 7–10 days, whereas the 14% C3F8 may remain for 2–3 weeks. The complications of C3F8 are probably due more to the physical properties of the gas than to toxicity. One study found the following rate of complications: cataract (67%), ocular hypertension (32%), fibrinous membrane formation (13%), keratopathy (6%), and corneal decompensation (4%). Lens opacities were more frequently found in diabetic patients because 93% of such patients developed significant posterior subcapsular cataracts.[29] The cause of cataracts is not thought to be secondary to the chemical effects of the gas but rather to the mechanical interference across the posterior capsule.[31, 32] Some studies found that these gas-induced cataracts were reversible.[33, 34] Increased IOP is a complication and is likely due to volume displacement caused by the scleral buckle,[35] expansion of the gas bubble anteriorly causing a flat anterior chamber,[36] or forward rotation of the ciliary body with resultant angle closure from buckling.[37] Expansion of the gas bubble during airplane travel is a potential problem that could increase IOP.[38, 39] Due to the possible forward expansion of the bubble, it is best to stress the importance of the patient's head being in the prone position. Fibrinous membrane formation was associated with increase in IOP, and the membrane makes visualizing the fundus difficult. These membranes clear up in a matter of weeks on topical steroid treatment.[29] Lastly, the keratopathy is believed to be secondary to the gas, having prolonged contact with the corneal endothelium.[40, 41] Posterior retinal folds (also called arcuate retinal folds) may develop after surgical repair of detachments with use of intraocular gas. These usually occur at the border between detached and attached retina and are probably the result of the gas bubble forcing the detached retina to fold at the border of the attached retina.[42-47] These folds are more likely to occur with wide or excessively tightened buckles.[44, 48] Buckle problems produce redundant retina,

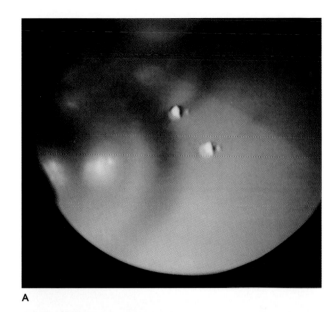

A

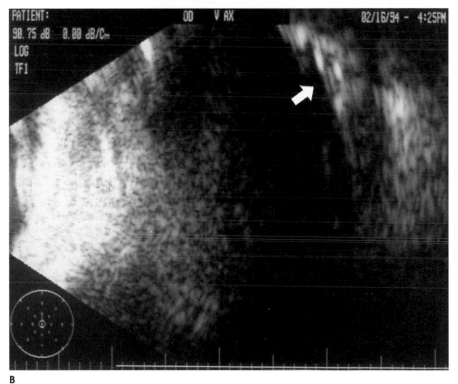

B

FIGURE 6-34
A. Bubbles of expandable gas that look very shiny immediately after injection for pneumatic retinopexy for a superior flap tear with localized detachment. B. B-scan ultrasonogram of superior gas bubbles (*arrow*).

which the gas bubble can push posteriorly against the attached border. If the fold involves the macula, metamorphopsia and decreased vision are likely to occur. Often, with time, the folds gradually flatten, and some even disappear.[48] Even with the stated complications, C3F8 is a very suitable temporary vitreous substitute for complex cases of retinal detachment. Choroidal detachment can also be a complication.[49, 50] Subconjunctival gas is possible after ocular injection, but it is a benign situation.[49] Frequent failures with intraocular gases are due to

detachments caused by inferior breaks (4 to 8 o'clock) because there is no comfortable position for patients to maintain to keep the bubble against the breaks.[51]

Pneumatic Retinopexy

Pneumatic retinopexy has been used to reattach selected types of retinal detachments. It was successful in 80% of 1,274 eyes in cases studied from 1985 to 1989.[49] Others report initial success rates of 63%, 75%, 82%, 91%, and 95%.[14, 50, 52, 53] Failed cases

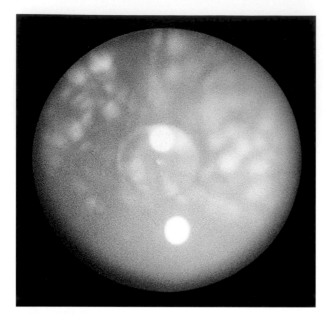

FIGURE 6-35
Silicone oil bead on the inferior laser-treated retina just posterior to the ora serrata. The silicone oil bead is in the center of the view through the indirect condensing lens and appears as a spherical magnifying lens.

were often successfully treated with a repeat injection, supplemental cryopexy or laser treatment, or modified head positioning. Failures were due to new breaks, missed breaks, reopened breaks, inadequate gas volume, PVR, and poor patient compliance.[49] Complications include retinal folds, subconjunctival gas, subretinal gas, malignant glaucoma, subretinal and peripheral hemorrhage, vitreous hemorrhage, iris incarceration, macular hole, macular pucker, neck pain, subretinal pigment, vitreal pigment, PVR, refractive changes, new breaks, retinal breaks never closed, retinal breaks reopened, shifting subretinal fluid into the macula, uveitis, and vitreous incarceration and loss.[49] In the case where gas bubbles are accidentally introduced into the break in the detachment ("fish eggs"), the patient can be positioned to allow the bubbles to collect at the superior pars plana. Finger-flick thumps to the superior bulbar conjunctiva may allow coalescing of the bubbles. Later, massaging with the scleral depressor may direct the bubble through the retinal break.[49]

Silicone Oil

Silicone oil has the advantage of being permanent and therefore able to seal future breaks even without further retinopexy or scleral buckling. Another advantage is that it may physically block fluid from entering a break. When the silicone oil produces a

poor tamponade of the inferior retina, the blockage effect may allow the macula to remain on even if complete reattachment of the inferior detachment is not achieved.[54] The retinal contact made by the inferior arc of the silicone is often poor and thus may allow for continued detachment or redetachment.[55] Silicone oil does not require special head positioning. It is sometimes necessary to perform reinjections to attain attachment. Sometimes silicone oil beads may be left over after removal (Figure 6-35).

Some significant complications are associated with the use of silicone oil. Silicone oil was originally thought to be toxic to the retina, but now it is believed to be not so toxic. It has been retained in some eyes for 2 years with signs of very little toxicity.[54, 56, 57] If the oil spills over into the anterior chamber in silicone-filled eyes, however, corneal decompensation ranging from 12% to 63%[58–61] and elevated IOP may result. The keratopathy is the direct result of endothelial touch, which may be irreversible.[62] It has been reported that there was little chance of the progression of the keratopathy after removal of the silicone oil.[63] An inferior peripheral iridectomy (PI) has been used to decrease the incidence of these complications in the anterior chamber[64–69] by allowing access of the aqueous into the anterior chamber. The incidence of keratopathy was reduced to 2–3% with an inferior PI.[65, 70] Subsequent closure of the PI may allow silicone to enter the anterior chamber.[59, 66, 68, 69] Cataract formation occurs in 30–100% of eyes and may appear as a late complication in 1–2 years.[60, 61, 71] A refractive shift in the eye with silicone injection may occur; this is due to the refractive index of silicone oil being 1.405, as compared to 1.336 for the aqueous and vitreous.[54, 72–74] In aphakic eyes, the refractive shift is more myopic, and in phakic eyes, the change is toward hyperopia. In one report, the mean refractive change for aphakes was –7.00 diopters, for phakic eyes it was +4.75 diopters, and for pseudophakes it was +1.75.[75] Silicone oil has been found to be superior to expandable gas in the treatment of retinal detachment due to PVR.[76, 77] Due to the inherent problems in the use of intraocular silicone oil, it would seem advisable to use it only when an eye has already had multiple surgical attempts and there is the residual prospect of maintaining some vision function.[62]

Silicone oil is also used for very difficult cases, such as retinal detachment in necrotizing retinitis in HIV infection. It has the benefit of possibly preventing detachment if future breaks occur.[54] Silicone oil has shown a high rate of reattachment in cases of necrotizing retinitis.[54, 78–83] The goal of this surgical treatment is palliative and aimed at preserving as much vision as possible before death because the mean survival rate is about 7 months after surgery.[54] This type of treatment is not as likely, however, to have the success rate of silicone oil. Small peripheral retinal detachments caused by cytomegalic retinitis may be surrounded by laser retinopexy to prevent them from progressing into symptomatic detachments.[78, 84, 85]

Scleral Buckle

A scleral buckle procedure is performed to approximate the retinal break to the RPE and thus to close the break in a chorioretinal scar produced by laserpexy, diathermy, or cryotherapy. All three modalities effect a thermal insult to the choroid or retinal tissue that results in inflammation and later scarring. The morphologic cellular response of the sensory retina and RPE is essentially the same, and within 2 weeks, it results in a retinal adhesive force.[86, 87] There are some differences, however, in the initial effects of treatment: Laser photocoagulation increases retinal adhesion in 24 hours, but cryotherapy reduces retinal adhesion for 1 week after treatment.[88] Cryotherapy is the treatment of choice for retinal tears during scleral buckling procedures.[89] The end point of cryotherapy is when whitening of the retina is seen; the clinician should not wait for formation of an ice ball.[90] Shortly after cryotherapy (approximately several minutes), there are white areas of retinal edema. If there is a bullous detachment, the appropriate areas of RPE from where the breaks settle back may be treated, or treatment may be deferred until the subretinal fluid drains. For a flap tear, the treatment should extend around the break anteriorly to the ora serrata.

The disadvantage of cryotherapy is the release of RPE cells, which may cause pigmentary changes beneath the reattached retina. These cells may be responsible for causing PVR. Therefore, it is best not to overtreat with cryotherapy and to avoid excessive scleral depression of the treated areas because it may lead to release of more pigment cells.[28] Cryotherapy does cause choroidal congestion and hyperemia, which may complicate drainage of subretinal fluid.[91] It produces a breakdown in the blood-ocular barrier, which is associated with the development of postoperative CME.[26]

Photocoagulation has these benefits: delivery with great precision, production of a localized burn to the RPE or outer sensory retina, less breakdown of the blood-ocular barrier, little effect on the choroid, and no effect on the sclera.[28] Diathermy achieves

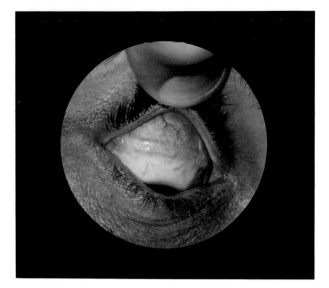

FIGURE 6-36
Anteriorly displaced encircling band after scleral buckling procedure.

effective RPE adhesion by thermal coagulation of the involved tissues. The disadvantage to diathermy is that it causes immediate scleral shrinkage, followed by scleral necrosis and choroidal and retinal bleeding.[92, 93] The goal of retinopexy is to surround the retinal break with 1–2 mm of continuous treatment.

Localization of the retinal breaks is performed with binocular indirect ophthalmoscopy using scleral depression and then diathermy. The wooden end of the cotton-tipped applicator (dehydrates the sclera) and special sterile marking ink are used to mark the external sclera so that the buckling material can be placed properly opposite the internal retinal breaks. In bullous detachments, external localization may be difficult to approximate; therefore, drainage of subretinal fluid may be necessary to move the detachment closer to the inner eye wall.

A scleral buckle sponge may be circular or radially oriented, depending on the characteristics of the retinal break and its location in the fundus. The sponge may be an explant sutured onto the external scleral surface or an implant sutured into a scleral bed cut out of the external sclera (Figure 6-36). The buckling element may have an encircling band attached to effect additional height. Greater height brings the break closer to the inner eye wall of a bullous detachment and decreases peripheral transvitreal traction (Figures 6-37 and 6-38). Often, the scleral buckle just flattens the inner eye wall (see Figure 6-45), but sometimes there is marked internal bowing of the inner wall. The encircling band is

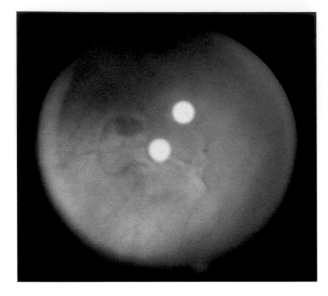

FIGURE 6-37
A lattice lesion with a flap tear on the lateral edge can be seen on a scleral buckle. The lattice lesion is well affixed to the buckle from cryopexy. Same patient as in Figure 3-77.

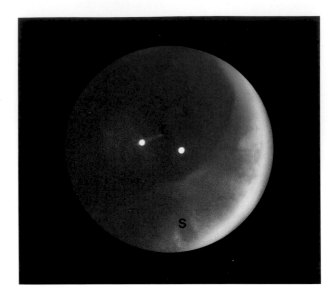

FIGURE 6-38
Scleral buckle (**s**) has indented the globe, and the internal buckle appears high and dry. Nonbuckled posterior retina (**r**).

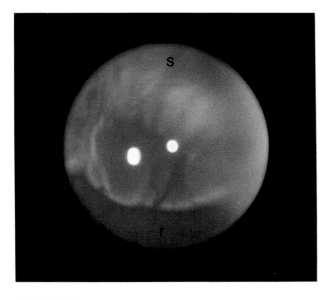

FIGURE 6-39
Note small bullous areas of detached retina on the posterior aspect of the scleral buckle (**s**). With time, the residual detached retina flattened back onto the buckle. Nonbuckled posterior retina (**r**). View is through the indirect condensing lens.

usually sutured onto the globe 12–14 mm posterior to the limbus at the equator. After a recent scleral buckling procedure, small billowing areas of retinal detachment (Figure 6-39) and radial folds of retina may be seen. These disappear as the retina flattens down against the buckle. The appearance is the same during reattachment, failure to acquire reat-

tachment, and redetachment of the buckle some time later. It is preferable to do a radial buckle because the detached retina tends to detach in a radial fashion from the disc to the ora serrata.

Radial buckles are usually used to treat retinal detachments with a single break, with closely spaced breaks less than 1 clock hour in total extent, and with posteriorly located breaks (Figure 6-40). In cases of multiple breaks, a radial sponge is required for each retinal break, provided that each break is 2 clock hours apart. Radial buckles are not practical for very large retinal breaks. Radial sponges produce little refractive error change. Encircling bands not only help in elevation of the buckle, but they also decrease vitreoretinal traction at the site of the break and in other peripheral retinal areas that may be the site of future breaks. Encircling bands are particularly indicated for eyes with multiple breaks in different quadrants and eyes with aphakia, pseudophakia, myopia, and diffuse vitreoretinopathy.[88] Circumferential bands tend to preserve the radial orientation due to the shortening of the circumference of the globe, and residual radial folds often extend to the break on the buckle, causing "fishmouthing."[10, 94, 95] Fishmouthing may lead to a persistent or recurrent retinal detachment. Fishmouthed tears can be closed by the use of intravitreal expandable gas.[88]

Modern scleral buckling material is composed of silicone rubber, silicone sponge, and biological materials consisting of donor sclera, fascia lata, and gelatin. All are well tolerated by the globe. The gelatin buckling material (composed mainly of hydrolyzed collagen) initially hydrates to produce greater height of the buckle, but over 3–6 months, it is broken down and the buckling effect is lost.[90, 96] Silicone rubber buckling material comes in many sizes and shapes.

Silicone sponges are made of silicone but have many air pockets that give them great compressible and elastic characteristics. Thin silicone rubber bands were first used as encircling material by Regan et al. in 1962.[97] Often, grooved pieces of silicone rubber or sponge are used along with the encircling element to obtain an enhanced circumferential or radial effect.[98] The buckling material is sutured onto the eye, and care must be taken with posterior suturing to avoid the vortex veins and their tributaries.[88] During the placement of the encircling band around the eye, the IOP may be markedly elevated, and the surgeon must periodically monitor the central retinal artery for adequate profusion. Although it is not known exactly how long the central retinal artery may remain closed before neurologic or retinal damage occurs, some surgeons suggest that it be no more than 5 minutes.[10] If the retinal artery does not reopen, it may be necessary to release the tension of the band on the eye. Sometimes, digital massage or paracentesis may reopen the central artery. A complication of circumferential scleral buckling is the formation of radial and circumferential folds after treatment of a bullous detachment. Radial folds are seen more frequently, and both are thought to be due to the redundant retinal tissue produced by the buckling elements. Radial folds start on top of the buckle and often involve the original tear, causing the tear to have a "fishmouth" appearance.[99, 100] Radial folds can decrease vision if there is macular involvement and even result in redetachment due to fluid leakage through the fishmouth tear.[45] Fortunately, radial buckles are rarely associated with radial folds.[101, 102]

One complication of a tight encircling band is the possible erosion through the sclera, choroid, retina, and into the vitreous cavity,[103] which may lead to vitreal and subretinal hemorrhage, retinal detachment, and phthisis bulbi. In some cases, there is no hemorrhaging or redetachment. This may be due to the slow progression of the eroding material, which may allow for scarring to seal retinal breaks. Such erosion with silicone bands occurs in only 3.8% of the cases in one report.[104] Risk factors that are associated with intrusion into the globe are high myopia, thin sclera, multiple operations, infections, and glaucoma.[104, 105] A reduction in eye wall erosion

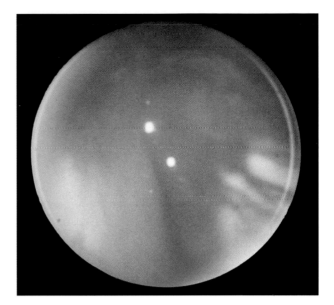

FIGURE 6-40
A radial buckle can be seen as a triangular elevation with the apex pointing toward the posterior pole. The retinal tear is located close to the apex of the buckle.

may be accomplished by using wider and softer explants.[105] Besides the encircling element and explants eroding into the globe, scleral suture intrusion may occur, which is usually found anterior at the edge of the buckle.[105] Suture intrusion may be caused by poor surgical technique, such as uncontrolled constriction of the globe, anchoring the sutures too deep, and using a narrow encircling band.[105] One study of a silicone band of 3-mm elastomer sponge used to constrict the globe found that more than 30% had complications, which included scleral thinning and intrusion of the encircling band (100%).[106] Newer encircling band technique uses polymethylmethacrylate belt loops for band, which can be fixed to the sclera with cyanoacrylate adhesive, thus negating the need for scleral sutures.[107] Subretinal and vitreous hemorrhage may be the result of blood vessels rubbing against the eroding explant or sutures. When erosion occurs, it may be better to cut the encircling band rather than remove the scleral buckle, which may lead to a reduced incidence of redetachment.[105] Erosion of the sutures may indicate future erosion of the buckle. There is no need to perform preventive surgery for suture erosion alone, but the patient should be followed closely for possible buckle erosion.[105] The discovery of subconjunctival or vitreous hemorrhage may indicate the need for silicone band cutting. Removal of scleral buckles that have eroded into the globe is

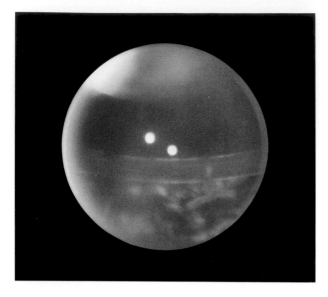

FIGURE 6-41
A polyethylene tube was used as an encircling band for a retinal detachment 22 years ago in this patient. With time, the tube eroded through the inferior third of the globe into the vitreous cavity. Note one nylon suture with knot still in place around the tube and another through the tube; these were used to secure the tube to the sclera. There is linear chorioretinal scarring with reactive pigment proliferation below the tube, the result of the healing process after the tube eroded through the globe. View is through the indirect condensing lens.

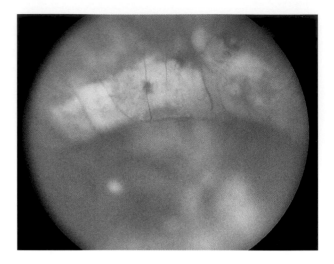

FIGURE 6-42
A polyethylene tube was used as an encircling band for a retinal detachment in this patient in 1971. With time, the tube eroded through the superior third of the globe into the vitreous cavity. There is linear chorioretinal scarring below the tube, which is the result of the healing process after the tube eroded through the globe. The degenerated retina can be seen draping over the eroding tube.

possible, but severe complications can follow such surgical procedures.[92] Retinal tacks may also erode into the globe and result in subretinal or vitreous hemorrhaging.[108]

In the distant past, the encircling elements were made of material such as silk, polyesters (Dacron and Mersiline), and nylon. If these were tied too tight, erosion could occur through the sclera, choroid, retina, and finally into the vitreous cavity.[92, 109] Approximately 20 years ago, polyethylene tubes were used as buckle material, but because they were less flexible and hardened with time, they occasionally eroded into the globe (Figures 6-41 and 6-42).[92, 110, 111] Such intraocular erosion occurred in 62.3% of eyes in one report.[104]

The placement of the scleral buckle is dictated to some degree by the presence of intraocular lenses (IOLs). Posterior chamber lenses pose the least difficulties in scleral buckling. Care must be taken when patients have anterior chamber, iris-fixed, or posterior chamber IOLs. The buckle should not be placed too far anterior in eyes with anterior chamber lenses because this may force the haptic into the angle and result in an anterior chamber bleed. Forward displacement of an iris-

fixed lens may cause corneal endothelial damage.[88] Due to poor visualization of the peripheral retina with IOL, encircling procedures are usually performed.[112]

SUBRETINAL DRAINAGE
Often, drainage of subretinal fluid is necessary to approximate the break onto the buckle. Less than 5% of retinal detachment patients require drainage of subretinal fluid. The other reason for drainage is to reduce the intraocular fluid volume so that there are few problems with increased IOP due to the elevation of the buckle into the vitreous cavity.[10] Some surgeons recommend the drainage of the subretinal fluid, and others prefer that the subretinal fluid be removed from the eye by the RPE-choroid complex.[90, 113–117] The success rate of reattachment in nondrainage is reported to be comparable to drainage procedures,[114, 117–119] and the primary advantages of nondrainage are fewer postsurgical complications. Nondrainage procedures require a longer period of time for reabsorption; subretinal fluid may persist for more than 1 week in 25% of studied cases.[115, 116] It has been reported that retinal detachments that are off for more than 2 weeks require a longer time for reabsorption.[115] Also, the closer the retinal break is to the buckle, the faster the reabsorption of subretinal

fluid.[114, 120] All eyes treated with diathermy should be drained because scleral shrinkage from the diathermy increases IOP. Other reasons to consider drainage are bullous detachments (to obtain faster approximation to the retinopexy site), inferior breaks (inferior breaks often take more time settle onto the buckle), PVR (may inhibit settling of the detached retina), highly myopic and aphakic eyes (vitreous degeneration may hinder the settling of the detached retina), chronic detachment (the subretinal fluid may be more viscous and more difficult to reabsorb), and eyes susceptible to damage from sustained IOP.[10]

It is not known how much fluid is actively transported by the RPE and how much is drawn through the RPE by the protein-rich underlying choroid.[28] The removal of fluid from the subretinal space decreases the hydrostatic pressure of the subretinal area relative to that of the vitreous. Because the barrier producing the resistance of water diffusion is the retina, the hydrostatic forces flatten the retina against the inner eye wall.[121] Drainage is often performed in glaucoma patients with a buckle because the elevated IOP may cause sustained closure of the central retinal artery. Procedures used to obtain drainage are diathermy, sclerotomy, and argon, carbon dioxide, and newer diode laser surgery.[92, 118, 122–131] Complications of subretinal drainage occur at a rate of 2.0–8.6%.[118, 124–127] They include choroidal detachment, vitreous and subretinal hemorrhage, retinal incarceration, choroidal neovascularization, and endophthalmitis.[12, 125, 126, 132–137] Choroidal hemorrhage, retinal perforation, and retinal incarceration occur in 5–10% of cases.[126] Subretinal hemorrhaging from sclerotomy occurs in 2.0–4.8%,[118, 124, 126, 127] and from argon laser it is 8.6%.[125] Carbon dioxide is reported to cause hemorrhaging in no patients in one study.[122] Retinal perforation may also occur but at a lower rate (0.2–3.3%).[118, 126, 127] Laser sclerotomies or choroidotomies have the advantage of not entering the choroid with a sharp object. Thus, there is no bleeding, and shallow detachments fare better for not having a sharp object potentially cutting the detached retina. The laser treatment does, however, result in some choroidal or retinal hemorrhage, but the hemorrhages tend to be smaller than those of needle drainage techniques.[130] Retinal incarceration at the sclerotomy site gives the retina a dimpled appearance.

POSTOPERATIVE VISUAL ACUITY

Even though the reattachment success rate is reported to be fairly high, the visual acuity outcomes are less impressive, with about 40–50% of the eyes having 20/50 or better vision.[138–141] Pseudophakic detachments have a 94–96% chance of achieving 20/50 or better vision.[112, 142, 143] Eyes with iris-fixed lenses have a 14–33% chance and eyes with an anterior chamber lens a 50% chance of obtaining 20/40 or better vision.[144, 145] A detached macula in a rhegmatogenous detachment is the most important prognostic indicator of postoperative vision; the most critical variable is the duration of detached macula and the preoperative visual acuity.[139, 146] Retinal detachments with the macula off have a poorer visual prognosis, likely because they are usually larger detachments that have been off longer. Reattachment of the retina results in some histologic reversal of retinal damage, but the amount of recovery depends on the extent and duration of the detachment.[88] In macula-off detachments, only about 37–39% have a final visual acuity of 20/50[140, 141, 147] despite a 90% reattachment rate.[140, 141] Even in detachments with the macula on, approximately 10% have some visual loss of two lines or more on Snellen acuity postoperatively.[88] Eyes with relatively poor preoperative acuity are less likely to obtain good postoperative acuity[148]; however, some have reported that pretreatment visual acuities have been obtained postoperatively in spite of the macula being off initially.[149] Preoperative acuities are the most consistent factor in predicting postoperative acuities.[140, 141] One study found that a preoperative acuity of 20/70, even if the macula was off for 26 weeks, generally retained this level of vision after reattachment. In eyes with preoperative vision less than 20/200 (even if only for 1 week), only 65% of the eyes regained 20/70 or better.[150] Another study found that only 48% of eyes with preoperative visual acuities of less than 20/200 regained 20/50 or better.[151] A third study found that if preoperative acuities were worse than 20/200, only 29% regained 20/50 or better, and if the preoperative vision was better than 20/200, 68% achieved 20/50 or better.[141] Age may also be a factor in postoperative visual acuities and may be related to older photoreceptors being more susceptible to damage during detachment and due to the higher prevalence of age-related macular disease.[141, 148] Other factors in decreased postoperative acuity are extent of detached retina and the presence of signs of PVR.[151] The presence of CME and macular epiretinal membranes tended to decrease postoperative acuities.[141, 148] The postoperative visual acuities of retinal detachments with posterior intraocular lenses are greater than those obtained in eyes with other types of IOLs.[151]

Postoperative Refractive Error

Fortunately, segmental buckles (implants or explants) have little effect on refractive error.[152] Large radial buckles that extend anteriorly to the ora serrata, however, may induce an irregular astigmatism due to changes in the corneal curvature.[153, 154] The placement of an encircling band may be associated with an induced myopic shift of the eye due to an increase in the axial length of the globe. Factors that are reported to produce this myopic shift are axial lengthening, shallowing of anterior chamber due to anterior displacement of iris or lens diaphragm, changes in corneal curvature, and increase in the thickness of the lens.[153, 155, 156] Whereas low and moderate buckles are responsible for an increase in axial length of 1.56–2.24 diopters in phakic eyes and 0.74–1.41 in aphakic eyes; high buckles (at least 5 mm) may actually decrease the axial length and cause a hyperopic shift of 0.35 diopters for phakic eyes and 0.59 diopters for aphakic eyes.[153, 155, 157] One study found that the average increase in axial length for scleral buckle placement was 0.99 mm and the average induced myopic shift was 2.75 diopters.[158] The degree of myopic shift probably depends most on the amount of equatorial constriction, and it usually measures 0.1–2.75 diopters.[106, 153, 157, 159, 160] Some have reported significant astigmatic changes.[12, 161, 162] There is an increase in lens thickness and shallowing of the anterior chamber for as long as 6 weeks after surgery,[155] but this effect is reported to return to within normal limits in 2 months.[156] Phakic eyes display a greater myopic shift than aphakic eyes; this is due to the anterior displacement of the iris or lens diaphragm.[153] Contact lenses are a very suitable means of correcting the induced axial refractive anisometropia, and they can be fit 1 week to 10 days after surgery.[159]

Success Rates

The overall success rate of retinal detachment surgery is reported to be around 90%.[10, 12, 119, 140, 141, 147, 148, 163–168] The success rate today has increased to nearly 100% in selected groups of patients having the macula-on detachments and detachments with only one retinal break.[146, 148, 168] The success rate of retinal reattachment after extracapsular cataract extraction is approximately the same as that found in phakic detachments.[112, 169, 170] Some have reported that the success rate for aphakic detachment is significantly lower than phakic,[140, 171] but others have found it to be about the same as phakic cases. The reattachment rate for eyes that undergo congenital cataract surgery is lower, at 50–75%.[172–174] The success rate

of retinal detachment repair depends on numerous factors: previous retinal surgery, previous ocular trauma, visual acuity of 20/60 or worse, patient more than 80 years of age, aphakia, myopia, choroidal detachment, uveitis, extent of detachment (total having a worse prognosis), pars plana detachment, number of retinal breaks, posterior location of breaks, structural degeneration of the vitreous, vitreous hemorrhage, preretinal or subretinal membrane proliferation, giant tear, more than 50 cryopexy applications, encircling scleral buckle, subretinal drainage technique, and postchoroidal detachment.[12, 140, 141, 161, 162, 164, 175–179] In one study, the most important causes of failure were choroidal detachment, significant vitreous opacification, intraoperative intravitreal injection, and postoperative sterile vitritis.[163] The success rate of reattachment of retinal detachments caused by holes in lattice degeneration was reported to be 98%.[180] The success rate of reattachment of a retinal tear caused by a retinal dialysis is excellent, except if a giant tear develops.[181] Reattachment of pseudophakic detachments is hampered by the difficulty in viewing the peripheral retina through a small pupil, the edge of the IOL, cortical remnants, and capsular opacification.[112, 144] Retinal breaks are not discovered in 20% of pseudophakic detachments.[144] Visualization of the fundus is reported to be even less in eyes without posterior chamber IOLs. It was found that an incomplete view of the ora serrata occurred in 44% of iris-fixed lenses and in 27% of anterior chamber lenses; therefore, there may be a slightly higher rate of surgical repair failure in these cases.[144] The success rate for posterior chamber IOL is higher than for other types of IOL at 95%;[112, 142] for iris-fixed eyes, it is 70–96%.[112, 143, 144]

Factors that have a negative effect on the success rate of reattachment are previous retinal detachment in the eye, a preoperative visual acuity of less than 20/60, a detachment involving more than three quadrants, no retinal breaks found, and cloudy media or poorly dilated pupils. Also, breaks located in more than one quadrant and at different distances from the ora are difficult to close and thus affect the success rate.[163] However, no association was found with the following preoperative conditions: open-angle glaucoma, an interval longer than 2 months after symptoms, aphakia, absence of demarcation lines, posterior breaks, hypotony, PVR, gender, and age.[182] In one study, factors that favored successful reattachment were preoperative visual acuity of 20/50 or better, detachment with tears located at or anterior to the equator, partial detachment, no giant tears, no preoperative hypertension or hypotony, fewer than 50 cryopexy applications, and single operation.[141]

FAILURE RATES

Failure rates are reported to be as high as 25%.[165] Even though a large number of failures are secondary to PVR, the majority of failed cases are not associated with membrane proliferation.[164, 165] Traditionally, failure of surgical repair was thought to be due to the surgery, but thought should be given to the possibility of progression of the underlying disease. Redetachment of the retina is defined as the reappearance of a detachment after initial reattachment, no matter how long the delay. The rate of redetachment in one study was 10.5%, and 50.5% of the redetachments occurred within less than 3 months.[183] Important risk factors for redetachment are retinal detachments due to tears rather than holes, bullous detachments, massive intraocular bleeding, and abnormal vitreous. Other reasons for failure of scleral buckles are missed retinal breaks, new breaks, and inaccurate buckle placement. Sometimes even when all retinal breaks have been recognized and with proper buckle placement, there is reattachment failure. This is likely due to continued vitreous traction and may indicate the presence of PVR.[88] Buckle revision, even only a few weeks postoperative, requires substantial cutting of scarred periocular tissue adjacent to the buckling elements, with the resulting longer reoperative time, more postoperative pain and inflammation, more scarring, and more potential complications.[184] There is a 20-fold increase in buckle extrusion secondary to periocular tissue scarring on revision surgery.[185] Buckle infection is more common after reoperations.[184] The removal of buckling elements under rectus muscles may result in diplopia.[186] During the revision surgery, further enhancement of buckling elements may produce ocular distortions that may induce a myopic shift in refraction and anisometropia.[153] Enhanced ocular compression due to reoperation may lead to choroidal detachment, chronic iritis, and anterior segment ischemia.[187] There is a higher incidence of PVR after revision operations.

COMPLICATIONS OF SCLERAL BUCKLING

Sometimes, an exudative retinal detachment follows a scleral buckling procedure due to the collection of subretinal fluid that usually occurs 48–72 hours after the surgery.[188, 189] The fluid may accumulate rapidly over a few days and even

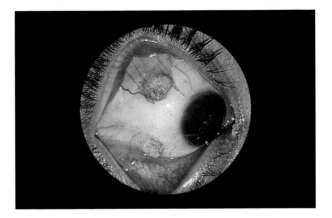

FIGURE 6-43
Eroding scleral sponge, causing pain and redness.

cause a total detachment where there was only a partial detachment initially.[88] The fluid is usually turbid, unlike the clear fluid seen under rhegmatogenous detachments. Another helpful clue to the diagnosis is that in rhegmatogenous detachments the subretinal fluid is associated with the location of the breaks, which is not the case in exudative detachments. Generally, exudative detachments spontaneously resolve in 2 weeks to 3 months, and in certain cases, systemic cortical steroids seem to hasten the resolution of the fluid.[88] Photocoagulation may worsen the condition by resulting in more fluid accumulation. The etiology of exudative detachment may be related to the compression of the vortex veins, causing venous obstruction.

An encircling element may migrate if it comes loose from the sutures used to anchor it in the scleral bed. Actual anterior extrusion (erosion) of the buckle can occur and may result in considerable ocular irritation (Figure 6-43). One of the most common causes of a scleral buckle extrusion is a secondary infection, which may be directly related to the surgery, or from an infectious agent gaining access through a small postoperative fistula. The rate of exposed or infected implants or explants is generally considered 1–3%,[190–193] and one author now reports that rate of infection of scleral buckles has now fallen to 0.5%.[194] There is usually marked pain, proptosis, chemosis, and conjunctival hyperemia (which is often followed by a mucopurulent discharge), vitritis, and scleral abscess.[195] The onset of infections usually occurs 4–9 days after surgery.[195] A localized exudate over a buckle may indicate early scleral necrosis and endophthalmitis.[196] The most common pathogens causing such infections are *Staphylococcus* species, *Proteus* species, and *Pseudomonas* species, with *Staphylococcus* being probably the most common of the three.[193, 195–197] Common sources of potential ocular contamination are the oral and nasal cavities.[198] If the infection is not responding to antibiotic therapy, the buckle must be removed. The two most common indications for removal of the exposed buckle are the spread of intraocular infection and pain. These types of infections are very difficult to treat because the buckling elements form a protective barrier against antibiotic penetration to the site of the infection and because the sclera is very avascular. Both factors make it difficult for antibiotics to reach a therapeutic level at the site of the infection. Studies have found that soaking the sponge explants in antibiotics greatly decreases the incidence of postoperative infections.[193, 199] Surgical draping is done to protect the surgical field from pathogens. The placement of multiple sponges and reoperations increases the incidence of extrusion and infection.[191, 193, 200]

The removal or cutting of the encircling band of a scleral buckle may lead to a redetachment of the retina (0–35% of cases).[191, 195, 197, 201–205] A more recent study found the redetachment rate after removal of buckling elements to be 29%.[206] The cases that are least likely to redetach are eyes in which the buckle has been in place for over a month or that display little vitreoretinal traction. If redetachment occurs, a scleral buckling procedure may be attempted after 1 week to allow the orbit to resterilize itself.[196] Reasons for buckle removal are infection, recurrent subconjunctival hemorrhage, vitreous hemorrhage, foreign body sensation, distortion of the macula, and impingement of the optic nerve.[105, 202]

A scleral buckle can cause embarrassment to the long posterior and anterior ciliary arteries and may lead to anterior segment ischemia syndrome, which is reported to occur in 3% of general retinal detachment cases.[207] The ischemia may result in corneal edema, bullous keratopathy, corneal scarring, iritis, iris necrosis, cortical lens opacities, posterior synechiae, rubeosis iridis, and glaucoma. Patients with diabetes and blood dyscrasias, such as sickle cell disease, are vulnerable to the development of anterior segment ischemia, which has been reported to occur in 71% of patients with sickle cell type retinopathy.[206] The damage caused by reattachment procedures can produce multiple abnormalities in the sympathetic and parasympathetic nerves innervating the eye.[208–211] A clinical picture similar to Adie's tonic pupil may occur and displays a mydriatic pupil, light-near dissociation, vermiform pupillary movements, and hypersensitivity to low concentrations of pilocarpine. Also after RD surgery, ciliary nerve dysfunction may result in a loss of up to 7 diopters of accommodation, but this usually resolves completely in about 5 weeks.[212]

Other Complications

Other ocular complications associated with retinal detachment operations are corneal damage, ptosis, diplopia, lagophthalmos, heterotropia, symblepharon, trichiasis, entropion, ectropion, implantation cyst, glaucoma, cataract, delayed intraocular hemorrhage, macular pucker, CME, macular hole,[213] central retinal artery occlusion, optic atrophy, sympathetic ophthalmia, and phthisis bulbi.[92, 214] The cause of postoperative CME seems to be related to a prostaglandin-mediated inflammation, which increases permeability of the perifoveal capillaries and causes fluid accumulation in the macula.[215] The incidence of angiographic CME 4–6 weeks after retinal detachment surgery in phakic patients is 25–28%, and in aphakes it increases to 40–60%.[25, 216–219] The incidence of clinically significant CME after surgery is reported to be around 3%.[220] The preoperative status of the macula and drainage of subretinal fluid does not seem to affect the occurrence of CME. Currently there is no treatment for postsurgical CME that has been found to be effective.

Macular pucker is caused by the RPE and glial cell proliferation,[221] and it has an incidence of 2–17%.[25, 121, 222, 223] Patients at risk for developing macular pucker are those who have total detachment, are older, have vitreous loss during drainage, or have PVR.[222, 223] Diplopia may occur if a large sponge is sutured beneath a rectus tendon, where adhesions can develop or trauma to the muscle may occur at the time of surgery.[88, 154, 224] Most cases of diplopia resolve spontaneously and completely.[224] Persistent cases may require surgical correction, but it is often difficult in these cases. Sometimes, prisms are beneficial. It has been reported that a 5-mm radial sponge eroded through a rectus tendon, causing diplopia.[10] The incidence of diplopia is low, at 3.3% in one study,[224] and the incidence increases with reoperations.[13, 186] Other complications are micropsia and metamorphopsia, which are likely due to spatial changes in the macular photoreceptors secondary to macular edema.[225] All complications occur more frequently after reoperations. Choroidal detachment has been reported to occur in approximately 40% of the cases in two separate studies.[226, 227]

PVR may be a complication (see Chapter 7, and Proliferative Vitreoretinopathy). Many of these complications of scleral buckling may be avoided by using temporary buckling with balloons.[228–230]

After retinopexy, retinal breaks may form at the edge of a previously treated area or at any location in the retina. A retinal tear may develop on a scleral buckle after the retina has been surgically reattached; this indicates continued vitreous traction (Figures 6-44 and 6-45). This complication may occur in the postoperative period, but it is more likely to be found years later. If the tear is on the posterior edge of the buckle, photocoagulation or cryopexy may be placed posterior to the break in an attempt to prevent a retinal detachment.

Vitrectomy

A newer technique in retinal reattachment surgery is the use of vitrectomy to reduce vitreous traction and vitreal or retinal traction bands and the associated use of endolaser photocoagulation and indirect ophthalmoscope laser delivery system for retinopexy of breaks. Also new is endodrainage retinotomy, which is the internal drainage of subretinal fluid through a surgical incision in the detached retina. One study reported an initial success rate of 78%.[184] Complications from this vitrectomy are cataracts,[231] iatrogenic retinal breaks 8%,[232, 233] glaucoma (typically

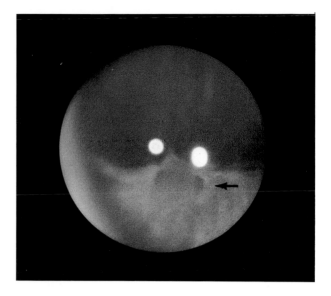

FIGURE 6-44
Scleral buckle for retinal detachment of patient seen in Figure 6-2 3 and a half years later. Note the horseshoe retinal tear in the middle of the buckle (*arrow*). View is of the inferior fundus seen through the indirect condensing lens.

secondary to vitreous hemorrhage or ghost cell obstruction),[234] and, rarely, endophthalmitis.[235] The complications found with endodrainage are rare and include epiretinal membranes, choroidal detachment, and recurrent detachment.[236]

FIGURE 6-45
B-scan ultrasonogram of a superior triangular scleral buckle shadow. Note that the eye wall is flattened straight by the buckle. On the center of the buckle is a small flap tear (*arrow*).

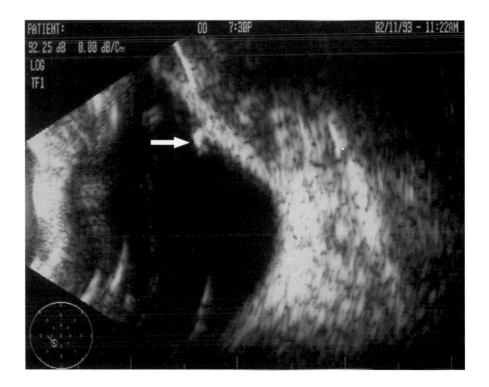

Surgical Anesthesia

Retinal detachment surgery can be done under general or local anesthesia. General anesthesia is clearly indicated for specific cases, but it carries significant risks and higher costs.[237–239] Local anesthesia is peribulbar or retrobulbar blocks, and because most surgical procedures can be completed in less than 2 hours, most cases can be done under local anesthesia. The major disadvantage of local anesthesia is inadequate analgesia in 4–10% of cases.[88] Retrobulbar injections may cause complications due to the blind insertion of the needle into the muscle cone that may result in venous or arterial retrobulbar hemorrhage (1–5%),[240] penetration of the globe, especially in myopes (<0.1%),[241–244] brainstem anesthesia (0.29%),[245] respiratory arrest,[245, 246] seizures,[246, 247] optic nerve trauma,[244, 248] and retinal vascular occlusions.[249, 250] Risk factors for perforation of the globe in retrobulbar injections are high axial length of the eye and previous detachment surgery.[241] To avoid many of these complications, many surgeons are performing peribulbar injections, which place the anesthesia fluid outside the muscle cone.[251, 252] With peribulbar injections there have been rare reported cases of perforation of the globe,[242, 243, 253] retrobulbar hemorrhage,[254] and extraocular paresis.[255] Many investigators have reported that peribulbar is a safer procedure and an effective means of obtaining ocular anesthesia.[252, 256–259]

Education

It is extremely important to educate the patient with retinal lesions that may predispose the patient to a retinal detachment. This is accomplished by giving the patient the symptoms of retinal tears and detachments and instructing the patient to have a dilated fundus examination as soon as possible if symptoms occur. A number of studies have shown that the fellow eye retinal detachment fared much better after surgery, which is likely due to the fact that the patient was aware of the potential ocular problem and returned much sooner for an eye examination. In one study of a large number of patients by Davis et al.,[260] it was found that in fellow phakic eye detachment, only 25% had a detached macula, compared to a large series of initial phakic detachments in which 65% had a detached macula.[261] In another study, Benson et al.[262] reported a reattachment success rate of 83% after intracapsular cataract surgery, with 45% retaining visual acuities of 20/50 or better. In the their series of the same type of patients with a fellow eye detachment the reattachment success rate was reported to be 96%, with 72% retaining 20/50 or better visual acuity.

References

1. Duke-Elder S, Dobree JH. Detachment and Folding of the Retina. In Duke-Elder S (ed), System of Ophthalmology. Vol. 10, Diseases of the Retina. St. Louis: Mosby, 1967:773.
2. Gonin J. Le Decollement de la Retine: Pathogenie-Traitement. Lausanne, Switzerland: Librairie Payot, 1934.
3. Gonin J. The treatment of the detached retina by searing the retinal tears. Arch Ophthalmol 1930;4:621–625.
4. Colyear BH Jr, Pischel DK. Preventative treatment of retinal detachment by means of light coagulation. Trans Pac Coast Oto Ophthalmol Soc 1960,41:193–215.
5. Halpern JI. Routine screening of the retinal periphery. Am J Ophthalmol 1966;6:99–202.
6. Meyer-Schwickerath G. Light Photocoagulation. St. Louis: Mosby, 1960.
7. Custodis E. Bedeutet die plombenaufnahung auf die sklera einen fortschritt in der operativen behanklung der netzhautablosung? Ber Dtsch Ophthalmol Ges 1953;58:102-105.
8. Custodis E. Beobachtungen bei der diathermischen behandlung der netzhautablosung und ein minweis zur therapie der amotio retinae. Berl Dtsch Ophthalmol Ges 1952;57:227–230.
9. Custodis E. Die behandlung der netzhautablosung durch umschriebene diathermiekoagulation und einer mettels plombenaufnahung erzeugten eindellung der sklera im bereich des risses. Klin Monatsbl Augenheilkd 1956;129:476–495.
10. Lincoff H, Kreissig. Management of Rhegmatogenous Retinal Detachment. In WR Freeman (ed), Practical Atlas of Retinal Disease and Therapy. New York: Raven, 1993:221–235.
11. American Academy of Ophthalmology Preferred Practice Patterns: Retinal Detachment. San Francisco: American Academy of Ophthalmology, 1990.
12. Wilkinson CP, Bradford RH Jr. Complications of draining subretinal fluid. Retina 1984,4:1–4.
13. Smiddy WE, Loupe D, et al. Extraocular muscle imbalance after scleral buckling surgery. Ophthalmology 1988;95:601.
14. Chen JC, Robertson JE, et al. Results and complications of pneumatic retinopexy. Ophthalmology 1977;84:641–644.
15. Jarrett WH. Retinal detachment. Trans Am Ophthalmol Soc 1988;86:307–320.
16. Ando F, Kondo J. A plastic tack for treatment of retinal detachment with giant tear. Am J Ophthalmol 1983;95:260–261.
17. DeJuan E, Hickingbotham D, et al. Retinal tacks. Am J Ophthalmol 1985;99:272–274.
18. DeJuan E, McCuen BW, et al. Mechanical fixation using tacks. Ophthalmology 1987;94:337–339.
19. Abrams GW, Williams GA, et al. Clinical results of titanium retinal tacks with pneumatic insertion. Am J Ophthalmol 1986;102:13–19.
20. O'Grady GE, Parel J-M, et al. Hypodermic stainless steel tacks and companion inserter designed for peripheral fixation of retina. Arch Ophthalmol 1988;106:271–275.
21. Algevere P, Stenkula S, et al. Sealing of retinal breaks with

metallic tacks: Evaluation of a new procedure in retinal reattachment surgery. Acta Ophthalmol 1986;64:421–424.

22. Machemer R, McCuen B, et al. Relaxing retinotomies and retinectomies. Am J Ophthalmol 1986;102:7–12.

23. De Juan E, McCuen B, et al. The use of retinal tacks in the repair of complicated retinal detachment. Am J Ophthalmol 1986;102:20–24.

24. Burke J, McDonald R, et al. Titanium retinal tacks with pneumatic insertion: Histological evaluation in rabbits. Arch Ophthalmol 1987;105:404–408.

25. Meredith TA, Reeser FH, et al. Cystoid macular edema after retinal detachment surgery. Ophthalmology 1990; 87:1090–1095.

26. Ackerman AL, Topilow HW. A reduced incidence of cystoid macular edema following retinal detachment surgery using diathermy. Ophthalmology 1985;92:1092–1095.

27. Campocguari PA, Kaden IH, et al. Cryotherapy enhances intravitreal dispersion of viable pigment epithelial cells. Arch Ophthalmol 1985;103:434–436.

28. Jaccoma EH, Conway BP, et al. Cryotherapy causes extensive breakdown of the blood-retinal barrier: A comparison of argon laser photocoagulation. Arch Ophthalmol 1985;103:1728–1730.

29. Sabetes NR, Tolentino FI, et al. The complications of perfluoropropane gas used in complex retinal detachments. Retina 1996;16:7–12.

30. The Silicone Study Group. Report 2: vitrectomy with silicone oil or perfluoropropane gas in eyes with severe proliferative vitreoretinopathy: Results of a randomized clinical trial. Arch Ophthalmol 1992;110:780–792.

31. Fineberg E, Machemer R, et al. SF6 for retinal detachment surgery. Mod Probl Ophthalmol 1974;12:173–176.

32. Schoch D, in discussion of Fineberg E, Machemer R, Sullivan P. SF6 for retinal detachment surgery. Mod Probl Ophthalmol 1974;12:345–368.

33. Lincoff H, Mardirossian J, et al. Intravitreal longevity of three perfluorocarbon gases. Arch Ophthalmol 1980;98: 1610–1611.

34. Lincoff H, Coleman J, et al. The perfluorocarbon gases in the treatment of retinal detachment. Ophthalmology 1983;90:546–551.

35. Thompson JT, Michels RG. Volume displacement of scleral buckles. Arch Ophthalmol 1985;103:1822–1826.

36. Whitacre MM. Principles and Applications of Intraocular Gas (2nd ed). Boston: Butterworth-Heinemann, 1997.

37. Bonnet B, Santamaria J. Intraoperative use of pure perfluoropropane gas in the management of proliferative retinopathy. Graefes Arch Clin Exp Ophthalmol 1987;225: 299–302.

38. Lincoff H, Weinberger D, et al. Air travel with intraocular gas. Arch Ophthalmol 1989;107:907–910.

39. Kokame GT, Ing MR. Intraocular gas and low-altitude air flight. Retina 1994;14:356–358.

40. Foulks GN, de Juan E, et al. The effects of perfluoropropane on the corneas in rabbits and cats. Arch Ophthalmol 1987;105:256–259.

41. Matsuda M, Tano Y, et al. Corneal endothelial cell damage associated with intraocular gas tamponade during pars plana vitrectomy. Jpn J Ophthalmol 1986;30:324–329.

42. Pavan PR. Retinal fold in macula following intraocular gas. Arch Ophthalmol 1988;106:83–84.

43. Pavan PR. Arcurate retinal folds after intraocular gas injection. Arch Ophthalmol 1988;106:164–165.

44. Pavan PR, Witherspoon D. Macular folds after retinal detachment repair. Vitreoretinal Surg Tech 1991;3:4–5.

45. Machemer R, Aaberg TM, et al. Giant retinal tears. II. Experimental production and management with intraocular air. Am J Ophthalmol 1969;68:1022–1029.

46. Lewen RM, Lyon CE, et al. Scleral buckling with intraocular air injection complicated by arcuate retinal folds. Arch Ophthalmol 1987;105:1212–1215.

47. Michels RG, Wilkinson CP, Rice TA. Retinal Detachment: Diagnosis and Management. St. Louis: Mosby, 1990.

48. Larrison WI, Frederick AR, et al. Posterior retinal folds following vitreoretinal surgery. Arch Ophthalmol 1993;111: 621–625.

49. Hilton GF, Tornambe PE, et al. Pneumatic retinopexy: An analysis of intraoperative and postoperative complications. Retina 1991;11:285–294.

50. Tornambe PE, Hilton GF. Pneumatic retinopexy: A multi-centered randomized controlled clinical trial comparing pneumatic retinopexy with scleral buckling. The Retinal Detachment Study Group. Ophthalmology 1989;96:772–783.

51. Blair NP, Shaw WE, et al. Retinal reattachment by continuous vitreous insufflation. Arch Ophthalmol 1989;107: 1217–1219.

52. Tornambe PE, Hilton GF, et al. Expanded indications for pneumatic retinopexy. Ophthalmology 1988;95:597–600.

53. Termote H. Pneumatic retinopexy: Analysis of the first 20 cases. Bull Soc Belge Ophtalmol 1989;231:107–116.

54. Davis JL, Serfass MS, et al. Silicone oil in repair of retinal detachments caused by necrotizing retinitis in HIV infection. Arch Ophthalmol 1995;113:1401–1409.

55. Fawcett IM, Williams RL, et al. Contact angles of substance used for internal tamponade in retinal detachment surgery. Graefes Arch Clin Exp Ophthalmol 1994;232:438–444.

56. Foerster MH, Esser J, et al. Silicone oil and influence on electrophysiological findings. Am J Ophthalmol 1985;99: 201–206.

57. Frumar KD, Gregor ZJ, et al. Electroretinographic changes after vitrectomy and intraocular tamponade. Retina 1985;5:16–21.

58. Pang MP, Peyman GA, et al. Early anterior segment complications after silicone oil injection. Can J Ophthalmol 1986;21:271–275.

59. Laganowski HC, Leaver PK. Silicone oil in the aphakic eye: The influence of a six o'clock peripheral iridectomy. Eye 1989;3:338–348.

60. Lucke K, Forster M, et al. Langzeiterfahrungen mit intraokularer silikonol-fulllung. Fortschr Ophthalmol 1987;84: 96–98.

61. Dimopoulos ST, Heimann K. Spatkomplikationen nach silikonolinjektion. Langzeitheobachfungen an 100 fallen. Klin Monatsbl Augenheilkd 1986;189:223–227.

62. Foulks GN, Hatchell DL, et al. Histopathology of silicone oil keratopathy in humans. Cornea 1991;10:29–37.

63. Skorpik C, Menapace R, et al. Silicone oil implantation in penetrating injuries complicated by PVR. Results from 1982 to 1986. Retina 1989;9:8–14.

64. Madreperla SA, McCuen BW. Inferior peripheral iridectomy in patients receiving silicone oil. Rates of postoperative closure and effect on oil position. Retina 1995;15:87–90.

65. Ando F. Intraocular hypertension resulting from pupillary block by silicone oil. Am J Ophthalmol 1985;99:87–88.

66. Federman JL, Schubert HD. Complications associated with use of silicone oil in 150 eyes after retina-vitreous surgery. Ophthalmology 1988;95:870–876.

67. Yeo JH, Glaser BM, et al. Silicone oil in the treatment of complicated retinal detachments. Ophthalmology 1987;94: 1109–1113.

68. Lemmen KD, Moter H, et al. Keratopathy following vitrectomy with silicone oil injection. Fortschr Ophthalmol 1989;86:570–573.
69. Reidel KG, Gabel VP, et al. Intravitreal silicone oil injection: Complications and treatment of 415 consecutive patients. Graefes Arch Clin Exp Ophthalmol 1990;228:19–23.
70. Beekhuis WH, Ando F, et al. Basal iridectomy at 6 o'clock in the aphakic eye treated with silicone oil: Prevention of keratopathy and secondary glaucoma. Br J Ophthalmol 1987;71:197–200.
71. Stilma JS, Koster R, et al. Radical vitrectomy and silicone-oil injection in the treatment of proliferative vitreoretinopathy following retinal detachment. Doc Ophthalmol 1986;64:109–116.
72. Cibis PA, Becker B, et al. The use of liquid silicone in retinal detachment surgery. Arch Ophthalmol 1981;68:590–599.
73. Stefansson E, Tiedeman J. Optics of the eye with air of silicone oil. Retina 1988;81:10–19.
74. Stefansson E, Anderson M, et al. Refractive changes from use of silicone oil in vitreous surgery. Retina 1988;81:20–23.
75. Dereklis DL, Lake SS, et al. Ocular Surgical News 1996; 14:65–67.
76. Lean J, Azen SP, et al. The prognostic utility of the silicone study classification system: silicone study report 9. Arch Ophthalmol 1996;114:286–292.
77. The Silicone Study Group. Vitrectomy with silicone oil or sulfur hexafluoride gas in eyes with severe proliferative vitreoretinopathy: Results of a randomized clinical trial: Silicone Study Report 1. Arch Ophthalmol 1992;110:770–779.
78. Freeman WR, Quiceno JI, et al. Surgical repair of rhegmatogenous retinal detachment in immunosuppressed patients with cytomegalovirus retinitis. Ophthalmology 1992;99:466–474.
79. Chuang EL, Davis JL. Management of retinal detachment associated with CMV retinitis in AIDS patients. Eye 1992;6:28–34.
80. Dugal PU, Liggett PE, et al. Repair of retinal detachment caused by cytomegalovirus retinitis in patients with the acquired immunodeficiency syndrome. Am J Ophthalmol 1991;112:235–239.
81. Irvine AR. Treatment of retinal detachment due to cytomegalovirus retinitis in patients with AIDS. Trans Am Ophthalmol Soc 1991;89:349–367.
82. Regillo CD, Vander JF, et al. Repair of retinitis-related retinal detachments with silicone oil in patients with acquired immunodeficiency syndrome. Am J Ophthalmol 1992; 113:21–27.
83. Kuppermann DB, Flores-Aguilar M, et al. A masked prospective evaluation of outcome parameters for cytomegalovirus-related retinal detachment surgery in patients with acquired immunodeficiency syndrome. Ophthalmology 1994;101:46–55.
84. Engstrom RE, Holland GN, et al. The progressive outer retinal layer syndrome: A variant of necrotizing herpetic retinopathy in patients with AIDS. Ophthalmology 1994;101:1488–1502.
85. Ross WH, Bryan JS, et al. Management of retinal detachments secondary to cytomegalovirus retinitis. Can J Ophthalmol 1994;29:129–133.
86. Lagua H, Machemer R. Repair and adhesion mechanisms of the cryotherapy lesions in experimental retinal detachment. Am J Ophthalmol 1976;81:833–846.
87. Kita M, Negi A, et al. Photothermal, cryogenic and diathermic effects on retinal adhesive force in vivo. Retina 1991;11:441–444.
88. Williams GA, Aaberg TM Sr. Techniques of Scleral Buckling. In W Tasman, EA Jaeger (eds), Clinical Ophthalmology. Vol. 6. Philadelphia: Harper & Row, 1994;39:1–40.
89. Welch RB. A survey of retinal detachment surgeons on the use of cryotherapy or diathermy. Am J Ophthalmol 1970;69:749–754.
90. Aaberg TM, Wiznia RA. The use of solid soft silicone rubber explants in retinal detachment surgery. Ophthal Surg 1976;7:98–105.
91. Oosterhuis JA, Brihaye M, et al. A comparative study of experimental transcleral cryocoagulation by solid carbon dioxide and diathermocoagulation of the retina. Ophthalmologica 1968;156:38–76.
92. Schepens CL. Retinal Detachment and Allied Diseases. Philadelphia: Saunders, 1983.
93. Norton EWD. Present status of cryotherapy in retinal detachment surgery. Trans Am Acad Ophthalmol Otolaryngol 1969;73:1029–1034.
94. Birchall CH. The fishmouth phenomenon in retinal detachment: Old concepts revisited. Br J Ophthalmol 1979;63:507–510.
95. Goldbaum MH, Smithline M, et al. Geometric analysis of radial buckling. Am J Ophthalmol 1975;79:958–965.
96. Borras A, Meerhoff A. Ten years' experience with intrascleral gelatin implants in retinal detachment. Am J Ophthalmol 1972;73:390–393.
97. Regan CDJ, Schepens CL, et al. The scleral buckling procedure. VI. Further notes on silicone in primary operation. Arch Ophthalmol 1962;68:313–328.
98. Michels RG. Scleral buckling methods for rhegmatogenous retinal detachments. Retina 1986;6:1–49.
99. Pruett RC. The fishmouth phenomenon. II. Wedge scleral buckling. Arch Ophthalmol 1977;95:1782–1787.
100. Pruett RC. The fishmouth phenomenon. I. Clinical characteristics and surgical options. Arch Ophthalmol 1977;95:1777–1781.
101. Lincoff H. The rationale for radial buckling. Mod Probl Ophthalmol 1974;12:484–491.
102. Lincoff H, Kreissig I. Advantages of radial buckling. Am J Ophthalmol 1975;79:955–957.
103. Regan CDJ, Schepens CL. Erosion of the ocular wall by circling polyethylene tubing: A late complication of scleral buckling. Trans Am Acad Ophthalmol Otolaryngol 1963;67:335–341.
104. Yoshizumi MD, Friberg T. Erosion of implants in retinal detachment surgery. Ann Ophthalmol 1983;15:430–434.
105. Weinberger D, Lichter H, et al. Intraocular intrusion of sutures after retinal detachment buckling surgery. Retina 1995;15:417–421.
106. Lincoff H, Kressig I, et al. Limits of constriction in the treatment of retinal detachment. Arch Ophthalmol 1976; 94:1473–1477.
107. Sternberg P, Tiedeman J, et al. Sutureless scleral buckle for retinal detachment with thin sclera. Retina 1988;8:247–249.
108. Lewis H, Aaberg TM, et al. Intrusion of retinal tacks. Am J Ophthalmol 1987;103:672–680.
109. Bietti GB, Pannarade MR. The Encircling Technique of Arruga and Various Substitutive Procedures. In A McPherson (ed), New and Controversial Aspects of Retinal Detachment. New York: Harper & Row, 1968:299–317.
110. Pischel DK. Retinal Detachment: A Manual (2nd ed). American Academy of Ophthalmology and Otolaryngology 1965;197–199.
111. Besada E, Jones WL. Eroding scleral polyethylene tube. J Clin Eye Vision Care 1992;3:123–125.

112. Wilkinson CP. Pseudophakic retinal detachment. Retina 1985;5:1–4.

113. O'Connor PR. External buckling without drainage. Int Ophthalmol Clin 1976;16:107–126.

114. Chignell AH. Retinal detachment surgery without drainage of subretinal fluid. Am J Ophthalmol 1974;77:1–5.

115. Leaver PK, Chester GH, et al. Factors influencing absorption of subretinal fluid. Br J Ophthalmol 1976;60:557–560.

116. Leaver PK, Chignell AH, et al. Role of nondrainage of subretinal fluid in re-operations of retinal detachment. Br J Ophthalmol 1975;59:252–254.

117. Lincoff H, Kreissig I. The treatment of retinal detachment without drainage of subretinal fluid: Modifications of the Custodis procedure: VI. Trans Am Acad Ophthalmol Otolaryngol 1972;76:1221–1233.

118. Hilton GF, Gizzard WS, et al. The drainage of subretinal fluid: A randomized controlled clinical trial. Retina 1981;1:271–280.

119. O'Connor PR. Absorption of subretinal fluid after scleral buckling without drainage. Am J Ophthalmol 1973;76:30–34.

120. Chignell AH, Talbot J. Absorption of subretinal fluid after nondrainage retinal detachment surgery. Arch Ophthalmol 1978;96:635–637.

121. Neumann E, Hyams S. Conservative management of retinal breaks. A follow up study of subsequent retinal detachment. Br J Ophthalmol 1972;56:482–486.

122. Engel JM, Blair NP, et al. Use of carbon dioxide laser in the drainage of subretinal fluid. Arch Ophthalmol 1989;107:731–734.

123. Freeman HM, Schepens CL. Innovations in the technique of drainage of subretinal fluid transillumination and choroidal diathermy. Mod Probl Ophthalmol 1975;15:119–126.

124. Gartner J. Release of subretinal fluid with the aid of the microscope: Report on 100 cases. Mod Probl Ophthalmol 1975;15:127–133.

125. Bovino JA, Marcus DF, et al. Argon laser choroidotomy for the drainage of subretinal fluid. Arch Ophthalmol 1985;103:443–444.

126. Meyer-Schwickerath G, Klein M. Drainage of subretinal fluid with a cathode needle. Mod Probl Ophthalmol 1975;15:154–157.

127. Humphrey WT, Schepens CL, et al. The Release of Subretinal Fluid and Its Complications. In RC Pruett, CDJ Regan (eds), Retina Congress. East Norwalk, CT: Appleton-Century-Crofts, 1972:383–390.

128. Kingham JD. Retinal reattachment surgery: The basic procedure and its modifications. Ophthalmic Surg 1978;9:51–80.

129. Martin B. Controlled release of subretinal fluid. Mod Probl Ophthalmol 1975;15:149–153.

130. Ibanez HE, Bloom SM, et al. External argon laser choroidotomy versus needle drainage technique in primary scleral buckle procedures: A prospective randomized study. Retina 1994;14:348–350.

131. Haller JA, Lim JL, et al. Pilot trial of transscleral diode laser retinopexy in retinal detachment surgery. Arch Ophthalmol 1993;111:952–956.

132. Gottlieb F, Fammartina JJ, et al. Retinal angiomatous mass: A complication of retinal detachment surgery. Retina 1984;4:152–157.

133. Guillaumat L. La ponction au cours des intervention pour decollement de la retine. Mod Probl Ophthalmol 1975;15:207–213.

134. Hilton GF. The drainage of subretinal fluid: A randomized controlled clinical trial. Trans Am Ophthalmol Soc 1981;79:517–540.

135. McLoed D. Monitored posterior transcleral drainage of subretinal fluid. Br J Ophthalmol 1985;59:433–434.

136. Fitzpatrick EP, Abott D. Drainage of subretinal fluid with the argon laser. Am J Ophthalmol 1993;115:755–757.

137. Burton RL, Carns TD, et al. Needle drainage of subretinal fluid: A randomized clinical trial. Retina 1993;13:13–16.

138. Dunnington JH, Macnie JP. Detachment of the retina: Operative results in 150 cases. Arch Ophthalmol 1935;13:191–200.

139. Burton TC. Recovery of visual acuity after retinal detachment involving the macula. Trans Am Ophthalmol Soc 1982;80:475–497.

140. Burton TC. Preoperative factors influencing anatomical success rates following retinal detachment surgery. Trans Am Acad Ophthalmol Otolaryngol 1977;83:499–505.

141. Tani P, Robertson DM, et al. Prognosis for central vision and anatomic reattachment of rhegmatogenous retinal detachment with macula detached. Am J Ophthalmol 1981;92:611–620.

142. Smith PW, Stark WJ, et al. Retinal detachment after extracapsular cataract extraction with posterior chamber intraocular lens. Ophthalmology 1987;94:495–504.

143. Greven CM, Sanders RJ, et al. Pseudophakic retinal detachment: Anatomic and visual results. Ophthalmology 1992;99:257–262.

144. Ho PC, Tolentino FI. Pseudophakic retinal detachment surgical success rate with various types of IOLs. Ophthalmology 1984;91:847–852.

145. Fuller DG, Hutton WL. Anterior chamber suture in pseudophakic retinal detachment requiring intraocular gas. Arch Ophthalmol 1980;98:1101.

146. Tani P, Robertson DM, et al. Rhegmatogenous retinal detachment without macular involvement treated with scleral buckling. Am J Ophthalmol 1980;90:503–508.

147. Grizzard WS, Hilton GF. Scleral buckling for retinal detachment complicated by periretinal proliferation. Arch Ophthalmol 1982;100:419–422.

148. Burton TC, Lambert RW Jr. A predictive model for visual recovery following retinal detachment surgery. Ophthalmology 1978;85:619–625.

149. Davis MD. Natural history of retinal breaks without detachment. Arch Ophthalmol 1974;92:183–194.

150. Grupposo SS. Visual acuity following surgery for retinal detachment. Arch Ophthalmol 1975;93:327–330.

151. Isernhagen RD, Wilkinson CP. Visual acuity after the repair of pseudophakic retinal detachments involving the macula. Retina 1989;9:15–21.

152. Jacklin HN. Refraction changes after surgical treatment of retinal detachment. South Med J 1971;64:148–150.

153. Rubin ML. The induction of refractive errors by retinal detachment surgery. Trans Am Ophthalmol Soc 1976;73:452–490.

154. Burton TC. Irregular astigmatism following episcleral buckle procedure with the use of silicone rubber sponges. Arch Ophthalmol 1973;90:447–448.

155. Burton TC, Herron BE, et al. Axial length changes after retinal detachment surgery. Am J Ophthalmol 1977;83:59–62.

156. Fiore JV, Newton JC. Anterior chamber changes following the scleral buckling procedure. Arch Ophthalmol 1970;84:284–287.

157. Harris JM, Blumenkranz MS, et al. Geometric alterations produced by encircling scleral buckles: Biometric and clinical considerations. Retina 1987;7:14–19.

158. Smiddy WE, Loupe DN, et al. Refractive changes after

scleral buckling surgery. Arch Ophthalmol 1989;107: 1469–1471.

159. Beekhuis H, Talsma M, et al. Changes in refraction after retinal detachment surgery corrected by extended wear contact lenses for early visual rehabilitation. Retina 1993;13:120–124.

160. Dalgleish R. Assessment of the intra-scleral silicone rubber implants with encircling band in retinal detachment surgery. Br J Ophthalmol 1966;50:245.

161. Morse PH. Fixed retinal star folds in retinal detachment. Am J Ophthalmol 1974;77:760–764.

162. The Retina Society Terminology Committee. The classification of retinal detachment with proliferative vitreoretinopathy. Ophthalmology 1983;90:121–125.

163. Sharma T, Challa JK, et al. Scleral buckling for retinal detachment. Predictors for anatomic failure. Retina 1994;14:338–343.

164. Rachal WF, Burton TC. Changing concepts of failures after retinal detachment surgery. Arch Ophthalmol 1979;97: 480–483.

165. Chignell AH, Fison LG, et al. Failure in retinal detachment surgery. Br J Ophthalmol 1973;57:525–530.

166. Kreiger AE, Hodgkinson J, et al. The results of retinal detachment surgery. Arch Ophthalmol 1971;86:385–394.

167. Tani P, Robertson DM, et al. Rhegmatogenous retinal detachment without drainage. Am J Ophthalmol 1980; 90:503–508.

168. Wilkinson CP. Visual results following scleral buckling for retinal detachments sparing the macula. Retina 1981;1: 113–116.

169. Cousins S, Boniuk I, et al. Pseudophakic retinal detachments in the presence of various IOL types. Ophthalmology 1986;93:1198–1207.

170. Ober RR, Wilkinson CR, Fiore JV, et al. Rhegmatogenous retinal detachment after neodymium-YAG laser capsulotomy in aphakic and pseudophakic eyes. Am J Ophthalmol 1986;101:1396–1402.

171. Norton EWD. Retinal detachment in aphakia. Trans Am Ophthalmol Soc 1963;61:770–779.

172. Jagger JD, Cooling RJ, et al. Management of retinal detachment following congenital cataract surgery. Trans Ophthalmol Soc UK 1983;103:103–107.

173. Kanski JJ, Elkington AR, et al. Retinal detachment after congenital cataract surgery. Br J Ophthalmol 1974;58:92–95.

174. Taylor BC, Tasman WS. Retinal detachment following congenital cataract surgery. Texas Medical Journal 1974; 70:83–87.

175. Cox MS, Freeman HM. Retinal detachment due to ocular penetration. I. Clinical characteristics and surgical results. Arch Ophthalmol 1978;96:1354–1361.

176. Seelenfreund MH, Kraushar MS, et al. Choroidal detachment associated with primary retinal detachment. Arch Ophthalmol 1974;94:254–258.

177. Gottlieb F. Combined choroidal and retinal detachment. Arch Ophthalmol 1973;88:481–486.

178. Norton EWD. Retinal detachment in aphakia. Am J Ophthalmol 1974;58:111–124.

179. Smith TR, Pierce LH. Idiopathic detachment of the retina: Analysis of results. Arch Ophthalmol 1953;49:36–44.

180. Tillery WV, Lucier AC. Round atrophic holes in lattice degeneration. Trans Am Acad Ophthalmol Otolaryngol 1976;81:509–518.

181. Hagler WS, North AW. Retinal dialysis and retinal detachment. Arch Ophthalmol 1968;79:376–388.

182. Tornquist R, Bodin L, et al. Retinal detachment. A study of a population-based patient material in Sweden 1971–1981. IV. Prediction of surgical outcome. Acta Ophthalmologica 1988;66:637–642.

183. Girard P, Bokobza Y, et al. Retinal detachment recurrences. I. Frequency and risk factors. J Fr Ophtalmol 1882; 5:99–102.

184. Friedman ES, D'Amico DJ. Vitrectomy alone for the management of uncomplicated recurrent retinal detachment. Retina 1995;15:469–474.

185. Flindall RJ, Norton EWD, et al. Reduction of extrusion and infection following episcleral silicone implants and cryopexy in retinal detachment surgery. Am J Ophthalmol 1971;71:835–837.

186. Sewell JJ, Knoblock WH, et al. Extraocular muscle imbalance after treatment for retinal detachment. Am J Ophthalmol 1974;78:321–323.

187. Hayreh SS, Bains JAB. Occlusion of the vortex veins: An experimental study. Br J Ophthalmol 1973;57:217–238.

188. Aaberg TM, Pawlowski GJ. Exudative retinal detachment following scleral buckling with cryotherapy. Am J Ophthalmol 1972;74:245–251.

189. Topilow HW, Ackerman AL. Massive exudative retinal and choroidal detachments following scleral buckling surgery. Ophthalmology 1983;90:143–147.

190. Hitchings RA, Levy IS, et al. Acute infection after retinal detachment surgery. Br J Ophthalmol 1974;58:588–590.

191. Wiznia RA. Removal of solid silicone rubber explants after retinal detachment surgery. Am J Ophthalmol 1983; 95:495–497.

192. Lincoff H. Discussion of Arribas NP, Olk RJ, et al. Preoperative antibiotic soaking of silicone sponges: Does it make a difference? Ophthalmology 1984;91:1689.

193. Arribas NP, Olk RJ, et al. Preoperative antibiotic soaking of silicone sponges: does it make a difference? Ophthalmology 1984;91:1684–1688.

194. Kreissig I, Lincoff H. Other advances in chorio-retinal surgery. A comparative study of sponge infections. Mod Probl Ophthalmol 1979;20:154–156.

195. Lincoff H, Nadel A, et al. The changing character of infected scleral implants. Arch Ophthalmol 1970;84: 421–423.

196. Benson WE (ed). Retinal Detachment: Diagnosis and Management. New York: Lippincott, 1987;9.

197. Ulrich RA, Burton TC. Infections following scleral buckling procedures. Arch Ophthalmol 1974;92:213–215.

198. Flindall RJ, Norton EWD, et al. Reduction of extrusion and infection following episcleral silicone implants and cryopexy in retinal detachment surgery. Am J Ophthalmol 1971;71:835–837.

199. Doft BH, Lipkowitz J, et al. An experimental model of the assessed factors associated with scleral buckle infection. Retina 1983;3:212–217.

200. Buettner H, Goldstein BG, et al. Infection prophylaxis with Silastic sponge explants in retinal detachment surgery. Dev Ophthalmol 1981;2:71–76.

201. Hahn YS, Lincoff A, et al. Infection after sponge implantation for scleral buckling. Am J Ophthalmol 1979;87: 180–185.

202. Hilton G, Wallyn R. The removal of scleral buckles. Arch Ophthalmol 1978;96:2061–2063.

203. Lindsey PS, Pierce LH, et al. Removal of scleral buckling elements. Arch Ophthalmol 1983;101:570–573.

204. Schwartz P, Pruett R. Factors influencing retinal detachment after removal of buckling elements. Arch Ophthalmol 1977;95:804–805.

205. Stratford TP. Fate of the Reattached Retina Following Removal of Silicone Elements. In CL Pruett, CDJ Regan (eds), Retina Congress. New York: Appleton-Century-Crofts, 1974:623.

206. Smiddy WE, Miller D, et al. Scleral buckling removal following retinal reattachment surgery: Clinical and microbiologic aspects. Ophthalmic Surg 1993;24:440–445.

207. Ryan SJ, Goldberg MF. Anterior segment ischemia following scleral buckling in sickle cell hemoglobinopathy. Am J Ophthalmol 1971;72:35–50.

208. Kronfield PC. Segmental impairment of pupillary motility after operations for retinal detachment. Trans Am Ophthalmol Soc 1961;59:239–251.

209. Lobes LA Jr, Bourgon P. Pupillary abnormalities induced by argon laser photocoagulation. Ophthalmology 1985;92:234–236.

210. Newsome DA, Einaugler RB. Tonic pupil following retinal detachment surgery. Arch Ophthalmol 1971;86:233–234.

211. Rogell GD. Internal ophthalmoplegia after argon laser panretinal photocoagulation. Arch Ophthalmol 1979;97:904–905.

212. Lerner BC, Lakhanpal V, et al. Transient myopia and accommodative paresis following retinal cryotherapy and panretinal photocoagulation. Am J Ophthalmol 1984;97:704–708.

213. Brown GC. Macular hole following rhegmatogenous retinal detachment surgery. Arch Ophthalmol 1988;106:765–766.

214. Tornquist R, Tornquist P. Retinal detachment. A study of a population-based patient material in Sweden 1971–1981. III. Surgical results. Acta Ophthalmol Scand 1988;66:630–636.

215. Miyake K, Miyake Y, et al. Incidence of cystoid macular edema after retinal detachment surgery and the use of topical indomethacin. Am J Ophthalmol 1983;95:451–456.

216. Preud'homme Y, Demolle D, et al. Metabolism of arachidonic acid in rabbit iris and retina. Invest Ophthalmol Vis Sci 1985;26:133–134.

217. Flach AJ. Cyclo-oxygenase inhibitors in ophthalmology. Surv Ophthalmol 1992;36:259–284.

218. Williams GA, Reeser F, et al. Prostacyclin and thromboxane A2 derivates in rhegmatogenous subretinal fluid. Arch Ophthalmol 1983;101:463–464.

219. Lobes LA Jr, Grand MG. Incidence of cystoid macular edema following scleral buckling procedure. Arch Ophthalmol 1980;98:1230–1232.

220. Bonnet M, LeNail B. Prophylaxis of operative macular complications of retinal detachment by microsurgery. J Fr Ophtalmol 1980;3:83–89.

221. Aaberg TM, Machemer R. Retinal Detachment. In A Gardner, GK Klintworth (eds), Pathophysiology of Ocular Disease: A Dynamic Approach, Part B. New York: Marcel Dekker, 1982.

222. Lobes LA Jr, Burton TC. The incidence of macular pucker after retinal detachment surgery. Am J Ophthalmol 1978;85:72–77.

223. Tanenbaum HL, Schepens CL, et al. Macular pucker following retinal detachment surgery. Arch Ophthalmol 1970;83:286–293.

224. Kanski JJ, Elkington AR, et al. Diplopia after retinal detachment surgery. Am J Ophthalmol 1973;76:38–40.

225. Sjostrand J, Anderson C. Micropsia and metamorphopsia in the re-attached macula following retinal detachment. Acta Ophthalmol 1986;64:425–432.

226. Packer AJ, Maggiano JM, et al. Serous choroidal detachment after retinal detachment surgery. Arch Ophthalmol 1983;101:1221–1224.

227. Valone J Jr, Moser D. Management of rhegmatogenous retinal detachment with macula detached: Steroids, choroidal detachment and visual acuity. Ophthalmology 1986;93:1413–1417

228. Lincoff H, Kreissig I, et al. A temporary balloon buckle for the treatment of small retinal detachments. Ophthalmology 1979;86:586–596.

229. Kreissig I. 10 years' experience with the balloon operation. Klin Monatsbl Augenheilkd 1989;194:145–151.

230. Kreissig I, Failer J, et al. Results of a temporary balloon buckle in the treatment of 500 retinal detachments and a comparison with pneumatic retinopexy. Am J Ophthalmol 1989;107:381–389.

231. Cherfan GM, Michels RG, et al. Nuclear sclerotic cataract after vitrectomy for idiopathic epiretinal membranes causing macular pucker. Am J Ophthalmol 1991;111:434–438.

232. Faulborn J, Conway BP, et al. Surgical complications of pars plana vitreous surgery. Ophthalmology 1978;85:116–125.

233. Oyakawa RT, Schachat AP, et al. Complications of vitreous surgery for diabetic retinopathy. Ophthalmology 1983;90:522–529.

234. Campbell DG, Simmons RJ, et al. Ghost cells as a cause of glaucoma. Am J Ophthalmol 1976;81:442–450.

235. Bacon AS, Davison CR, et al. Infective endophthalmitis following vitreoretinal surgery. Eye 1993;7:529–534.

236. McDonald HR, Lewis H, et al. Complications of endodrainage retinotomies created during vitreous surgery for complicated retinal detachments. Ophthalmology 1989;96:358–363.

237. Bosomworth PP, Ziegler CH, et al. The oculo-cardiac reflex in eye muscle surgery. Anesthesiology 1958;19:7–10.

238. Kirsh RE, Samet P, et al. Electrocardiographic changes during ocular surgery and their prevention by retrobulbar injection. Arch Ophthalmol 1957;58:348–356.

239. Snow JC, Sensel S. Cataract extraction under local and general anesthesia. Anesth Analg 1966;45:742.

240. Feibel RM. Current concepts in retrobulbar anesthesia. Surv Ophthalmol 1985;30:102–110.

241. Ramsay RC, Knobloch WH. Ocular perforation following retrobulbar anesthesia for retinal detachment surgery. Am J Ophthalmol 1978;86:61–64.

242. Gizzard WS, Kirk NM, et al. Perforating ocular injuries caused by anesthesia personnel. Ophthalmology 1991;98:1011–1016.

243. Hay A, Flynn WH, et al. Needle perforation of the globe during retrobulbar and peribulbar injections. Ophthalmology 1991;98:1017–1024.

244. Ramsay RC, Knobloch WH. Ocular perforation following retrobulbar anesthesia for retinal detachment surgery. Am J Ophthalmol 1978;86:61–64.

245. Wittpenn JR, Rapoza P, et al. Respiratory arrest following retrobulbar anesthesia. Ophthalmology 1986;93:867–870.

246. Ahn JC, Stanley JA. Subarachnoid injection as a complication of retrobulbar anesthesia. Am J Ophthalmol 1987;103:225–230.

247. Ravin MB. Medications supplementing local anesthesia in ophthalmic surgery. Surv Ophthalmol 1974;18:275–277.

248. Carrol FD. Optic nerve complications of cataract extraction. Trans Am Ophthalmol Otolaryngol 1973;77:623–628.

249. Sullivan KL, Brown GC, et al. Retrobulbar anesthesia and retinal vascular obstruction. Ophthalmology 1983;90:373–377.

250. Morgan MD, Schatz H, et al. Ocular complications associated with retrobulbar injections. Ophthalmology 1988;95:660–665.
251. Kelman CD. Parachute Cataract Surgery. In EA Klein (ed), Transactions of the New Orleans Academy of Ophthalmology (Symposium on Cataract Surgery). St. Louis: Mosby, 1983:159–163.
252. Davis DB II, Mandel MR. Posterior peribulbar anesthesia: An alternative to retrobulbar anesthesia. J Cataract Refract Surg 1986;12:182–184.
253. Kimble JA, Morris RE, et al. Globe perforation from peribulbar anesthesia. Arch Ophthalmol 1987;105:749.
254. Puustjarvi T, Purhonen S, et al. Permanent blindness following retrobulbar hemorrhage after peribulbar anesthesia for cataract surgery. Ophthalmic Surg 1992;23:450–452.
255. Esswein MB, Von Noorden Gk. Paresis of a vertical rectus muscle after cataract extraction. Am J Ophthalmol 1993;116:424–430.
256. Hamilton RC, Gimbel HV, et al. Regional anesthesia for 1200 cataract extraction and intraocular lens implantation procedures. Can J Ophthalmol 1988;35:615–623.
257. Weiss JL, Deichman CB. A comparison of retrobulbar and peribulbar anesthesia for cataract surgery. Arch Ophthalmol 1989;107:96–98.
258. Arnold PN. Prospective study of single-injection peribulbar technique. J Cataract Refract Surg 1992;18:157–161.
259. Schriver PA, Sinha S, et al. Prospective study of the effectiveness of retrobulbar and peribulbar anesthesia for anterior segment surgery. J Cataract Refract Surg 1992;18:162–165.
260. Davis MD, Segal PP, et al. A Natural Course Followed by the Fellow Eye in Patients with Rhegmatogenous Retinal Detachment. In RC Pruett, CDJ Regan (eds), Retina Congress. New York: Appleton-Century-Crofts, 1972:643–660.
261. Ashrafzadeh MT, Schepens CL, et al. Aphakic and phakic retinal detachment. Arch Ophthalmol 1973;89:476–483.
262. Benson WE, Grand MG, Okun E. Aphakic retinal detachment. Arch Ophthalmol 1975;93:245–249.

Chapter 7

Proliferative Vitreoretinopathy

Proliferative vitreoretinopathy (PVR), also known as massive periretinal proliferation, massive preretinal retraction, and massive vitreous retraction syndrome, is a malignant form of retinal detachment (RD) characterized by large, fixed retinal folds. PVR is the pathologic growth of cells that are capable of forming cellular and collagenous membranes on intraocular structures, such as the retinal surface and the vitreous (particularly the posterior cortical face).[1–6] PVR generally occurs after a retinal tear or detachment and is most often associated with the treatment of these entities. In one retrospective study of 1,180 consecutive eyes operated on for RD, the finding of vitreous traction on the tear was the determining factor in developing PVR.[7] Twenty percent of the aphakic eyes developed PVR after retinal detachment, as did 25.8% of senile myopic eyes and 44.2% of eyes with senile myopic aphakia; 78.1% of the patients had giant tears.[7] Posterior involvement includes the inner and outer retinal surface, and anterior involvement includes the vitreous base, ciliary body, posterior iris, and pupillary margin.[8, 9] The cells proliferate and migrate along the surface of the retina and the vitreous face of the detached posterior vitreous. On the retinal surface these areas of proliferation become organized and cause contraction on the retina that forms fixed and irregular folds (Figure 7-1).[3, 4, 6, 10–14] Focal areas on the retinal surface can cause contraction stars, and over broader areas, fixed and irregular folds develop.[15] Epiretinal membranes are more commonly seen in the inferior fundus, which is likely due to gravitational forces causing settling of the migrating cells inferiorly. The tractional forces generated by the epiretinal and transvitreal membranes can produce new breaks, which may lead to a recurrent rhegmatogenous detachment or produce a pure tractional detachment.

Subretinal membranes have been found in 47% of eyes and may need to be removed through one or many retinotomies.[16] On the posterior layer of detached retina there can be cellular proliferation, which is mostly composed of retinal pigmented epithelium (RPE) cells and only rarely of glial cells. The cells result in a membrane that is usually very transparent and may develop numerous holes that give the membrane a "moth-eaten" appearance.[1–4, 13, 17] As the holes enlarge and the membranes roll up, strands or bands of white or pigmented, fibrotic-looking tissue form.[18–20] These "clothesline" bands stretch for a considerable distance under the detached retina, and sometimes the band forms a narrow ring around the detached retina close to the apex of the funnel and is called a napkin ring (Figure 7-2). The pigmentation of the bands depends on the amount of melanin in the cells composing the band, and the white-yellow appearance is due to the collagen produced.[21] Deposition of RPE cells on the posterior surface of a detached retina can be found within 1 week of the detachment.[1, 22] The earliest sign of proliferative membrane formation is white subretinal precipitates, which are presumed to be pigment epithelial macrophages.[4, 22] The precipitates are irregularly distributed, with most being found on the inferior retina.

Further contraction of the proliferative membranes across the posterior cortical vitreous face in the equatorial region may pull the retina off centrally, causing a "funnel" detachment.[23] Anterior proliferation may occur, especially after a vitrectomy. Because the vitreous base is difficult to remove, remnants often remain after a vitrectomy, and this tissue is believed to contribute to continued progress of the PVR. The contraction of the circular vitreous base with attachment to the anterior peripheral retina causes the peripheral retina to be pulled anteriorly and centrally. This results in zones of elevated peripheral retina that appear smooth and may form a circular trough and posterior radiating retinal folds.[8, 23] The anterior PVR can extend to involve the pars plana, ciliary processes, and posterior iris. Pulling on the ciliary processes can cause them to stretch and may produce hypotony; in advanced cases the iris may be retracted.[24]

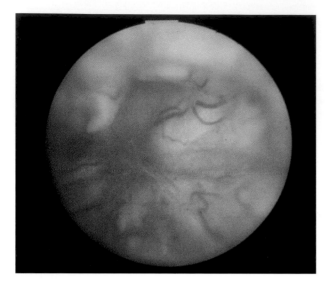

FIGURE 7-1
Proliferative vitreoretinopathy has pulled the retina off into a mass located in the center of the vitreous cavity.

The ophthalmoscopic appearance is that of an RD with triangular folds with rounded corners, with the apex of the triangle close to the optic disc. Folds can be circular, and there may be isolated star-shaped retinal folds (contraction stars) (Figure 7-3). Generally, the entire retina is pulled off due to contraction of a transvitreal membrane located in the equatorial zone and preretinal membranes. The transvitreal membrane forms across the posterior vitreous face of a PVD.[25] The transvitreal prolifera-

tive membrane may occur as a rather solid fibrous membrane spanning the anterior region of the funnel detachment (Figure 7-4) or as a "napkin ring" strand of 360 degrees of encircling proliferative material that contracts and pulls the retina centrally into a funnel detachment (see Figure 7-3). The RD that forms is a funnel-shaped structure with the narrow end posterior. In the early developmental stages, the optic disc can be seen at the bottom of the funnel, but as the process advances, the optic disc is hidden from view with continued collapse and adhesion near the apex of the funnel. Sometimes, areas of the fundus previously treated with photocoagulation or cryopexy do not become detached during PVR.

The pathophysiology includes RPE cells, glial cells (fibrous astrocytes), macrophages, fibrocytes, and myofibrocyte-like cells in the vitreous and on the inner and outer layers of a detached retina.[3, 4, 26–28] The exact origin of these cells is controversial, but they are likely secondary to RPE cells and glial cells that have the potential to transform into myofibroblast-like cells, which can produce collagen.[1, 3, 5, 10, 26, 29–36] It is widely believed that the primary effector cell is the RPE cell,[1, 4, 23] and ultrastructural studies have found that the tissue of epiretinal and subretinal membranes removed from eyes with PVR have shown mostly RPE cell types,[2, 5, 9, 17–20, 37] with additional cell types being glial cells (fibrous astrocytes), macrophages, fibrocytes, and myofibroblast-like cells. The metaplastic RPE cells produce collagen, which can cause a great

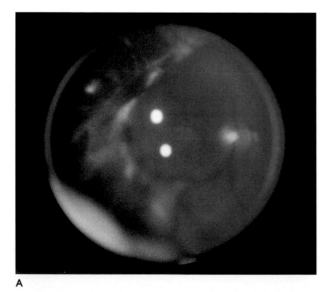

A

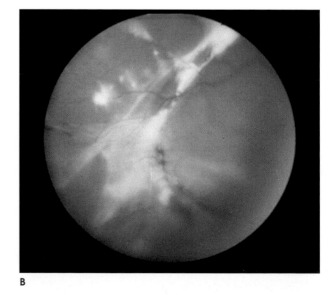

B

FIGURE 7-2
A. Proliferative vitreoretinopathy has produced a fibrotic equatorial band (a "napkin ring") underneath the detached retina that contracted and pulled the retina off. This occurred after retinal detachment repair of a rhegmatogenous detachment. View is through the indirect condensing lens. B. A magnified view of the napkin ring. Note the grayish detached retina draped over the fibrotic band with areas of pigment proliferation.

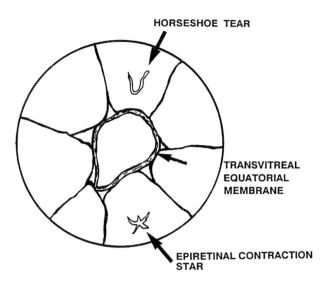

FIGURE 7-3
Cross-sectional drawing. A proliferative transvitreal membrane has contracted and pulled the retina off centrally into a narrow funnel detachment.

deal of retraction of the vitreous body. A small number of these cells can produce a large degree of contraction, in what is known as "hypocellular gel contraction."[24, 38] The proliferating glial cells found in PVR probably derive from Müller cells. These glial cells seem to be able to grow through both inner and external limiting membranes of the retina and then form membranes on the epiretinal and retroretinal surfaces. Glial cell proliferation occurs around the third week after the RD.[24] Thus, an overall proliferation of RPE and glial cells is responsible for contractile membranes that form in PVR.

The process begins with RPE cells dislodging from exposed pigment epithelium under an RD and the glial cells migrating from the detached sensory retina.[2, 5, 32, 39–42] They float in the subretinal space and then migrate through the break in the retina

into the vitreous cavity, and it has been found that RPE cells are the principal cell type in both the subretinal and epiretinal proliferative membranes.[20] The increase in the number of pigment cells in the vitreous may be the harbinger of PVR. The freeing of the RPE cells (up to fourfold) is exacerbated by the use of cryotherapy, which weakens the bonding between the basal lamina and the RPE.[39, 41, 43–45] Therefore, it is advisable not to overtreat with cryotherapy to reduce the possibility of PVR.[46] The further release of RPE cells can be enhanced by the use of scleral depression after cryotherapy, thus, it is best to perform scleral depression before cryotherapy.[41, 46, 47] To minimize the release of RPE cells, it may be better to use photocoagulation rather than cryopexy.[48] Cryotherapy may also disrupt the blood-retina barrier (BRB), which enhances the formation of PVR.[49] The freed RPE cells in the vitreous milieu are stimulated to proliferate and make a morphologic change from an epithelium-like appearance to that of a fibroblast or mesenchymal cell.[50, 51] The RPE cells that remain viable can produce chemoattractants that can attract glial cells, and the RPE cells can produce platelet-derived growth factor (PDGF) that can attract both RPE and glial cells.[52–55] RPE cells can also produce transforming growth factor-beta (TGF-β), which stimulates fibroblasts to proliferate and synthesize collagen and fibronectin (a chemical that attracts monocytes).[56–58] Macrophages in the vitreous on eyes with PVR can attract RPE cells.[59, 60]

The breakdown of the BRB allows the release of serum into the vitreous cavity, which contains PDGF, TGF-β, and components of inflammation that can stimulate the formation of PVR.[49] The BRB is found at two locations: the outer BRB at the level of the RPE and inner BRB at the endothelium of the retinal vessels. Patients with PVR demonstrate clinical signs of BRB breakdown early in the disease

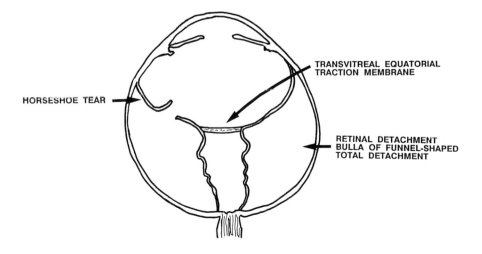

FIGURE 7-4
Drawing of an anterior view of a total rhegmatogenous retinal detachment caused by a transvitreal equatorial membrane that has pulled the retina off as 7 bullae. Note the horseshoe tear and the epiretinal contraction star.

course.[15] The breakdown of the BRB stimulates basic cellular processes of growth, migration, chemotaxis, and proliferation.[61, 62] Serum itself has been found to be a potent attractant to RPE cells and other retina-derived cells types,[63, 64] and the primary agents seems to be fibronectin and PDGF.[45, 53, 63, 65–67] Fibronectin has been found to be a powerful chemical for cellular migration and proliferation of a variety of cell types.[68–70] Cryotherapy is associated with an increase in the breakdown of the BRB, along with the increase in the release of RPE cells; thus, cryotherapy is a major contributor to PVR.[71] A vicious cycle is thus set into play, where RPE cells are released into the subretinal space and vitreous; the RPE cells and the breakdown in the BRB produce chemotactic agents, which increase the number of RPE and glial cells; and this process results in more chemoattractants and more vitreous cells.[59] It has been found in an animal model of PVR that the leakage through the BRB was greater in eyes that developed a detachment as compared to eyes without a detachment. The role of inflammation in the pathogenesis remains to be defined, but some have suggested that the complement system, macrophages, and some types of lymphocytes may be involved in the production of PVR.[72–74] The role of macrophages is not fully known, but it has been found that a macrophage-conditioned medium in vitro has the ability to induce metaplastic changes in RPE cells.[75, 76] Because one of the functions of the vitreous is to inhibit cellular invasion,[76] the changes brought on by the freed RPE and glial cells and the breakdown of the BRB somehow alter this protective function to allow for cell migration and proliferation (PVR). It is believed that all these changes in the microenvironment of the vitreous collectively influence the development of PVR.[2, 11, 70, 77] It is thought that even the hyalocytes secrete inhibitors of RPE cell proliferation.[78]

Predisposing factors in the development of PVR are chronic RD (>1 month), pre- and postoperative vitreous hemorrhage, increasing size of retinal breaks (>3 disc diameters), horseshoe tears, aphakia, poor visual acuity, PVR before surgery, pre- and postoperative choroidals, use of air tamponade, sulfur hexafluoride, cryopexy, diathermy, and vitrectomy. Also, patients with a giant tear (>3 clock hours) with a folded-over posterior edge are at a high risk for PVR.[41, 46, 79–96] Some have reported that aphakia is not a risk factor.[79, 80] The most common type of PVR is related to RD surgery and is associated with scleral buckling, pneumatic retinopexy, or vitrectomy.[24] However, PVR is sometimes seen in long-standing detachments and rarely found in cases of PVR, such as diabetic retinopathy.[24] PVR can be secondary to severe penetrating injuries to the posterior segment of the eye.[11, 97–102] Even the successful sealing of all breaks in the treatment of an RD does not provide total protection against the development of PVR.[86, 103] High myopia does not appear to be associated with PVR.[87, 104, 105] Also, the drainage of subretinal fluid is not a risk factor for PVR.[106, 107]

PVR may rarely occur in patients with a rhegmatogenous RD without previous RD surgery, but it is generally seen in patients who have undergone retinal surgery. It is most likely to develop in cases of rhegmatogenous RD associated with Wagner's vitreoretinal degeneration, lattice retinal degeneration, giant retinal tear, penetrating ocular injury, massive vitreous hemorrhage, and surgical aphakia with vitreous loss. In traumatic cases it was found that there was proliferation of RPE on the posterior retinal surface as soon as 1 week after the trauma.[13] It sometimes occurs in eyes with a nonrhegmatogenous detachment after severe intraocular inflammation.[108] The treatment of retinal tears alone may result in PVR, and it has been stated that this may occur in 7% of the cases of treated tears.[109] PVR has been occasionally seen with Coats' disease,[110] choroidal melanoma,[27, 111] and subretinal fibrosis and uveitis syndrome.[112–114]

The onset of PVR is acute, and it can produce large areas of RD overnight; within weeks the process can become well established. The condition seems to occur some 6–12 weeks after successful reattachment, but in all likelihood, the process was probably on-going for some time. When sufficient traction has developed, there can be a sudden detachment.[25] This, coupled with strong vitreal traction, can cause the rapid development of an RD. Early in the process, the fundus reflex changes to a gray color and fundus detail becomes indistinct due to vitreous haze. This haze results from a marked outpouring of serum protein into the vitreous gel with the resultant Tyndall effect. Retinal vessels become dilated and tortuous, and intraretinal hemorrhages are not unusual, especially at the equator.

Folds are the primary finding in PVR, and the disease process is classified according to the presence and severity of retinal folds (Table 7-1). Grade A PVR is the earliest form of the disease and shows vitreous pigment clumps, vitreous haze, and pigment clumps on the inferior retina. Grade B has wrinkling of the inner retinal surface without full-thickness retinal folds, vessel tortuosity, and retinal stiffening. There may be retinal holes with rolled and irregular margins, and there is decreased movement of the vitreous on eye movements. Grade C demonstrates full-thickness retinal folds. It is divided into posterior and anterior types. The posterior form includes membrane proliferation and contraction posterior to the equator, and the anterior type demonstrates proliferation and contraction anterior to the equator. Grading of the PVR is also done on clock hours of involvement by proliferation.

Histopathology

Preretinal and equatorial membranes are composed of fibrocellular tissue with collagen-like fibers (myofibroblasts), which mature, contract, and produce strong tractional forces.

Clinical Significance

The prognosis for patients with PVR is poor. Signs of PVR are found in 10% of RDs, but fortunately progression to PVR that requires vitrectomy occurs in only 25% of these cases.[115, 116] The Multicenter Randomized Controlled Clinical Trial Comparing Pneumatic Retinopexy and Scleral Buckling found that PVR occurred in 5% of the cases of RD treated with scleral buckling and 3% with pneumatic retinopexy.[117] There is a 2% failure rate due to PVR in RDs that do not undergo subretinal drainage.[118] In pneumatic retinopexy, there is a failure rate of 4% due to PVR.[48] Another report gives the incidence of PVR and excessive fibrosis as 7% in patients who were treated for retinal tears.[109] Surgery for rhegmatogenous RD is successful in more than 90% of cases. PVR is the most frequent cause of failure (7–10%),[11, 47, 119–122] and it is seen in a higher percentage of reoperations.[80] The primary reason for permanent surgical failure (>90%) of RD is PVR.[47] Aphakic intracapsular cataract extractions are associated with a higher incidence of PVR, and eyes with RD and vitreous incarceration in the wound site are more than twice as likely to show some signs of PVR compared to eyes without vitreous incarceration.[123–125]

Rarely, mild forms of PVR resolve spontaneously, but some type of ocular surgery is usually necessary. Treatment requires vitrectomy, scleral buckling with an encircling band, complete drainage of subretinal fluid, membrane segmentation, retinal tamponade, and retinal tacks to reattach the retina.[3, 126] Star-shaped retinal folds should be included on the buckle. Sometimes multiple surgical procedures are necessary to achieve total final success.[121, 127–129] Surgical segmentation or removal of the membranes may lead to successful reattachment, but reprolifer-

Table 7-1. Retina Society Classification of Proliferative Vitreoretinopathy

Group	Name	Clinical Findings
A	Minimal	Vitreous haze, vitreous cellular clumps
B	Moderate	Wrinkling of the retina, retinal stiffness, rolled edges of breaks, vessel tortuosily
C	Marked	Full-thickness fixed retinal folds
C-1		One quadrant
C-2		Two quadrants
C-3		Three quadrants
D	Massive	Fixed folds in four quadrants
D-1		Wide funnel
D-2		Narrow funnel (anterior margin of funnel is visible with BIO using 20-diopter condensing lens)
D-3		Closed funnel (optic nervehead not visible)

ation with redetachment is a frequent complication.[130, 131] In some limited cases, scleral buckling is sufficient to reattach the retina in PVR.[132] However, sometimes it is necessary to inject air, silicone, or sulfur hexafluoride (SF6) into the vitreous cavity to flatten out the retina against the RPE. The Silicone Oil Study and other reports have recently confirmed the importance of perfluoropropane (C3F8) in the surgical reattachment of retinas in PVR.[77, 133] It may be necessary to perform vitrectomy, segmentation, and peeling of the preretinal membranes with microscissors (a hazardous procedure) to unfold areas of the retina that seem to be incorporated into a strong, fixed membrane.[11] Silicone oil injection may result in reproliferation with recurrent RD.[134–136] The goal of vitreous surgery is to convert a PVR RD into a rather "routine" rhegmatogenous detachment and then to repair the "routine" detachment.[21]

Vitrectomy is not indicated for grades A and B PVR, and eyes with grade C may be treated with scleral buckling. Vitrectomy is usually indicated for eyes in which adequate relief of traction is not anticipated to achieve reattachment with scleral buckling.[24] During vitrectomy it is important to remove as much as possible of the vitreous in the area of the vitreous base so as to lessen the chances of anterior PVR. Retinotomies and retinectomies are done to relieve retinal surface traction to achieve reattachment.[137] They are usually reserved for the treatment of anterior retinal contraction, which cannot be adequately relieved by membrane dissection. Silicone oil long-term tamponade offers the best prognosis for eyes with PVR, and it is usually reserved for eyes scheduled for repeat vitrectomy and retinotomy or retinectomy.[24] In eyes that require the removal of a scleral buckle, those with PVR carry a very high risk of redetachment[138] (see Treatment in Chapter 6 on Retinal Detachment).

Subretinal membrane formation is believed to be modulated by the RPE cells.[4, 17] The surgical treatment for subretinal membranes is limited because most cases of retrolental membranes do not interfere with retinal reattachment.[139] Surgical procedures include scleral buckle with encircling band, drainage of subretinal fluid, relaxing incisions of subretinal bands, and partial or complete removal of bands.[139–141]

The postoperative period is extremely important in determining the status of the PVR eye. It is also important for (1) careful control of the intraocular pressure (IOP), (2) adequate retinal tamponade, (3) control of inflammation, (4) elimination of hemorrhage or fibrin, and (5) detection of recurrent detachment.[24] Early recurrent detachment usually indicates the existence of untreated retinal breaks or excessive vitreous traction; the most common reason for it is the presence of anterior vitreous traction that opens an anterior retinal break.[24] However, a recurrent detachment may be caused by residual posterior epiretinal membranes.

Postoperative complications of PVR surgery are an elevated IOP, which is not uncommon in patients who have undergone extensive intraocular surgery. Intraocular fibrin formation may act as a scaffold for subsequent proliferation and may cause pupillary block. Intraocular hemorrhage in the immediate postoperative period is most frequently seen in eyes with extensive relaxing retinotomies.[126, 142] A late complication of PVR surgery is hypotony (IOP <5 mm Hg).[127–129, 143] Keratopathy (epithelial, stromal, or bullous) is another frequent complication.[128, 129] Macular pucker is one of the most notable long-term complications (12–30% of eyes).[144, 145] It is associated with poor visual acuity results, but epiretinal peel surgery can be found to result in a significant increase in central vision.[146] Subretinal strands in the posterior pole have been observed in 8.6% of eyes.[144] Disc edema has been seen on fluorescein angiography.[144] Recurrent RD is common,[128, 129] the primary reason being the continued proliferative process with recurrent contraction membranes. These membranes may form new breaks or reopen old breaks. The most common location of the new breaks is on the scleral buckle (63.5%) or posterior to the buckle (22.2%).[147] A more recent study found most new breaks on the posterior border of the buckle adjacent to a chorioretinal scar; therefore, it is important to examine the cryoscars on buckles for retinal breaks in recurrent detachments secondary to PVR.[148] Most of the recurrent detachments occurred after 4–8 weeks postsurgery; reoperation success rates of reattachment are 55–71% (visual results are poor).[129] The use of vitrectomy has made it possible to do retinal detachment surgery on formerly inoperable cases of PVR with detached retinas. Even though great advances have been made in the surgical techniques for the treatment for RD secondary to PVR, about 50% of the eyes that have been successfully treated with vitrectomy develop a recurrent detachment.[129, 149] Another complication of surgical treatment of PVR is rubeosis iridis;[150–155] however, neovascular glaucoma is not a common finding (11%).[150]

One recommended preventative is to treat rhegmatogenous detachments as soon as possible (no later than 1 month) to lessen the intraocular stimulating events that lead to PVR.[79] There has been active research in the development of pharmacologic agents that inhibit the vitreoretinal scarring response. It is hoped that these agents will retard the reactive intraocular membrane proliferation in PVR. The following is a list of possible agents: naturally occurring peptides arg-gly-asp-ser (RGDS),[156] naturally occurring complex polymeric glycoproteins (heparin),[157] anti-inflammatory agents (triamcinolone acetonide, indomethacin),[157, 158] and synthetic and naturally occurring antimetabolites (5-fluorouracil, daunorubicin).[157, 159–169] Anti-inflammatory therapy works in these cases by direct inhibition of cellular proliferation and the prevention of attachment of the proliferating cells to collagen. Corticosteroids appear to reduce reproliferation by decreasing the inflammatory response and inhibiting miotic cellular activity.[24] Nonsteroidals may be used, but they are not as effective as corticosteroids. An important aspect in the development of PVR is the attachment of the proliferating cells to collagen and fibronectin, which is secreted from fibroblasts. Therefore, agents that interfere with the attachment of fibronectin to various ligands (e.g., heparin and RGDS) may be beneficial in treating this condition. Also, the ability to reduce fibrin may be helpful, and a fibrolytic agent, such as tissue plasminogen activator (t-PA), may be used after vitrectomy.[24] A major problem with the use of these antiproliferative agents is the toxic side effects.[160]

In the past, the reported success rates of reattachment of eyes with grade C-1 to D-2 PVR was 35%,[132] which seems to be fairly representative of most reports, but in recent reports the rate has risen to 65–80%.[121, 129, 145, 170–176] Even though advances in surgical techniques have improved anatomic success rates of reattachment, visual results are still suboptimal.[121, 128, 129, 145, 170–176] Poor visual results are likely secondary to late complications of the surgery. The main causes for poor visual outcome are recurrent PVR, posterior PVR with macular pucker, and hypotony,[177] but it may be related to any of the complications of PVR surgery mentioned above. The results of surgery for cases with previous vitrectomies are not as good as for those without vitrectomy. Visual acuity of 5/200 or better was obtained in 85% of eyes that had achieved total reattachment.[24] Another study found that 82.7% of such eyes had a final acuity of 20/400 or better, and 29.3% had 20/70 or better.[144] The severity of vision loss was related to the grade of PVR and the postoperative status of the macula. In eyes with grade C-2 to C-3 PVR, 42.8% had visual acuities of 20/70 or better, but only 8.6% of the eyes with D-1 to D-3 had such acuities.[144] Postoperative cases had observable macular changes on fluorescein angiography in 79.3% of eyes, and 51.7% demonstrated cystoid macular edema (CME).[144] Factors that may predispose to the development of CME are more than one operation and preoperative macular detachment.[178–180] Angiographic improvement in CME (along with an improvement in visual acuity) occurred in 30% of eyes within 12–30 months.[144]

In eyes with redetachment, cellular proliferation and traction with anterior PVR occurred in half of the cases. In PVR induced by perforating ocular injuries the use of silicone oil tamponade is reported to have a total reattachment rate of 52–64% and a partial reattachment rate of 9–27%.[127, 134, 181–183] In one report, useful vision was achieved in 67% of patients, 37% had vision from 1/60 to 20/400, and 30% had 20/300 to 20/20.[181] One of the major reasons for failure of PVR surgery is the development of anterior PVR, which is usually the result of leaving remnants of the vitreous base to use as a scaffolding for proliferation.[9, 170, 174, 184] The anterior PVR causes anterior retinal traction that leads to recurrent RD. This condition is difficult to treat due to the tight adherence of the vitreous by collagenous fibers to the retina and pars plana.[185] The removal of the entire vitreous base during vitrectomy would greatly decrease the incidence of anterior PVR.[8, 9, 170, 184]

References

1. Machemer RG. Pathogenesis and classification of massive periretinal proliferation. Br J Ophthalmol 1978;62:737–747.
2. Machemer RG, Laqua H. Pigment epithelial proliferation in retinal detachment (massive periretinal proliferation). Am J Ophthalmol 1975;80:1–23.
3. Laqua H, Machemer RG. Glial cell proliferation in retinal detachment (massive periretinal proliferation). Am J Ophthalmol 1975;80:602–608.
4. Laqua H, Machemer RG. Clinical-pathological correlation in massive periretinal proliferation. Am J Ophthalmol 1975;80:913–929.
5. Machemer RG, van Horn D, et al. Pigment epithelial proliferation in human retinal detachment with massive periretinal proliferation. Am J Ophthalmol 1978;85:181–191.
6. van Horn D, Aaberg TM, et al. Glial cell proliferation in human retinal detachment with massive periretinal proliferation. Am J Ophthalmol 1977;84:383–393.
7. Malbrain E, Dodds RA, et al. Retinal break type and proliferative vitreoretinopathy in nontraumatic retinal detachment. Graefes Arch Clin Exp Ophthalmol 1990; 228:423–425.
8. Lewis H, Asberg TM. Anterior proliferative vitreoretinopathy. Am J Ophthalmol 1988;105:277–284.
9. Elner SG, Elner VM, et al. Anterior proliferative vitreoretinopathy: Clinicopathologic, light microscopic and ultrastructural findings. Ophthalmology 1988;95:1349–1357.
10. Constable IJ, Tolentino FI, et al. Clinico-Pathologic Correlation of Vitreous Membrane. In RC Pruett, CDJ Regan (eds), Retina Congress. New York: Appleton-Century-Crofts, 1974:245–257.
11. Ryan SJ. The pathophysiology of proliferative vitreoretinopathy and its management. Am J Ophthalmol 1985;100:188–193
12. Smith TR. Pathologic Findings after Retinal Surgery. In CL Schepens, CDJ Regan (eds), Importance of the Vitreous Body in Retinal Surgery with Special Emphasis on Reoperations. St. Louis: Mosby, 1960:61–75.
13. Wilkes SR, Mansour AM, et al. Proliferative vitreoretinopathy: Histopathology of retroretinal membranes. Retina 1987;7:94–101.
14. Wilson DJ, Green WR. Histopathologic study of the effect of retinal detachment surgery on 49 eyes obtained at post mortem. Am J Ophthalmol 1987;103:167–179.
15. The Retina Society Terminology Committee. The classification of retinal detachment with proliferative vitreoretinopathy. Ophthalmology 1983;90:121–125.
16. Lewis H, Aaberg TM, et al. Subretinal membranes in proliferative vitreoretinopathy. Ophthalmology 1989;96: 1403–1414.
17. Sternberg P Jr, Machemer RG. Subretinal proliferation. Am J Ophthalmol 1984;98:456–462.
18. Fleury J, Bonnet M. Retinal detachment and massive periretinal proliferation: clinical study of 60 cases. Bull Soc Ophtalmol Fr 1990;90:433–435.
19. Matsummura M, Yamakawa R, et al. Subretinal strands: Tissue culture and histologic study. Graefes Arch Clin Exp Ophthalmol 1987;225:341–345.
20. Trese MT, Chandler DB, et al. Subretinal strands: Ultrastructural features. Graefes Arch Clin Exp Ophthalmol 1985;223:35–40.
21. Antoszyk AN, McCuen BW. Vitreous Surgery in Proliferative Vitreoretinopathy. In W Tasman, EA Jaeger (eds), Clinical Ophthalmology. Vol. 6. Philadelphia: Lippincott, 1994;58:1–28.
22. Wilkes SR, Glaser BM, et al. Proliferative vitreoretinopathy: histopathology of retroretinal membranes. Retina 1987;7:94–101.
23. Machemer RG, Aaberg TM, et al. An updated classification of retinal detachment with proliferative vitreoretinopathy. Am J Ophthalmol 1991;112:159–165.

24. Abrams GW, Glazer LC. Proliferative Vitreoretinopathy. In WR Freeman (ed), Practical Atlas of Retinal Disease and Therapy. New York: Raven, 1993;17:279–297.

25. Michaels RG. Surgery of retinal detachment with proliferative vitreoretinopathy. Retina 1984;4:63–83.

26. Clarkson JG, Green WR, et al. A histopathologic review of 168 cases of preretinal membranes. Am J Ophthalmol 1977;84:1–17.

27. Wallow IHL, Tso MOM. Proliferation of the retinal pigment epithelium over malignant choroidal tumors. Am J Ophthalmol 1972;73:914–926.

28. Engel HM, Green WR, et al. Diagnostic vitrectomy. Retina 1981;1:121–149.

29. Hiscott PS, Grierson I, et al. Retinal pigment epithelial cells in epiretinal membranes: an immunohistochemical study. Br J Ophthalmol 1984;68:708–715.

30. Nguyen-Tan JQ, Thompson JT. RPE cell migration into intact vitreous body. Retina 1989;9:203–209.

31. Raymond MC, Thompson JT. RPE-mediated collagen gel contraction. Inhibition by colchicine and stimulated by TGF-beta. Invest Ophthalmol Vis Sci 1990;31:1079–1086.

32. Mandelcorn M, Machemer RG, et al. Proliferation and metaplasia of intravitreal retinal pigment epithelial cell autotransplants. Am J Ophthalmol 1975;80:227–237.

33. Michels RG. A clinical and histopathologic study of epiretinal membranes affecting the macula and removed by vitreous surgery. Trans Am Ophthalmol Soc 1982; 80:580–656.

34. Mueller-Jensen K, Machemer RG, et al. Autotransplanation of retinal pigment epithelium in intravitreal diffusion chambers. Am J Ophthalmol 1975;80:530–537.

35. Newsome DA, Rodrigues MM, et al. Human massive periretinal proliferation. Arch Ophthalmol 1981;99: 873–880.

36. Wallow IHL, Stevens TS, et al. Actin filaments in contracting preretinal membranes. Arch Ophthalmol 1984; 102:1370–1375.

37. Schwartz D, De La Cruz, et al. Proliferative vitreoretinopathy: ultrastructural study of 20 retroretinal membranes removed by vitreous surgery. Retina 1988;8:275–281.

38. Grierson I, Rahi AHS. Structural basis of contraction in vitreous fibrous membranes. Br J Ophthalmol 1981;65:737–749.

39. Singh AK, Glaser BM, et al. Gravity-dependent distribution of retinal pigment epithelial cells dispersed into the vitreous cavity. Retina 1986;6:77–80.

40. Michels RG. Surgery of retinal detachment with proliferative vitreoretinopathy. Retina 1984;4:63–83.

41. Camprochiaro PA, Kaden IH, et al. Cryotherapy enhances intravitreal dispersion of viable retinal pigment epithelial cells. Arch Ophthalmol 1985;103:434–436.

42. Kroll AJ, Machemer R. Experimental retinal detachment of the owl monkey. III. Electron microscopy of retina and pigment epithelium. Am J Ophthalmol 1968;66:410–427.

43. Hilton GF. Subretinal pigment migration: Effects of cryosurgical retinal detachment. Arch Ophthalmol 1974;91:445–450.

44. Sudarsky RD, Yannuzzi LA. Cryomarcation line and pigment migration after retinal cryosurgery. Arch Ophthalmol 1970;83:375–401.

45. Camprochiaro PA, Bryan JA, et al. Intravitreal chemotactic and mitogenic activity. Arch Ophthalmol 1986;104: 1685–1687.

46. Singh AK, Michels RG, et al. Scleral indentation following cryotherapy and repeat cryotherapy enhance release of viable retinal pigment epithelial cells. Retina 1986;6: 176–178.

47. Williams GA, Aaberg TM Sr. Techniques of Scleral Buckling. In W Tasman, EA Jaeger (eds), Clinical Ophthalmology. Vol. 6. Philadelphia: Lippincott, 1994;59:1–40.

48. Hilton GF, Tornambe PE, et al. Pneumatic retinopexy. An analysis of intraoperative and postoperative complications. Retina 1991;11:285–294.

49. Jaccoma EH, Conway BP, et al. Cryotherapy causes extensive breakdown of the blood-retinal barrier: A comparison with argon laser photocoagulation. Arch Ophthalmol 1985;103:1728–1730.

50. Vidaurri-Leal JS, Hohman R, et al. Effect of vitreous on morphologic characteristics of retinal pigment epithelial cells: a new approach to the study of proliferative vitreoretinopathy. Arch Ophthalmol 1984;102:1220–1223.

51. Israel P, Masterson E, et al. Retinal pigment epithelial cell differentiation in vitro. Invest Ophthalmol Vis Sci 1980; 19:720–727.

52. Rowen SL, Glaser BM. Retinal pigment epithelial cells release a chemoattractant for astrocytes. Arch Ophthalmol 1985;103:704–707.

53. Camprochiaro PA, Glaser BM. Platelet-derived growth factor is chemotactic for human retinal pigment epithelial cells. Arch Ophthalmol 1985;103:576–579.

54. Uchihori Y, Puro DG. Mitogenic and chemotactic effects of platelet-derived growth factor on human retinal glial cells. Invest Ophthalmol Vis Sci 1991;32:2689–2695.

55. Shimakado K, Raines E, et al. A significant part of macrophage-derived growth factor consists of at least two forms of KPDGF. Cell 1985;43:277–286.

56. Connor TB Jr, Roberts AB, et al. Correlation of fibrosis and transforming growth factor-b type 2 levels in the eye. J Clin Invest 1989;83:1611–1666.

57. Wahl SM, Hunt DA, et al. Transforming growth factor type beta induces monocyte chemotaxis and growth factor production. Proc Natl Acad Sci USA 1987;84:5788–5792.

58. Glaser BM, Lemor M. Pathobiology of Proliferative Vitreoretinopathy. In SJ Ryan (ed), Retina. Vol. 3. St. Louis: Mosby, 1989:380.

59. Burke JM, Twining S. Vitreous macrophage elicitation-generation of stimulant for pigment epithelium in vitro. Invest Ophthalmol Vis Sci 1987;28:1100–1107.

60. Camprochiaro PA, Jerdan JA, et al. The extracellular matrix of human retinal pigment epithelial cells in vivo and its synthesis in vitro. Invest Ophthalmol Vis Sci 1986;27:1615–1621.

61. Sen HA, Robertson TJ, et al. The role of breakdown of the blood-retinal barrier in cell-injection models of proliferative vitreoretinopathy. Arch Ophthalmol 1988;106:1291–1294.

62. Champrochiaro PA, Sen HA, et al. The role of breakdown of the blood-retinal barrier in proliferative vitreoretinopathy. In Proliferative Vitreoretinopathy. Heidelberg, Germany: Kadon, 1989:45–49.

63. Camprochiaro PA, Jerdan JA, et al. Serum contains chemoattractants for human retinal pigment epithelial cells. Arch Ophthalmol 1984;102:1830–1833.

64. Gauss-Muller V, Kleinman H, et al. Role of attachment and attractants in fibroblast chemotaxis. J Lab Clin Med 1980;96:1071–1080.

65. De Juan E Jr, Dickson J, et al. Serum is chemotactic for retinal-derived glial cells. Arch Ophthalmol 1988;106:986–990.

67. Kato H, Lansing M, et al. Experimental traction retinal detachment (TRD) after intravitreous injection of combinations of platelet-derived growth factor (PDGF), transforming growth factor-beta (TGF-β) and fibronectin (FN). Invest Ophthalmol Vis Sci 1988;29(Suppl):307.

68. Yamada KM. Fibronectin in Cell Interactions. In KM Yamada (ed), Cell Interactions and Development. New York: Wiley, 1983:231–249.

69. Tsukamoto Y, Heisel W, et al. Macrophage production of fibronectin, a chemoattractant for fibroblasts. J Immunol 1981;127:673–678.

70. Camprochiaro PA, Jerdan JA, et al. Vitreous aspirates from patient with proliferative vitreoretinopathy stimulate retinal pigment epithelial cell migration. Arch Ophthalmol 1985;103:1403–1405.

71. Grisanti S, Wiedeman P, et al. The significance of complement in proliferative vitreoretinopathy. Invest Ophthalmol Vis Sci 1991;32:2711–2717.

72. Baudouin C, Fredj-Reygrobellet D, et al. Immunohistologic study of proliferative vitreoretinopathy. Am J Ophthalmol 1989;108:387–394.

73. Baudouin C, Fredj-Reygrobellet D, et al. Immunohistologic study of epiretinal membranes in proliferative vitreoretinopathy. Am J Ophthalmol 1990;110:593–598.

74. Martini B, Wang H, et al. Synthesis of extracellular matrix by macrophage-modulated retinal pigment epithelium. Arch Ophthalmol 1991;109:576–580.

75. Kirchhof B, Kirchhof E, et al. Human retinal pigment epithelial cell cultures. Phenotypic modulation by vitreous and macrophages. Exp Eye Res 1988;47:457–463.

76. Sebag J. The Vitreous: Structure, Function and Pathobiology. New York: Springer-Verlag, 1989:60–61.

77. Glaser BM, Cardin A, et al. Proliferative vitreoretinopathy: the mechanism of development of vitreoretinal traction. Ophthalmology 1987;94:327–332.

78. Lazarus HS, Schoenfeld CL, et al. Hyalocytes synthesize and secrete inhibitors to retinal pigment epithelial cell proliferation in vitro. Arch Ophthalmol 1996;114:731–736.

79. Yoshino Y, Ideta H, et al. Comparative study of clinical factors predisposing patients to proliferative vitreoretinopathy. Retina 1989;9:97–100.

80. Bonnet M. Clinical factors predisposing to massive proliferative vitreoretinopathy in rhegmatogenous retinal detachment. Ophthalmologica 1984;188:148–152.

81. Schepens CL. Ophthalmoscopic Observations Related to the Vitreous Body. In CL Schepens (ed), Importance of the Vitreous Body in Retina Surgery with Special Emphasis on Reoperations. St. Louis: Mosby, 1960:94–123.

82. Tolentino FI, Schepens CL, et al. Massive preretinal retraction: a biomicroscopic study. Arch Ophthalmol 1967;78:16–22.

83. Machemer R. Allen AW, et al. Retinal tears 180 degrees and greater: management with vitrectomy and intravitreal gas. Arch Ophthalmol 1976;94:1340–1346.

84. Freeman HM, Castillejos ME. Current management of giant retinal tears: results with vitrectomy and total air-fluid exchange in 95 cases. Trans Am Ophthalmol Soc 1981;179:89–100.

85. Bonnet M. The development of severe proliferative vitreoretinopathy after retinal detachment surgery. Grade B. A determining risk factor. Graefes Arch Clin Exp Ophthalmol 1988;226:201–205.

86. Cowley M, Conway BP, et al. Clinical risk factors for proliferative vitreoretinopathy. Arch Ophthalmol 1989;107:1147–1151.

87. Girard P, Mimoun G, et al. Clinical risk factors for proliferative vitreoretinopathy after retinal detachment surgery. Retina 1994;14:417–424.

88. Laatikainen L, Harju H, et al. Postoperative outcome in rhegmatogenous retinal detachment. Acta Ophthalmol 1985;63:647–655.

89. Chignell AH, Fison LG, et al. Failure in retinal detachment surgery. Br J Ophthalmol 1973;57:525–530.

90. Malbran E, Dodds RA, et al. Retinal break type and proliferative vitreoretinopathy in nontraumatic retinal detachment. Graefes Arch Clin Exp Ophthalmol 1990;228:423–425.

91. Tornqvist R, Tornqvist P. Retinal detachment. a study of a population-based patient material in Sweden (1971– 1981). III. Surgical results. Acta Ophthalmol 1988; 66:630–636.

92. Nagasaki H, Ideta H, et al. Comparative study of clinical factors that predispose patients to proliferative vitreoretinopathy in aphakia. Retina 1991;11:204–207.

93. Grizzard WS, Hilton GF, et al. A multivariate analysis of the anatomic success of retinal detachments treated with scleral buckling. Graefes Arch Clin Exp Ophthalmol 1994; 232:1 7.

94. Kroerner F, Merz E, et al. Proliferative vitreoretinopathy: correlation with extent of retinal detachment, size of retinal break, and area of coagulation. Klin Monatsbl Augenheilkd 1988;192:465–467.

95. Gerhard JP, Annonier P, et al. Choroidal detachment after chorioretinal surgery: frequency and correlation with proliferative vitreoretinopathy. Klin Monatsbl Augenheilkd 1989;190:321–323.

96. Cangemi FE, Pitta CG, et al. Spontaneous resolution of massive periretinal proliferation. Am J Ophthalmol 1982;93:92–95.

97. Kroll P, Schiller B. Zur Amotio-Prophylaxe bei der Versorgung perforierender Verletzung. Fortschr Ophthalmol 1984;81:105–108.

98. Atkinson A, Faulborn J. Vitreous morphology after perforating injury treated by primary vitrectomy. Trans Ophthalmol Soc UK 1978;98:43–46.

99. Faulborn J, Topping TM. Proliferations in the vitreous cavity after perforating injuries. Graefes Arch Clin Exp Ophthalmol 1978;205:157–166.

100. Winthrop SR, Cleary PE, et al. Penetrating eye injuries: a histopathological review. Br J Ophthalmol 1980;64:809–817.

101. Cleary PE, Ryan SI. Vitrectomy in penetrating eye injury. Arch Ophthalmol 1981;99:287–292.

102. Gregor Z, Ryan SJ. Complete and core vitrectomies in the treatment of experimental posterior penetrating eye injury in the rhesus monkey. II. Histologic features. Arch Ophthalmol 1983;101:446–450.

103. Bonnet M. Clinical factors predisposing to massive proliferative vitreoretinopathy in rhegmatogenous retinal detachment. Ophthalmologica 1984;188:148–152.

104. Glazer LC, Mieler WF, et al. Complications of primary scleral buckling procedures in high myopia. Retina 1990;10:170–172.

105. Rodrigues FJ, Lewis H, et al. Scleral buckling for rhegmatogenous retinal detachment associated with severe myopia. Am J Ophthalmol 1991;111:595–600.

106. Hilton GF. The drainage of subretinal fluid. A randomized controlled clinical trial. Trans Am Ophthalmol Soc 1981; 79:517–540.

107. Wildinson CP, Bradford RH. Complications of draining subretinal fluid. Retina 1984;4:1–4.

108. Machemer R, Norton EWD. Experimental retinal detachment in owl monkey. I. Methods of production and clinical picture. Am J Ophthalmol 1968;66:388–396.

109. Hilton G, Machemer R, et al. The classification of retinal detachment with proliferative vitreoretinopathy. Ophthalmology 1983;90:121–125.

110. Manschot WA, De Bruijn WC. Coats' disease. Definition and pathogenesis. Br J Ophthalmol 1967;51:145–157.

111. Pitts RE, Awan KJ, et al. Choroidal melanoma with massive retinal fibrosis and spontaneous regression of retinal detachment. Surv Ophthalmol 1976;20:273–280.

112. Palestine AG, Nussenblatt RB, et al. Progressive subretinal fibrosis and uveitis. Br J Ophthalmol 1994;68:667–673.

113. Palestine AG, Nussenblatt RB, et al. Histopathology of the subretinal fibrosis and uveitis syndrome. Ophthalmology 1985;92:838–844.

114. Cantrill HL, Folk JC. Multifocal choroiditis associated with progressive subretinal fibrosis. Am J Ophthalmol 1986;101:170–180.

115. Kampik A, Kenyon KR, et al. Epiretinal and vitreous membranes. Arch Ophthalmol 1981;99:1445–1454

116. Morse PH. Fixed retinal star folds in retinal detachment. Am J Ophthalmol 1974;77:760–764.

117. Tornambe PE, Hilton GF. Pneumatic retinopexy. A multicentered randomized controlled clinical trial comparing pneumatic retinopexy with scleral buckling. The Retinal Detachment Study Group. Ophthalmology 1989;96: 772–783.

118. Lincoff H, Kreissig I. Management of Rhegmatogenous Retinal Detachment. In WR Freeman (ed), Practical Atlas of Retinal Disease and Therapy. New York: Raven, 1993;13:221–235.

119. The Silicone Study Group. Proliferative vitreoretinopathy. Am J Ophthalmol 1985;99:593–595.

120. Rachal WF, Burton TC. Changing concepts of failures after retinal reattachment surgery. Arch Ophthalmol 1979;97: 480–483.

121. Lewis H, Aaberg TM, et al. Causes of failure after initial vitreoretinal surgery for severe proliferative vitreoretinopathy. Am J Ophthalmol 1991;111:8–14.

122. Lewis H, Aaberg TM, et al. Causes of failure after repeat vitreoretinal surgery for severe proliferative vitreoretinopathy. Am J Ophthalmol 1991;111:15–19.

123. Benson WE. Retinal Detachment: Diagnosis and Management (2nd ed). New York: Lippincott, 1987:33–52.

124. Kraff MC, Sanders DR, et al. Secondary intraocular lens implantation. Ophthalmology 1983;90:324–326.

125. le Mesurier R, Vickers S, et al. Aphakic retinal detachment. Br J Ophthalmol 1985;69:737–741.

126. Algvere P, Stenkula S, et al. Sealing of retinal breaks with metal tacks. Evaluation of a new procedure in retinal reattachment surgery. Acta Ophthalmol Scand 1986;64: 421–424.

127. McCuen BW II, Landers MB III, et al. The use of silicone oil following failed vitrectomy for retinal detachment with advanced proliferative vitreoretinopathy. Ophthalmology 1985;92:1029–1033.

128. The Silicone Study Group. Vitrectomy with silicone oil or sulfur hexafluoride gas in eyes with severe proliferative vitreoretinopathy: results of a randomized clinical trial. Silicone Study Report 1. Arch Ophthalmol 1992;110: 770–779.

129. The Silicone Study Group. Vitrectomy with silicone oil or perfluoropropane gas in eyes with severe proliferative vitreoretinopathy: results of a randomized clinical trial. Silicone Study Report 2. Arch Ophthalmol 1992;110: 780–792.

130. Machemer R. Massive periretinal proliferation: a logical approach to therapy. Trans Am Ophthalmol Soc 1977; 75:556–586.

131. Sternberg P, Machemer R. Result of conventional vitreous surgery for proliferative vitreoretinopathy. Am J Ophthalmol 1985;100:141–146.

132. Grizzard WS, Hilton GF. Scleral buckling for retinal detachment complicated by periretinal proliferation. Arch Ophthalmol 1982;100:419–422.

133. Sabetes NR, Tolentino FI, et al. The complications of perfluoropropane gas use in complex retinal detachments. Retina 1996;16:7–12.

134. Cox MS, Trese MT, et al. Silicone oil for advanced proliferative vitreoretinopathy. Ophthalmology 1986;93:646–650.

135. Gonvers M. Temporary silicone oil tamponade in the management of retinal detachment with proliferative vitreoretinopathy. Am J Ophthalmol 1985;100:239–245.

136. Fastenberg DM, Diddie KR, et al. Intraocular injection of silicone oil for experimental proliferative vitreoretinopathy. Am J Ophthalmol 1983;95:663–667.

137. Machemer R, McCuen BW, et al. Relaxing retinotomies and retinectomies. Am J Ophthalmol 1986;102:7–12.

138. Lindsey PS, Pierce LH, et al. Removal of scleral buckling elements: causes and complications. Arch Ophthalmol 1983;101:570–573.

139. Federman JL, Folberg R, et al. Subretinal cellular bands. Trans Am Ophthalmol Soc 1983;81:172–181.

140. Wallyn RH, Hilton GF. Subretinal fibrosis in retinal detachment. Arch Ophthalmol 1979;97:2128–2129.

141. Machemer R. Surgical approaches to subretinal strands. Am J Ophthalmol 1980;90:81–85.

142. Abrams GW. Retinotomies and Retinectomies. In SJ Ryan (ed), Retina. Vol. 3. St. Louis: Mosby, 1989:343–344.

143. Lambrou FH, Burke JM, et al. Effect of silicone oil on experimental traction retinal detachment. Arch Ophthalmol 1987;105:1269–1272.

144. Bonnet M. Macular changes and fluorescein angiographic findings after repair of proliferative vitreoretinopathy. Retina 1994;14:404–410.

145. Lopez R, Chang S. Long-term results of vitrectomy and perfluorocarbon gas for the treatment of severe proliferative vitreoretinopathy. Am J Ophthalmol 1992;113: 424–428.

146. Rice TA, DeBistros S, et al. Prognostic factors in vitrectomy for epiretinal membranes of the macula. Ophthalmology 1986;93:602–610.

147. De Bustros, Michels RG. Surgical treatment of retinal detachment complicated by proliferative vitreoretinopathy. Am J Ophthalmol 1984;98:694–699.

148. Moisseiev J, Glaser BM. New and previously unidentified retinal breaks in eyes with recurrent retinal detachment with proliferative retinopathy. Arch Ophthalmol 1989; 107:1152–1154.

149. McCuen BW II, De Juan E Jr, et al. Silicone oil in vitreoretinal surgery. II. Results and complications. Retina 1985;5:198–205.

150. van Meurs JC, Bolt BJP, et al. Rubeosis of the iris in proliferative vitreoretinopathy. Retina 1996;16:292–295.

151. Decorral LR, Peyman GA. Pars plana vitrectomy and intravitreal silicone oil injection in eyes with rubeosis iridis. Can J Ophthalmol 1986;21:10–12.

152. Federman J, Eagle RC, et al. Extensive peripheral retinectomy combined with posterior 360 degree retinotomy for retinal reattachment in advanced proliferative retinopathy cases. Ophthalmology 1990;97:1305–1320.

153. Tanaka S, Ideta H, et al. Neovascularization of the iris in rhegmatogenous retinal detachment. Am J Ophthalmol 1991;112:632–634.

154. Comaratta MR, Chang S, et al. Iris neovascularization in proliferative vitreoretinopathy. Ophthalmology 1992; 99:898–905.

155. Barr CC, Lai MY, et al. Postoperative intraocular pressure abnormalities in the silicone oil study: Silicone Oil Report 4. Ophthalmology 1993;100:1629–1635.

156. Avery RL, Glaser BM. Inhibition of retinal pigment epithelial cell attachment by a synthetic peptide derived from the cell binding domain of fibronectin. Arch Ophthalmol 1986;104:1220–1222.

157. Blumenkranz MS, Hartzer MK. The Mechanism of Action of Drugs for the Treatment of Vitreoretinal Scarring. In SJ Ryan (ed), Retina. Vol. 3. St. Louis: Mosby, 1989:401–411.

158. Chandler DB, Rozakin G, et al. The effect of triamcinolone acetonide on a refined experimental model of proliferative vitreoretinopathy. Am J Ophthalmol 1985;90:686–690.

159. Radtke ND, Weinsieder AD, et al. Pharmacological therapy for proliferative vitreoretinopathy. Graefes Arch Clin Exp Ophthalmol 1986;224:230–233.

160. Sunalp M, Weidemann P, et al. Effects of cytotoxic drugs on proliferative vitreoretinopathy in the rabbit cell injection model. Curr Eye Res 1984;3:619–623.

161. Wiedemann P, Kirmani M, et al. Control of experimental massive periretinal proliferation by daunomycin: dose-response relation. Graefes Arch Clin Exp Ophthalmol 1983;220:233–235.

162. Weller M, Heimann K, et al. Cytotoxic effects of daunomycin on retinal pigment epithelium in vitro. Graefes Arch Clin Exp Ophthalmol 1987;225:235–238.

163. Wiedemann P, Lemmen K, et al. Intraocular daunorubicin for the treatment and prophylaxis of traumatic proliferative vitreoretinopathy. Am J Ophthalmol 1987;104:10–14.

164. Heath TD, Brown CS, et al. Ocular cicatricial disease. Drug effects in vitro on cell proliferation, contraction, and viability. Invest Ophthalmol Vis Sci 1990;31:1245–1251.

165. Blumenkranz M, Hernandez E, et al. 5-fluorouracil. new applications in complicated retinal detachment for an established antimetabolite. Ophthalmology 1984;91:122–130.

166. Blumenkranz M, Ophir A, et al. Fluorouracil for the treatment of massive preretinal proliferation. Am J Ophthalmol 1982;94:458–467.

167. Stern WH, Lewis GP, et al. Fluorouracil therapy for proliferative vitreoretinopathy after vitrectomy. Am J Ophthalmol 1983;96:33–42.

168. Tano Y, Sugita G, et al. Inhibition of intraocular proliferation with intravitreal corticosteroids. Am J Ophthalmol 1983;96:131–136.

169. Kirmani M, Santana M, et al. Antiproliferative drugs in the treatment of experimental proliferative vitreoretinopathy. Control by daunomycin. Retina 1983;3:269–272.

170. Aaberg TM. Management of anterior and posterior proliferative vitreoretinopathy. XLV Edward Jackson Memorial Lecture. Am J Ophthalmol 1988;106:519–532.

171. Federman JL, Schubert HD. Complications associated with the use of silicone oil in 150 eyes after retina-vitreous surgery. Ophthalmology 1988;95:870–876.

172. Fisher YL, Shakin JL, et al. Perfluorocarbon gas, modified panretinal photocoagulation, and vitrectomy in the management of severe proliferative vitreoretinopathy. Arch Ophthalmol 1988;106:1255–1260.

173. Hanneken AM, Michels RG. Vitrectomy and scleral buckle methods for proliferative vitreoretinopathy. Ophthalmology 1988;95:865–869.

174. De Juan E, McCuen B. Management of anterior vitreous traction in proliferative vitreoretinopathy. Retina 1989;4:258–262.

175. Fleury J, Bonnet M. Le C3F8 dans le tritement des cecollements de la retine associes a une proliferation vitreoretininenne. J Fr Ophtalmol 1989;12:89–94.

176. Yang CM, Cousins SW. Quantitative assessment of growth stimulating activity of the vitreous during PVR. Invest Ophthalmol Vis Sci 1992;33:2436–2442.

177. Cousins SW, Rubsamen PE. Comparison of flow cytometry with the surgeon regarding ability to predict the ultimate success of surgery for proliferative vitreoretinopathy. Arch Ophthalmol 1994;112:1554–1560.

178. Meredith TA, Reeser FH, et al. Cystoid macular edema after retinal detachment surgery. Ophthalmology 1980;87:1090–1095.

179. Lobes LA, Grand MG. Incidence of cystoid macular edema following scleral buckling procedure. Arch Ophthalmol 1980;98:1230–1232.

180. Bonnet M, Bievelez B, et al. Fluorescein angiography after retinal detachment microsurgery. Graefes Arch Clin Exp Ophthalmol 1983;221:35–40.

181. Skorpik C, Menapace R, et al. Silicone oil implantation in penetrating injuries complicated by PVR. Results from 1982–1986. Retina 1989;9:8–13.

182. Zivojnovic R, Mertens DAE, et al. Das flussige Silikon in der Amotiochirurgie. II Bericht uber 280 Falle-weitere Entwicklung der technik. Klin Monatsbl Augenheilkd 1982;181:444–452.

183. Heimann K, Dimopoulos ST, et al. Silikonolinjektion in der Behandlung komplizierter Netzhautablosungen. Klin Monatsbl Augenheilkd 1984;185:505–508.

184. Charles S. Vitreous Microsurgery. Baltimore: Williams & Wilkins, 1981:1221–1225.

185. Spencer WH. Vitreous in Ophthalmic Surgery. In WH Spencer (ed), Ophthalmic Surgery: An Atlas and Textbook. Philadelphia: Saunders, 1985:548–554.

Chapter 8

Choroidal Detachment

Choroidal detachments are also known as choroidal edema and effusion. These terms are often used interchangeably, but fluid accumulation alone is best called edema or effusion. When there is actual cleavage of the fibers that connect the choroid or ciliary to the sclera, it is more appropriate to denote this as a detachment. Choroidal detachments are usually large bullous elevations in the peripheral fundus that commonly involve the pars plana and the peripheral retina; however, they may be rather flat due to choroidal areas that limit fluid accumulation. Sometimes they are located in the posterior pole, or they may have an annular appearance when the detachment is of the ciliary body behind the iris. Their appearance is that of a normal retinal and choroidal pattern that seems darker than usual. The dark appearance is produced by the pigment epithelium in place beneath the retina on the choroidal detachment. They do not undulate on eye movements, as do recent retinal detachments (Table 8-1). Intraocular pressure (IOP) tends to be low in eyes containing choroidal detachments. The ora serrata and the pars plana can be seen without the aid of scleral depression because of the bullous elevation of the detachment. There may be the acute onset of myopia due to anterior displacement of the lens.[1]

Multiple choroidal detachments in a single eye tend to be found in quadrants because of the vortex veins firmly anchoring the choroid at specific locations.[2] Two bullous detachments in adjacent quadrants may actually touch each other ("kissing" choroid detachments; Figure 8-1), and retinal adhesions may develop if these bullae remain in contact for several days. Choroidal detachments can affect a small localized area or, when they are massive, can involve the entire peripheral fundus and ciliary body. A very bullous detachment may be seen in the pupil and be mistaken for a melanoma (Figure 8-2; see Table 8-1). Persons at greatest risk for developing a choroidal detachment are the elderly and those with glaucoma.

A choroidal detachment is the result of fluid accumulation in the potential space between the sclera and the choroid or ciliary body.[3–5] The fluid is usually located between the fibrous strands that connect the choroid or ciliary body to the sclera.[6] Because the suprachoroid has very few capillaries and lymphatic channels, any fluid that accumulates in this area must exit through the choroidal vessels or seep through openings in the sclera.[7, 8] There are two principal types of choroidal detachments: hemorrhagic and transudative. The hemorrhagic form involves leakage of blood from a choroidal vessel into the choroidal space. This can follow trauma, but it usually occurs during or after intraocular surgery. It is generally caused by the accidental rupturing of a choroidal vessel, often after a scleral puncture to release subretinal fluid during retinal detachment surgery. The blood is slowly reabsorbed, and the choroid detachment decreases in size over weeks to months. A hemorrhagic detachment may be diagnosed by performing external scleral transillumination beneath the lesion. Because the choroid is engorged with blood, little if any illumination is seen through the pupil. A unilateral case of icteric (yellow) sclera is also a possible sign of a hemorrhagic choroidal detachment and results from degeneration of blood corpuscles that causes bilirubin to accumulate in the choroid and later to percolate into the sclera. A hemorrhagic choroidal detachment may exhibit blood along its margin, and blood may even slowly enter the vitreous.[9] Fluorescein angiography can be used to differentiate the two types of effusion. In the serous detachment, the dye study shows a characteristic background fluorescence, pigment epithelium abnormalities, and leakage from the large choroidal vessels, but all these findings are obscured in the hemorrhagic type.[10, 11]

Ultrasonography can be used to differentiate a choroidal detachment from a choroidal tumor, as Coleman did in more than 60% of cases.[12] Choroidal

TABLE 8-1. Choroidal Detachment vs. Malignant Melanoma vs. Retinal Detachment

Choroidal Detachment	Malignant Melanoma	Retinal Detachment
Usually very elevated	May be fairly flat to markedly elevated	Shallow to markedly elevated
Fairly darkly pigmented	Usually fairly pigmented but may be amelanotic	Whitish if recent
Retinal vessels visible on surface	Retinal vessels on surface unless tumor has broken through basal lamina into vitreous cavity	Retinal vessels visible on surface
Usually recent history of ocular trauma or surgery, especially retinal detachment repair with encircling band	Usually no history of preceding trauma	May have history of recent trauma but usually not
Often spontaneously resolves	Rarely resolve spontaneously	Rarely resolve spontaneously
Ora serrata may be easily seen without scleral depression	Ora serrata not usually seen without scleral depression	Ora serrata not usually seen without scleral depression
Does not undulate on eye movements	Does not undulate on eye movements	Recent detachments undulate on eye movements
Intraocular pressure may be low	Intraocular pressure may be low, high, or normal	Intraocular pressure may be low
May be multicentric	Rarely multicentric but may be lobulated	Rarely multicentric but may be lobulated
No folds seen on surface	A few retinal folds visible above or adjacent to tumor	Many folds, both small and large
Ultrasonography shows a rounded mass with acoustic shadowing	Ultrasonography may show a slightly to dramatically elevated mass in the vitreous cavity, high reflective signal, and often prominent underlying acoustic scleral excavation	Obvious vitreous membrane with folds and significant acoustic height (greater than retinoschisis) seen on ultrasonography
Negative ^{32}P test	^{32}P test usually positive	Negative ^{32}P test
Transillumination of the globe is reduced if the fluid causing the choroidal detachment is blood but not much effect if it is serous	Transillumination of the globe is reduced in the involved area	Transillumination of the globe is normal in the involved area
In serous detachment, dye study shows characteristic background fluorescence, pigment epithelium abnormalities, and leakage from the large choroidal vessels, but all these findings are obscured in hemorrhagic type	Late hyperfluorescence on fluorescein angiography	Fluorescein angiography usually not performed but would likely show no hyperfluorescence and a blurred view of fundus

detachments can be differentiated from retinal detachments during ultrasonography by noting that choroidal detachment has an acute angle of acoustic shadowing and extension anterior to the ora serrata. A choroidal detachment has a very smooth and convex surface, is limited posteriorly by the vortex veins and anteriorly by the base of the iris, and does not undulate on eye movements (see Table 8-1). Both choroidal and retinal detachments are very reflective and sometimes not easily differentiated on ultrasonography,[13] but the difference in thickness can be measured with digital techniques.[14] A thickening of the posterior sclera may indicate such conditions as posterior scleritis, intraocular tumor, and choroidal inflammation, which may be associated with a choroidal detachment.[15] A clear space beneath the choroidal detachment may indicate serous fluid, and numerous echoes indicate hemor-

rhage. CT scanning has been used to distinguish between hemorrhagic choroidal detachment and serous effusions.[16]

A transudative choroidal detachment is caused by leakage of serous proteinaceous fluid into the choroid. It is often seen after intraocular surgery[17, 18] and seems to be the result of prolonged hypotony when the globe is open. Intraocular surgery dramatically reduces IOP, and the low pressure is transmitted to the choroid, where it may result in vascular engorgement and transudation. This may partially explain the formation of choroidal detachments secondary to surgery or trauma.[19, 20] An increase in permeability of choroidal vessels can result from intraocular inflammation or vascular incompetence. Vortex vein compression by thickened sclera has been implicated in the development of choroidal detachments and is sometimes found in

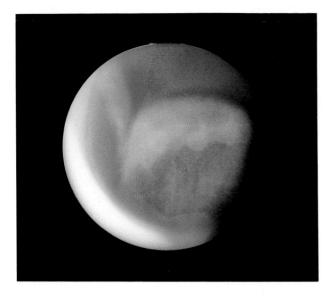

FIGURE 8-1
"Kissing" choroidal detachments are seen after retinal detachment surgery with a scleral buckle and an encircling band. Note the brown pars plana, the ora serrata, and the white-with-pressure appearance of the retina just posterior to the ora serrata. View is through the indirect condensing lens.

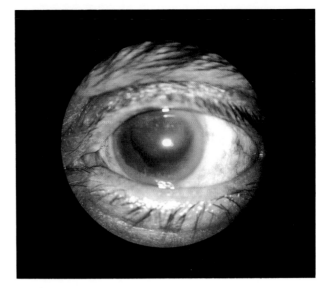

FIGURE 8-2
A dark brown choroidal detachment can be seen through the pupil of a patient who had cataract surgery 2 months ago. Note the smooth margin of the choroidal detachment.

nanophthalmic eyes.[21–23] Decompression of vortex veins in nanophthalmic eyes has met with some improvement.[24] Fluid in the suprachoroidal space increases in protein content, which causes a reduction in the intravascular colloid osmotic force that is responsible for reabsorption. Thus, a cycle develops that tends to sustain fluid in the space.[25–27]

Relative hypotony can result from choroidal detachment, perhaps because of increased uveoscleral outflow.[28–30] Other reasons for choroidal detachments from venous problems are increased venous pressure[31] and arteriovenous fistula.[32, 33] The lower limit of IOP is usually recognized as 8–10 mm Hg, and a pressure below 2 mm Hg is generally regarded as hypotony. The range of 2–8 mm Hg is considered low pressure.[34] Although low IOP could be an ominous sign, an eye with such pressure could remain viable indefinitely. Prolonged low IOP may lead to phthisis bulbi, a condition where the eye becomes shrunken and dysfunctional. A condition called prephthisis may be used to describe an eye in an intermediate stage before phthisis, in which the soft globe may be surgically saved. This stage is characterized by a pressure below 4 mm Hg, foreshortened anterioposterior length on ultrasonography (around 16–18 mm), thickened choroidoscleral walls, a cyclitic membrane, and ciliary body detachment.[35] Reattachment of the ciliary body generally results in a loss of the hypotony state.

A choroidal detachment frequently occurs after retinal detachment surgery (23%)[36–43] and seems to be related to the use of diathermy, cryopexy, and encircling bands. A 360-degree encircling band is linked with significant frequency of choroidal detachment, which seems to be due to the trauma or compression of the vortex veins or disturbance of the choroidal vasculature during retinal surgery.[40] Hypotony is also related to choroidal detachment formation in retinal detachment surgery and is often associated with drainage of subretinal fluid.[36, 38, 40–42] Ultrasound biomicroscopy has found that ciliary body detachment occurs frequently after retinal detachment surgery using scleral buckling.[44] Cataract surgery is known to cause suprachoroidal edema and lead to choroidal detachment.[3, 11, 18, 45–55] Sometimes, expulsive choroidal effusion may mimic an expulsive choroidal hemorrhage during cataract surgery (especially in with patients with prominent episcleral veins in Sturge-Weber syndrome).[31, 51, 52, 56, 57] Iridectomy and glaucoma filtering procedures can lead to choroidal detachment.[3, 11, 28, 31, 45, 58, 59] Postoperative choroidal detachments can occur weeks to months and sometimes years after surgery.[50] Laser panretinal photocoagulation of the retina can produce this type of detachment, which is likely due to a thermally damaged choroidal vessel.[60, 61]

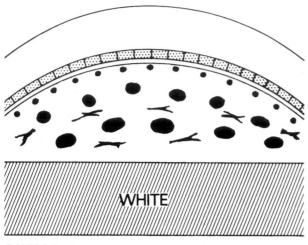

WHITE

FIGURE 8-3
Fluid has accumulated in the choroid, resulting in a choroidal detachment. Note that the vessels in the choroid have been spread apart by the increased fluid content in the choroidal space.

Blunt, penetrating eye trauma and perforating corneal ulcers are both known to be associated with choroidal edema.[3, 62] Pre-existing vascular disease[63] and very rigid sclera may also be associated with choroidal edema. Choroidal detachment may be secondary to one of the following conditions: idiopathic[43, 64]; arteriovenous fistula[32, 33]; myxedema[65]; multiple myeloma[64] after spontaneous remission of acute angle-closure glaucoma[59]; secondary to occlusive vasculitis, Wegener's granulomatosis, rheumatoid arthritis, or polyarteritis nodosa; and myopia.[64, 65–68] Other vascular diseases associated with a transudative choroidal detachment include hypertension, toxemia of pregnancy, and chronic nephritis.[45] Eye conditions that have been associated with choroidal detachments are subconjunctival abscess,[69] orbital pseudotumor,[70] episcleritis,[71–73] vasculitis,[66–68] scleritis,[45, 64, 65, 74, 75] uveitis,[76–79] Vogt-Koyanagi-Harada syndrome (VKH),[80] sympathetic ophthalmia,[64, 81] pars planitis,[82, 83] toxoplasmic retinochoroiditis,[64] and syphilitic posterior uveitis.

Pigmented blotches and streaks (Verhoeff streaks) are often noted in the fundus as a result of a past choroidal detachment.[84] They are a result of reactive hyperplasia of the pigment epithelium and may indicate the previous existence of a choroidal detachment. The pigmented streaks may look like the arteriosclerotic lines of Siegrist or be confused with angioid streaks.

Differential diagnosis of choroidal detachment includes several entities. A retinal detachment can be differentiated by its whitish color, wrinkled surface that undulates on eye movements, and poor view of the underlying choroid. The presence of a tear also implicates the existence of a rhegmatogenous retinal detachment. A choroidal detachment is a smooth, bullous lesion that does not undulate on eye movements and shows a clear choroidal pattern. Tumors such as melanoma and choroidal hemangioma can be confused with a choroidal detachment. Ferry[85] found that ciliochoroidal effusions are the second most frequent lesion mistaken for a choroidal melanoma. A choroidal detachment shows obvious normal-appearing retinal blood vessels, whereas malignant melanomas that have broken through the retina do not show vessels on the anterior surface. Scleral transillumination, ultrasonography, fluorescein angiography, and tests using chromic phosphate P 32 (^{32}P) can help to differentiate these tumors from a choroidal detachment. Increased transillumination due to ciliochoroidal effusions is known as Hagen's sign,[86] but sometimes ciliary body melanomas (especially nonpigmented tumors) readily transilluminate (see Table 8-1).

Ultrasonography can accurately differentiate tumors from benign lesions, such as choroidal detachments, in more than 60% of cases[12] and can distinguish a choroidal effusion by the acute angle of the acoustic shadow and the extension anterior to the ora serrata.[6] If the ultrasonographic findings show a thickening of the sclera opposite the suspected choroidal detachment, then posterior scleritis, choroidal inflammation, and intraocular tumors must be ruled out.[15] Choroidal edema is sometimes mistaken for a choroidal detachment.[6] Other entities include Harada's disease, leukemia, reactive lymphoidal hyperplasia of the choroid, posterior scleritis, and idiopathic central serous choroidopathy.[33]

Histopathology

Choroidal detachments are produced by the accumulation of either blood or serous fluid within the choroid. Fluid seems to collect more readily in the suprachoroidal space, and this is where the detachment usually begins. The fluid percolates throughout the choroid, causing the vessels to spread out and the choroid and retina to elevate into the vitreous cavity (Figure 8-3).

Clinical Significance

Fortunately, most transudative choroidal detachments spontaneously regress with time, which can vary from weeks to months. In cataract surgery, the choroidal detachment generally occurs within 1–2 weeks after surgery and resolves in 1–2 weeks.[8] Thus, no treatment is usually required; however, a detachment that persists longer than 6 months may require aspiration of fluid to effect regression. A persistent detachment occurs in less than 1% of patients after cataract surgery.[2] Today, with better wound-sealing surgical techniques, this complication is fairly rare.[87] Transudative choroidal detachments are sometimes treated with oral or retrobulbar injections of steroids. Hemorrhagic choroidal detachments in a surgical setting may be catastrophic, requiring immediate posterior sclerotomy to release the increased pressure and blood to avoid an irreparable expulsive hemorrhage. Occasionally, a choroidal detachment has an associated retinal detachment, a more frequent finding in older patients with a history of ocular surgery.[88–90] A retinal hole may be difficult to find in such cases because it may be hidden in the folds of the choroidal detachment. These patients may have improved vision due the apposition of the choroid to the detached retina.[6]

A complication of a ciliochoroidal detachment is the formation of a shallow anterior chamber and possible production of angle-closure glaucoma. This is produced by the anterior rotation of the ciliary body on its attachment to the scleral spur.[91, 92] The formation of a shallow anterior chamber often indicates the need for drainage of suprachoroidal fluid, because a flat chamber that persists longer than 7 days greatly increases the likelihood of peripheral anterior synechiae.[48, 93] Other complications are low-grade uveitis (which may result in a secondary cataract and cyclitic membrane), retinal adhesions due to apposition from kissing choroidals (choroidal detachments that abut each other), or corneal decompensation from anterior displacement of the lens. Persistent choroidal detachments can ultimately cause phthisis bulbi.[6]

Treatment in persistent cases of choroidal detachment is usually a sclerotomy in which a 6- to 8-mm incision is made behind the limbus opposite the area where most of the internal fluid has accumulated.[6] Slow release of the internal fluid is suggested to avoid rebound hypotony and the reaccumulation of choroidal fluid.[94] If intraocular inflammation is present, then treatment with topical and systemic steroids is indicated to reduce choroidal vascular leakage.[90]

Treatment of an expulsive hemorrhagic choroidal detachment is the immediate closure of the wound, which allows IOP to increase and tamponade the detachment back onto the internal scleral wall.[57] If the intraocular contents prolapse through the surgical wound, which cannot be reposited due to the

choroidal detachment, it may be necessary to perform a sclerotomy to rapidly decrease the volume of choroidal fluid.[95] Any wound leak after surgery may result in a continued low IOP and formation of a choroidal detachment; therefore all postoperative leaks should be sealed or somehow patched to reduce intraocular fluid egress to avoid choroidal detachment formation. If no leak is found and the anterior chamber remains flat for 2 weeks, then a cyclodialysis may have begun during surgery.[6, 96] In such cases, external pressure opposite the site of internal leakage may help to reform the anterior chamber.[52] Argon laser treatment to the site of the cyclodialysis,[97, 98] penetrating diathermy around the leaking site, and suturing the ciliary body to the sclera have met with some success in sealing the leak.[94]

In toxemia of pregnancy, treatment may require the induction of labor; retinal diseases must be diagnosed and appropriately treated; collagen vascular disease, rheumatoid arthritis and VHK may require treatment with steroids; and pars planitis should be treated with short-acting mydriatics to prevent synechiae formation.[6, 84] In eyes with thickened sclera (nanophthalmos), a localized partial-thickness resection and unroofing of the vortex vein has been helpful in some cases.[23, 24]

References

1. Hyman BN, Hagler WS. Bilateral annular detachment and myopia. Am J Ophthalmol 1970;70:853–858.
2. Brubaker RF, Pederson JE. Ciliochoroidal detachment. Surv Ophthalmol 1983;27:281–289.
3. Spaeth EP, de Long P. Detachment of the choroid: A clinical and histopathologic analysis. Arch Ophthalmol 1944; 32:217–238.
4. Brav SS. Serous choroidal detachment. Surv Ophthalmol 1961;6:395–415.
5. Von Graefe A. Zur diagnose des beginnenden intraocularen Krebses. Graefes Arch Clin Exp Ophthalmol 1858; 4:218–229.
6. Finlay AE, Fogle JA, et al. Choroidal Effusion. In WE Tasman, FA Jaeger FA (eds), Clinical Ophthalmology. Vol 4. Philadelphia: Harper & Row, 1986;52:1–19.
7. Weiter JJ, Ernest JT. Anatomy of the choroidal vasculature. Am J Ophthalmol 1974;78:583–590.
8. Bill A. Intraocular pressure and blood flow through the uvea. Arch Ophthalmol 1962;67:336–348.
9. Bell FC, Stenstrom WJ. Atlas of the Peripheral Retina. Philadelphia: Saunders, 1983:52–53.
10. Kimbrough RL, Tremple CS, et al. Angle-closure glaucoma in nanophthalmos. Am J Ophthalmol 1979;88:572–579.
11. Rosen E. Uveal effusions. I. A clinical picture. Am J Ophthalmol 1968;65:509–518.
12. Coleman DJ. Ocular Diagnosis. In DJ Coleman, FL Lizzi, RL Jack (eds), Ultrasonography of the Eye and Orbit. Philadelphia: Lea & Febiger, 1977.
13. Coleman DJ, Wilcox LM. The Choroid. Its Function, Eval-

uation, and Surgical Management. In Symposium on Medical and Surgical Diseases of the Retina and Vitreous. Transactions of the New Orleans Academy of Ophthalmology. St. Louis: Mosby, 1983:1–24.

14. Wu G, Silverman RH, et al. In vivo thickness of human detached retina by ultrasonic signal processing. Graefes Arch Clin Exp Ophthalmol 1989;227:21–25.

15. Wing GL, Schepens CL, et al. Serous choroidal detachment and the thickened-choroid sign detected by ultrasonography. Am J Ophthalmol 1982;94:499–505.

16. Peyman GA, Mafee M, et al. Computerized tomography in choroidal detachment. Ophthalmology 1984;91:156–162.

17. O'Brien CS. Further observations on detachment of the choroid after cataract extraction. Arch Ophthalmol 1936;16:655–656.

18. Swyers EM. Choroidal detachment immediately following cataract extraction. Arch Ophthalmol 1972;88:632–634.

19. Moses RA. Detachment of the ciliary body: Anatomic and physical considerations. Invest Ophthalmol 1965;4:935–941.

20. Capper SA, Leopold IH. Mechanism of serous choroidal detachment. Arch Ophthalmol 1956;55:101–113.

21. Gass JDM, Jallow S. Idiopathic serous detachment of the choroidal, ciliary body and retina (uveal effusion syndrome). Ophthalmology 1982;89:1018–1032.

22. Brockhurst RJ. Nanophthalmos with uveal effusion. Trans Am Ophthalmol 1974;72:371–403.

23. Brockhurst RJ. Nanophthalmos with uveal effusion. A new clinical entity. Arch Ophthalmol 1975;93:1989–1999.

24. Brockhurst RJ. Vortex vein decompression for nanophthalmic uveal effusion. Arch Ophthalmol 1980;98:1987–1990.

25. Chylack LT Jr, Bellows AR. Molecular sieving in suprachoroidal fluid formation in man. Invest Ophthalmol 1978;17:420–427.

26. Wilson RS, Hanna C, et al. Idiopathic chorioretinal effusions: An analysis of extraocular fluids. Ann Ophthalmol 1977;9:647–653.

27. Lam WK, Lee PF, et al. Albumin-bound bilirubin in subchoroidal fluid. Arch Ophthalmol 1979;97:149–151.

28. Pederson JE, Gasterland DE, et al. Experimental ciliochoroidal detachment. Effect on intraocular pressure and aqueous humor flow. Arch Ophthalmol 1979;97:536–541.

29. Bill A. The aqueous humor drainage mechanism in the cynomolgus monkey (Macaca irus) with evidence for unconventional routes. Invest Ophthalmol 1965;4:911–919.

30. Inomata H, Bill A, et al. Unconventional routes of aqueous humor outflow in cynomolgus monkey (Macaca irus). Am J Ophthalmol 1972;73:893–907.

31. Bellows AR, Chylack LT Jr, et al. Choroidal effusion in glaucoma surgery in patients with prominent episcleral vessels. Arch Ophthalmol 1979;97:493–497.

32. Harbison JW, Guerry D, et al. Dural arteriovenous fistula and spontaneous choroidal detachment. New cause of an old disease. Br J Ophthalmol 1978;62:483–490.

33. Woillez M, Dufour ABD. Decollement annulaire anterieure de la chorio-retine apres fistule cartidocaverneuse. Bull Soc Ophtalmol Fr 1967;67:819–822.

34. Coleman DJ. Evaluation of ciliary body detachment in hypotony. Retina 1995;15:312–318.

35. Coleman DJ, Smith ME. Ultrasonic criteria for surgically salvageable prephthisical eyes. Ultrasound Med Biol 1978;4:297–298.

36. Chignell AH. Choroidal detachment following retinal surgery without drainage of subretinal fluid. Am J Ophthalmol 1972;73:860–862.

37. Swan KC, Christensen L, et al. Choroidal detachment in the surgical treatment of retinal separation. Arch Ophthalmol 1956;55:240–245.

38. Hawkins WR, Schepens CL. Choroidal detachment and retinal surgery. Am J Ophthalmol 1966;62:813–819.

39. Hayreh SS, Baines JAB. Occlusion of the vortex veins. An experimental study. Br J Ophthalmol 1973;57:217–238.

40. Packer AJ, Maggiano JM, et al. Serous choroidal detachment after retinal detachment surgery. Arch Ophthalmol 1983;101:1221–1224.

41. Kishimoto M. Choroidal detachment after retinal detachment surgery. Folia Ophthalmol Jpn 1966;17:569–579.

42. Topilow HW, Ackerman AL. Massive exudative retinal and choroidal detachments following scleral buckle surgery. Ophthalmology 1983;90:143–147.

43. Michels RG, Wilkenson CP, Rice TA. Retinal detachment. St. Louis: Mosby, 1995:1005–1011.

44. Maruyama Y, Yuuki T, Kimura Y, et al. Ciliary body detachment surgery after retinal detachment surgery. Retina 1997;17:7–11.

45. Hertz V. Choroidal detachment with notes on scleral depression and pigmented streaks in the retina. Acta Ophthalmol Scand Suppl 1954;41:3–256.

46. Fuchs E. Ablosung der aderhaut nach staaroperation. Arch Ophthalmol 1900;51:199.

47. Bard LA. Eyes with choroidal detachments removed for suspected melanoma. Arch Ophthalmol 1965;73:320–323.

48. Cotlier E. Aphakic flat anterior chamber. III. Effect of inflation of the anterior chamber and drainage of choroidal detachments. Arch Ophthalmol 1972;88:16–21.

49. McClure HL. Massive bilateral choroidal detachment occurring in an aphakic patient six years and nine months postoperatively. Am J Ophthalmol 1967;63:295–297.

50. Shah RR. Flat anterior chamber and choroidal detachment in aphakia: Study of 500 cataract extractions. Br J Ophthalmol 1971;55:48–49.

51. Villaseca A. Late emptying of anterior chamber and choroidal detachment in cataract operations. Arch Ophthalmol 1954;52:250–263.

52. Ruiz RS, Salmonsen PC. Expulsive choroidal effusion: A complication of intraocular surgery. Arch Ophthalmol 1976;94:69–70.

53. Savir H. Expulsive choroidal effusion during cataract surgery. Ann Ophthalmol 1979;11:113–115.

54. Rosengren B. Aqueous leakage through the uveal vessels a factor in choroidal detachment? Acta Ophthalmol Scand 1970;48:901–904.

55. Janotka H, Huczynska B. Choroidal detachment following cataract extraction. Klin Oczna 1972;42:743–746.

56. Campbell JK. Expulsive choroidal hemorrhage and effusion. A reappraisal. Ann Ophthalmol 1980;12:332–340.

57. Maumenee AE, Schwartz MF. Acute intraoperative choroidal effusion. Am J Ophthalmol 1985;100:147–154.

58. Sakai T, Tamashita S. Choroidal detachment after glaucoma surgery. Folia Ophthalmol Jpn 1968;19:174–184.

59. Ursin KY. On spontaneous choroidal detachment after acute glaucoma in the light of an exceptional case. Acta Ophthalmol Scand 1965;43:751–760.

60. Huamonte FU, Peyman GA, et al. Immediate fundus complications after retinal scatter photocoagulation. Ophthalmic Surg 1976;7:88–99.

61. Weiter JJ, Brockhurst JJ, et al. Uveal effusion following panretinal photocoagulation. Ann Ophthalmol 1979;11:1723–1727.

62. Dotan S, Oliver M. Shallow anterior chamber and uveal effusion after nonperforating trauma to the eye. Am J Ophthalmol 1982;94:782–784.

63. Friedman E, Smith TR, et al. Choroidal vascular patterns in hypertension. Arch Ophthalmol 1964;71:842–850.
64. Green WR. The Uveal Tract. In WH Spencer (ed), Ophthalmic Pathology. Vol 3. Philadelphia: Saunders, 1986:1778–1791.
65. Hurd ER, Snyder WM, et al. Choroidal nodules and detachments in rheumatoid arthritis. Am J Med 1970; 48:273–278.
66. Austin D, Green WR, et al. Peripheral corneal degeneration and occlusive vasculitis in Wegener's granulomatosis. Am J Ophthalmol 1978;85:311 317.
67. Nanjiani MR. Ocular manifestations of polyarteritis nodosa. Br J Ophthalmol 1967;51:696–697.
68. Vancea P, Popa G, et al. Periarterite noususe a localisation oculaire. Ann Ocul 1962;195:632–651.
69. Muirfield WM. Diseases of the conjunctiva: case of subconjunctival abscess associated with a detachment of the choroid. Trans Ophthalmol Soc UK 1934;54:578–579.
70. Ryan SJ, Zimmerman LE, et al. Reactive lymphoid hyperplasia: an unusual form of intraocular pseudotumor. Trans Am Acad Ophthalmol Otolaryngol 1972;76:652–671.
71. Preisler E. Spontaneous choroidal detachment. Acta Ophthalmol Scand 1964;42:657–664.
72. Simpson ER, Adams ST. Spontaneous uveal effusion. Can J Ophthalmol 1970;5:41–45.
73. Van Alphen GWHM. On emmetropia and ametropia. Ophthalmologica 1961;142(Suppl):40–92.
74. Velzeboer J Jr. Spontaneous choroidal detachment. Am J Ophthalmol 1960;49:898–903.
75. Sears ML. Choroidal and retinal detachment associated with scleritis. Am J Ophthalmol 1964;58:764–766.
76. Woillez M, Dufour ABD, et al. Le decollement annulaire inflammatoire. Bull Soc Ophthalmol Fr 1967;67:822–827.
77. McGrand JC. Choroidal detachment in aphakic uveitis. Br J Ophthalmol 1969;53:778–781.
78. Kanter PJ, Goldberg MF. Bilateral uveitis with exudative retinal detachment. Arch Ophthalmol 1974;91:13–19.
79. Gramringer H, Schreck E, et al. Zur Pathogenese und Therapie der cyclitis annularis ersudative Pseudotumorosa. Klin Monatsbl Augenheilkd 1959;135:638–646.
80. Kimura R, Sakai M, et al. Transient shallow anterior chamber as initial symptom of Harada's syndrome. Arch Ophthalmol 1981;99:1604–1606.
81. de Veer JA. Sympathizing eye in sympathetic ophthalmia. A pathological study. Arch Ophthalmol 1952;48:723–737.
82. Brockhurst RJ, Schepens CL, et al. Uveitis. II. Peripheral uveitis: clinical description, complications and differential diagnosis. Am J Ophthalmol 1960;49:1257–1266.
83. Brockhurst RJ, Schepens CL, et al. Uveitis. III. Peripheral uveitis: etiology and treatment. Am J Ophthalmol 1961; 51:19–26.
84. Verhoeff FH. The nature and origin of the pigmented streaks caused by separation of the choroid. JAMA 1931;92:1873–1877.
85. Ferry AP. Lesions mistaken for malignant melanoma of the posterior uvea. Arch Ophthalmol 1964;72:463–469.
86. Hagen S. Die serose postoperative Choroideallablosung und ihre pathogenese. Klin Monatsbl Augenheilkd 1921; 66:161–211.
87. Charlton JF, Weinstein GW. Cataract Surgery. In WE Tasman, EA Jaeger (eds), Clinical Ophthalmology. Vol 4. Philadelphia: Harper & Row, 1986;6:1–46.
88. Gottlieb F. Combined choroidal and retinal detachment. Arch Ophthalmol 1972;88:481–486.
89. Graham PA. Unusual evolution of retinal detachment. Trans Ophthalmol Soc UK 1958;78:359–371.
90. Seelenfreund MH, Kraushar MF, et al. Choroidal detachment associated with primary detachment. Arch Ophthalmol 1974;91:254–458.
91. Scheie HG, Morse PH. Shallow anterior chamber as a sign of nonsurgical choroidal detachment. Ann Ophthalmol 1974;6:317–319.
92. Schepens CL, Brockhurst RJ. Uveal diffusion. I. Clinical picture. Arch Ophthalmol 1963;70:189–201.
93. Bellows AR, Chylack LT Jr, et al. Choroidal detachment. Ophthalmology 1981;88:1107–1115.
94. Shea M, Medrick EB. Ciliary body reattachment in ocular hypotony. Arch Ophthalmol 1981;99:278–281.
95. Verhoeff FH. Scleral puncture for expulsive subchoroidal hemorrhage following sclerostomy: scleral puncture for postoperative separation of the choroid. Ophthalmic Res 1915;24:55–59.
96. Grant WM, Chandler PA. An arrangement for gonioscopy during surgery. Arch Ophthalmol 1954;52:454–455.
97. Harbin TS Jr. Treatment of cyclodialysis clefts with argon laser photocoagulation. Ophthalmology 1982;89: 1082–1083.
98. Partamian LG. Treatment of cyclodialysis clefts with argon laser photocoagulation in a patient with a shallow anterior chamber. Am J Ophthalmol 1985;99:5–7.

Index